Physiotherapy in Respiratory Care

For Roger

Physiotherapy in Respiratory Care

A problem-solving approach to respiratory and cardiac management

Second edition

ALEXANDRA HOUGH

Freelance lecturer, Senior Physiotherapist, Whittington Hospital, London, former Senior Lecturer, North London School of Physiotherapy

Stanley Thornes (Publishers) Ltd

First edition published by Chapman & Hall in 1991
Second edition published by Chapman & Hall in 1996
(ISBN 0-412-62320-X)

Reprinted in 1997 by:
Stanley Thornes (Publishers) Ltd
Ellenborough House
Wellington Street
CHELTENHAM
GL50 1YW
United Kingdom

98   99   00   01   /   10   9   8   7   6   5   4   3   2

A catalogue record for this book is available from the British Library.

ISBN 0–7487–3284–5

Typeset by Photoprint, Torquay, S. Devon
Printed and bound in Great Britain by Scotprint, Musselburgh

Contents

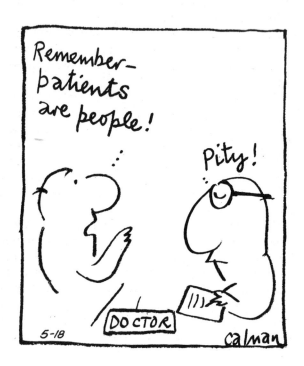

Preface

Respiratory care is an immensely satisfying branch of physiotherapy. It challenges our intellect, exploits our handling skills and employs our humanity to the full.

Respiratory physiotherapy is both art and science. It is not an exact science, and effective treatment therefore depends on problem-solving. Analytic problem-solving requires the ability to define a problem and the knowledge to address it. Creative problem-solving requires a clear perspective of the individual patient's need. These are the aims of this book.

Clinicians now expect explanations that are referenced and physiologically sound, meticulous attention to detail of technique and a patient-centred approach. This book is written for such readers and those who question fundamental assumptions and traditional rituals.

Evaluation of practice is emphasized so that we are equipped to justify our protocol to ourselves and others. Carefully reasoned explanations and updated physiotherapy techniques are covered in precise detail. There is integration of theory and practice and emphasis on the hands-on aspect of physiotherapy.

The glossary serves as a quick reference guide and an explanation of abbreviations, which are usually defined once only in the text. It has been greatly extended for the second edition and can be read in its own right as an extra physiology chapter.

The text is enthusiastically written, highly readable and enlivened by quotations from patients whose experiences are a central theme throughout.

The book is suitable for physiotherapists from student level to accomplished clinician because problem-solving requires thinking rather than experience. It is also aimed at specialist respiratory nurses. All readers will benefit from the patient quotations which enrich the text throughout. The clinician will find here the opportunity to achieve clarity of thought, breadth of vision and mastery in respiratory care. Enjoy it.

Acknowledgements

Profound thanks to the patients who have taught me much over the years. I am also indebted to Veronica Bastow for her perceptive insights, Clare Pain for her wisdom, John Widdicombe for his meticulous scrutiny of the physiology and Mel Calman for his cartoons.

Heartfelt thanks also to Alison Brown, Fiona Bryden, Joy Conway, Diana Davis, Stephanie Enright, Nicky Harvey, Bernadette Henderson, Avril Imison, Sue Pirrie, Marylin Place, Carolyn Roskell, Irene Rowbottom and Judith Sweeney, for their specialist advice.

And to the students with whom it has been my privilege to work and learn, thank you.

*Royalties from this publication to be donated to
the Campaign Against the Arms Trade.*

1. Overview of physiology in relation to clinical practice

1.1 INTRODUCTION

Breathing is the basic rhythm of life.
Hippocrates

Breathing is unique. Most of us give it little thought, yet it can be automatic or voluntary, and is preserved in unconsciousness. It is associated with a respiratory system of remarkable ingenuity, and an understanding of how this respiratory system works creates a foundation for logical practice. This chapter places less emphasis on the textbook lungs of hefty young male medical students and more on the lungs of patients who may smoke, be overweight, past middle-age and spend time slumped in hospital beds. Liberal use of the glossary should be made in this chapter.

1.2 DEFENCE

Every day, the 300 million alveoli in an adult lung will expose a surface area of 80 square metres, or nearly the size of a tennis court, to a volume of air and pollutants that could fill an average swimming pool (Hanley and Tyler 1987). It is only by means of a sophisticated biological barrier that the body does not succumb to this onslaught of inhaled insults. Indeed, so effective is the pulmonary defence system that the lung is normally sterile from the first bronchial division downwards. Protection is based on a network of filters, secretions, reflexes and specialized cell-mediated defences.

People who most need a strong defence system are often those who are most compromised. The physiotherapist treats patients whose noses are evaded by mouth-breathing or artificial airways, whose cilia are damaged by smoking or disease, and whose cough is inhibited by pain.

1.2.1 Nose

The nose is the gatekeeper of the respiratory tract, providing the first line of defence by means of:

- smelling suspicious aromas,
- sneezing in response to irritating substances,
- filtering large particles through an extensive labyrinth of passageways,
- protecting against cold dry air by its warm humid environment.

1.2.2 Pharynx

The entrance to the oropharynx is encircled by tonsils and adenoids whose phagocytes guard against infection. The lower pharynx houses the epiglottis, which snaps shut over the larynx during swallowing to prevent aspiration into the trachea.

1.2.3 Bronchoconstriction

If irritant particles are inhaled, normal bronchoconstrictor tone is increased reflexly in order to narrow and protect the airway. In diseases such as asthma, this mechanism is exaggerated and counter-productive, becoming known as bronchospasm and acting to obstruct airflow and increase the work of breathing.

1.2.4 Mucociliary escalator

Small particles that escape filtration in the nose are trapped on a sticky mucus blanket

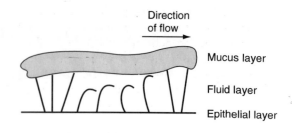

Figure 1.1 The mucociliary escalator. Claws on the tips of the cilia grip the mucus and a whip-like movement propels it mouthwards.

that is carried by cilia, against gravity, from the terminal bronchioles to the throat over a period of several hours (Pavia 1991). This moving staircase (Fig. 1.1) propels secretions to the pharynx and larynx, from where the debris is swallowed or, if excessive, expectorated. 10–100 ml secretions are cleared every day, or up to 300 ml when the airways are irritated (Hodgkin 1993, p. 469). This finely co-ordinated mechanism is compromised by dehydration, smoking, hypoxia, inflammation or pathological conditions that affect the viscosity of mucus or function of cilia. The mucus also defends the lungs from drying out.

1.2.5 Cough

Sputum clearance depends primarily on mucociliary transport and secondarily on cough. The cough is the body's strongest physiological reflex and is used as a reserve mechanism to expel secretions when mucociliary clearance is damaged or overwhelmed. It is initiated by inflammatory, chemical, mechanical or thermal stimulation of receptors that are located anywhere from the oropharynx to lung tissue. It can be voluntary or involuntary, and comprises:

- an inspiratory gasp to 90% of total lung capacity,

- closure of the glottis and trapping of air in the lungs at powerful positive pressures of up to 300 mmHg, narrowing the trachea and main bronchi by 60% (Rees 1987).
- sudden opening of the glottis, causing air to explode outwards at up to 70 mph (Brannon *et al* 1993), thus shearing secretions off the airway walls.

Coughing is accompanied by violent swings in intrapleural pressure and blood pressure (BP), which cause long segments of airway to collapse. For most people, the airways re-open with a subsequent deep breath, but for those unable to take a deep breath, they stay closed for lengthy periods (Nunn *et al* 1965). Despite high pressures, the lung is protected from overdistension and barotrauma by muscle action to buttress the chest wall.

The beneficial effects of coughing are to expel sputum and inhaled irritants from large airways as far as the 10th generation (Pavia 1991). Beyond this, airflow cannot attain sufficient speed to expel secretions. Adverse effects, such as bronchospasm and exhaustion, may follow sustained bouts of coughing. The cough mechanism is inefficient in people with obstructive airways disease because they have poor expiratory flow rates and airways that collapse on expiration. Coughing may fail in the presence of coma, neuromuscular disease or postoperative pain. It is weakened if the glottis is bypassed by intubation or tracheostomy.

1.2.6 Other lung defences

Further mechanisms await pollutants that evade the above defences. They include an immunoglobulin in respiratory secretions called IgA, 600 million scavenger macrophages (multiplied fourfold in smokers), which engulf unwanted particles, and alpha$_1$-antitrypsin, a plasma protein that combats proteolytic enzyme activity which would otherwise destroy alveoli. Asbestos particles circumvent these and other defences because of their peculiar shape.

Soluble particles enter the bloodstream and are thereby cleared from the lungs, along with other unsavoury substances picked up by venous blood from peripheral vascular beds. The entire blood volume passes through the lungs, which detoxify foreign substances, perform a range of metabolic functions and act as a filter to protect the arterial system, particularly the vulnerable coronary and cerebral circulations, from unwanted chemicals.

1.3 CONTROL

Breathing is normally controlled with such exquisite sensitivity that oxygen and CO_2 in the blood are maintained within precise limits despite unpredictable inputs. Clusters of neurones in the pons and medulla receive and integrate a multitude of stimuli from the rib cage, lungs, chemoreceptors, metabolic and other systems, then discharge impulses to the respiratory muscles. Exercise and postural change are two of the disturbances that are perceived by the respiratory centre, with immediate responses. Respiratory control occurs at a subconscious level, but can be overridden by reflexes or voluntary action, such as speech, laughter, emotion, pain, sudden cold, some pathological states and breathing exercises.

1.4 MECHANICS

1.4.1 The respiratory muscles

Every breath is as essential to life as every heart beat, but only recently have the respiratory muscles been granted the same respect as heart muscle. Attention is now focused not only on gas exchange through the lungs, but also on the respiratory pump which ventilates the lungs. The respiratory pump comprises the respiratory muscles, chest wall, nerves and respiratory centre.

Inspiration

The diaphragm separates two compartments of markedly different densities, the thorax and abdomen, and provides 70% of the work of inspiration (Rochester 1991). It was thought to be the seat of the soul by the ancient Greeks, but despite this distinction, its exact mechanism is still a source of some mystery. It is a dome-shaped sheet of muscle attached to the bottom of the rib cage, which, at rest, allows the dome to extend upwards almost to nipple level. Contraction flattens it, displacing the abdominal viscera downwards (by 5–7 cm with a deep breath), creating negative intrathoracic pressure and sucking air into the lungs. The contracting diaphragm presses down against the fulcrum of the abdominal contents and outwards against the lower rib cage, causing expansion of the lower chest. The abdominal contents help stabilize the diaphragm, but the abdomen protrudes out on inspiration unless prevented voluntarily.

Other inspiratory muscles stabilize the chest wall so that diaphragmatic action can create pressure changes in the chest. Pharyngeal muscles prevent collapse of the upper airway, and accessory muscles (mainly the scalenes and sternomastoid) stabilize the upper rib cage to prevent it being pulled downwards. The accessory muscles become major inspiratory muscles when there is airflow obstruction, and arm and trunk muscles are recruited when breathing becomes especially difficult.

Expiration

Normal expiration is largely passive, elastic recoil providing the driving pressure. 'Elastic recoil' is due, first, to surface tension acting throughout the vast gas/liquid interface lining the alveoli and, secondly, to elasticity of lung tissue which has been stretched during inspiration. This recoil pressure of the lung decreases at low lung volume. Normal airflow resistance and continued low-grade inspiratory muscle activity act as necessary brakes on expiratory flow. If airway resistance is increased by obstructive disease, abdominal and internal intercostal muscles are recruited in an attempt to augment passive recoil.

1.4.2   Pressures

Alveolar pressure pressure inside the lung.
Pleural (intrathoracic) pressure pressure in the pleural space.
Transpulmonary (transmural) pressure difference between the above two pressures, i.e. distending pressure across the lung, representing the driving pressure responsible for inflating the lungs (increases with greater lung volume).

Alveolar pressure is slightly negative on inspiration and slightly positive on expiration. Pleural pressure is normally negative in relation to alveolar pressure because the elastic recoil of the lung pulls inwards and the elastic recoil of the chest wall pulls outwards, creating an average pleural pressure of minus 2 cmH_2O at end-expiration and minus 7 cmH_2O at end-inspiration (Kam *et al* 1993). The two forces of inward and outward pull are at equilibrium at the end of a quiet exhalation (functional residual capacity). The eagerness of the ribs to spring out, due to elastic recoil of the chest wall, assists inspiration. These pressures are disturbed by:

- fractured ribs with a pneumothorax, which destabilize the chest wall so that elastic recoil is unopposed and the lung shrivels inwards,
- emphysema, which causes loss of lung elastic recoil, so that the outward pull of the chest wall is unopposed and the lung hyperinflates.

A change in alveolar pressure of only 1 cmH_2O is usually enough for airflow, but is greater with high airflow resistance.

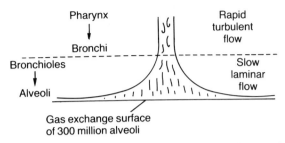

Figure 1.2 Increase in total cross-sectional area of airways as they subdivide.

1.4.3 Resistance

Resistance is present whenever there is airflow through a vessel because gas slides against the vessel walls and over itself. Airflow resistance depends mainly on the calibre of the airway. The site of greatest airflow resistance is the upper respiratory tract, where total cross section is narrowest and airflow most turbulent (Fig. 1.2). The nasal route resists airflow more than the oral route, which is why we breathe through the mouth when breathless or exercising.

1.4.4 Compliance

Compliance = change in volume / change in distending pressure

Compliance is the ease with which the lung inflates. It is represented by the relationship between pressure and volume, which is curved rather than linear (Fig. 1.3). The lung is least compliant, i.e. stiffest, at either extreme of lung volume, as is a balloon, so it is difficult to inflate alveoli that are closed or hyperinflate those that are fully open.

Compliance is related partly to tissue elasticity but mostly to surfactant in alveolar fluid. This acts like detergent to decrease surface tension and prevent the alveolar walls sticking together after being deflated, as happens when a plastic bag is wet inside. Surfactant stabilizes the lungs by preventing small alveoli collapsing and emptying their contents into large alveoli. Regular deep breaths

stimulate surfactant production and help maintain compliance.

Conditions of low compliance include bronchospasm, stiff lungs, a stiff chest wall, low lung volume and disorders of surfactant production, such as the neonatal and adult respiratory distress syndromes.

Static compliance is measured during a breath-hold so that equilibrium is achieved between alveolar pressure and mouth pressure, alveoli being filled to a volume determined by their regional compliance. **Dynamic compliance** is measured during breathing and normally approximates static compliance, but may be less in diseased lungs if regional variations in compliance and resistance mean that alveolar filling is not completed within the inspiratory period.

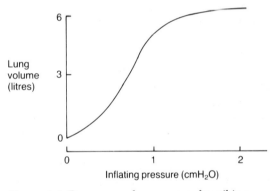

Figure 1.3 Pressure–volume curve describing lung compliance, showing how more pressure is needed to increase lung volume at either extreme of inflation. Examples are atelectasis for a low volume state and emphysema for hyperinflation.

1.4.5 Work of breathing

Work is done during inspiration to overcome the resistive, elastic and inertial forces of airflow, lungs and chest wall. Work of breathing (WOB) can be defined in several ways:

- amount of pressure generated to move a certain volume of gas,
- transpulmonary pressure × tidal volume

- oxygen consumed by the respiratory muscles.

Normally, breathing is surprisingly efficient, helped by the slippery fluid which lines moving surfaces such as the alveoli and pleura. WOB uses 1–4% of total body oxygen consumption at rest, but up to 40% in people with chronic obstructive pulmonary disease (COPD) during exercise (Pilbeam 1992, p. 80).

Deep breathing at double tidal volume can quadruple the elastic WOB (Haas and Axen 1991, p. 17), while rapid shallow breathing increases the resistive work, i.e. WOB against air flow resistance (Nunn 1987, p. 109). Most patients find the right balance, but some need assistance to find the optimal breathing pattern to minimize their WOB.

WOB can be assessed by measuring the oxygen cost of breathing (Tobin and Yang 1990), which is the oxygen consumed by the respiratory muscles.

1.4.6 Inspiratory muscle weakness and fatigue

Inspiratory muscle fatigue is less common than systemic muscle fatigue because the diaphragm has a large reserve capacity. It differs from other skeletal muscles in its automatic function and capacity for a lifetime of sustained action against elastic and resistive loads instead of irregular action against inertial loads. It is equipped for this by a high proportion of fatigue-resistant fibres and the unusual way in which perfusion increases instead of decreases during contraction (Anzueto 1992). But it is thought that fatigue may occur if energy demand exceeds supply, as when WOB is increased by severe airways obstruction. Fatigue serves a protective function to avoid depletion of enzymes, and procedures that encourage patients to overuse fatigued muscles can cause damage (Goldstone and Moxham 1991). People with COPD may have inspiratory muscle fatigue or weakness, both of which impair muscle contractility. The signs of fatigue and weakness are similar (p. 27), but the distinction is important because treatment is different.

Weakness is failure to generate sufficient force in an otherwise fresh muscle, as occurs in neuromuscular disorders, disuse atrophy or malnourishment. It is associated with a chronic decrease in strength and sometimes a chronic increase in $PaCO_2$. It is not reversible by rest, but is treated by addressing the cause and, if appropriate, encouraging activity.

Fatigue is defined as reduced force generated by a muscle after it has been overloaded. It is associated with a relatively abrupt decrease in respiratory muscle strength and sometimes abrupt increase in $PaCO_2$. It is treated by rest. Loss of tension generation in muscle can be due to failure of any of the links in the physiological chain. Failure within the central nervous system (CNS) is called central fatigue and failure beyond the CNS is called peripheral fatigue.

Fatigue differs from weakness in that even a normal muscle can become fatigued with sufficient effort. Both fatigue and weakness may occur in respiratory failure or during weaning from mechanical ventilation.

1.5 VENTILATION

Breathing (or ventilation) is the act of moving gas in and out of the lungs, i.e. inspiration and expiration.

Respiration is (a) the exchange of gases between the environment and tissue cells (external respiration at alveolar/capillary level and internal respiration at capillary/tissue level), and (b) regulation of acid-base, metabolic and defence functions of the respiratory system.

Gas that moves in and out of the lungs is made up of alveolar ventilation, which is the fresh air that gets into the alveoli and participates in gas exchange, and dead space ventilation (V_D), which does not contribute to gas exchange. Most dead space is made up of **anatomical dead space** (Fig. 1.4), which is air

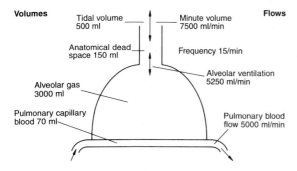

Figure 1.4 Lung unit with average volumes and flows of gas and blood for both lungs. (From West, J.B. (1995) *Ventilation/blood flow and gas exchange*, 5th edn Blackwell, Oxford, with permission.)

in the conducting passages that does not reach the alveoli, i.e. that which is last in and first out. It comprises one-third of tidal volume (V_1) in an average human, more in the giraffe. **Alveolar dead space** represents air that reaches the alveoli but not the blood, due to insufficient perfusion. It is minimal in normal lungs but increases in most forms of lung disease. The sum of anatomical and alveolar dead space is called **physiological dead space**. The presence of dead space is one reason why it is more economical to increase ventilation by breathing deeper rather than faster. Dead space is most usefully expressed in relation to tidal volume (V_D/V_T).

Quiet breathing moves a V_T of only one-tenth the vital capacity, but oscillations in V_T and involuntary sighs every 5–10 minutes help prevent alveolar collapse. Patients who are drowsy or sedated lose this mechanism.

Ventilation is not distributed evenly within the lungs (Fig. 1.5). In most spontaneously-breathing adults, dependent regions are better ventilated for two reasons:

1. Alveoli in upper regions are already more inflated because expanding stress is exerted by the lung hanging within the frame of the chest. Alveoli in lower regions are squashed by the weight of lungs (heavy with blood) above and around them. The sponge-like properties of the lungs mean that change in volume, and therefore ventilation, is greater in dependent regions because there is more potential to expand.

2. In the horizontal position, the excursion of the dependent portion of the diaphragm is twice that of the upper portion because the lower fibres are more stretched by abdominal pressure and therefore contract from a position of mechanical advantage (Nunn 1987, p. 103). Fig. 1.6 shows the relevance of this in the side-lying position. This ventilation gradient is reversed in children (p. 288), obese people (p. 16) and those on ventilators (p. 221).

Side-lying augments the ventilation gradient because of a greater vertical distance, the lower lung receiving twice the ventilation of the upper (Nunn 1987, p. 103).

Points of relevance for the physiotherapist are:

- deep breathing encourages basal ventilation and increases diffusion (Prabhu *et al* 1990),
- deep breathing increases lung compliance by stretching alveoli and encouraging surfactant production,
- a sustained deep breath reduces dead space by mixing dead space gas with alveolar gas, and improves the distribution of ventilation by using collateral channels (Cormier *et al* 1991),
- shallow breathing is inefficient because more V_T is lost to dead space since the same air is going in and out more often,
- deep breathing can cause bronchospasm in people with hyperreactive airways,
- external breathing apparatus, such as a ventilator circuit, increases dead space.

1.6 DIFFUSION

Diffusion occurs in both gaseous and liquid states, leading to equilibration of gases

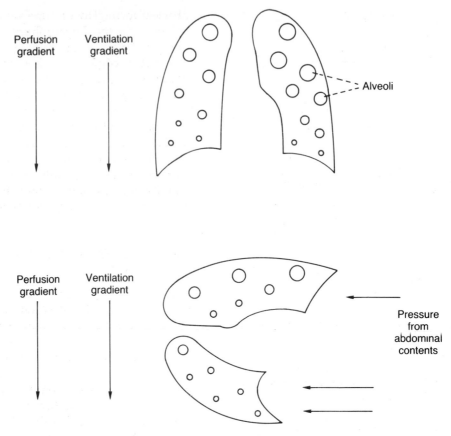

Figure 1.5 Effect of gravity on the distribution of ventilation and perfusion on the lung.

between air and blood. In the peripheral airways, where total cross-section widens dramatically (Fig. 1.2), airflow essentially ceases, and gas exchange from the respiratory bronchioles to the alveoli only continues by gaseous diffusion.

Gases then have to diffuse through an obstacle course of membranes and fluid in order to locate the haemoglobin, but the process is so efficient that oxygen tension is equalized in one-third of the time that the blood spends in the capillary, while CO_2 diffuses 20 times as easily (Widdicombe and Davies 1991, p. 51). Diffusion defects therefore do not play a major role in gas exchange abnormalities. Diffusion is measured by the carbon monoxide diffusing capacity (p. 49).

1.7 PERFUSION

Along with ventilation and diffusion, a further component needed for gas exchange in the lung is perfusion. The lungs have a dual circulation but, because they are normally awash with blood from the dominant **pulmonary** circulation, the **bronchial** circulation, which services lung tissue itself, is less vital, as shown by the survival of lung after transplantation, in which the bronchial vessels are tied.

The pulmonary circulation differs from the systemic circulation in three ways:

1. Pulmonary vessels have thinner walls, and in order to match the enormous surface area of the alveoli, the pulmonary circulation forms a dense network that

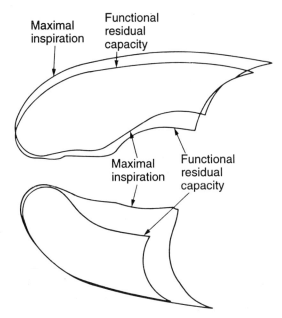

Figure 1.6 Lung volumes in the lateral position, showing greater volume change, i.e. greater ventilation, in the lower lung on inspiration. (From Nunn, J.F. (1987) Applied Respiratory Physiology, 3rd edn, Butterworth-Heinemann, Oxford, with permission.)

functions as a sheet of blood enwrapping the air sacs.

2. The pulmonary circulation has only one-tenth the resistance of the systemic circulation, yet it has the unusual ability to further reduce resistance, in response to a rise in pressure, by increasing the calibre of capillaries and recruiting others that are closed (West 1994). Such a low pressure system is very responsive to gravity, and there is a steep perfusion gradient from top to bottom of the lung (Fig. 1.5). In the base of the upright lung, the greater volume of blood may lead to some airway closure. In the apex, arterial pressure barely overrides alveolar pressure. The vulnerable vessels collapse in upper lung regions if this balance is disturbed, as when hypovolaemic shock reduces arterial pressure, or mechanical ventilation increases alveolar pressure. Perfusion is affected by lung volume, the vessels being stretched in the hyperinflated state and partly collapsed in low volume states. The distribution of perfusion is susceptible to pathological change, e.g. COPD causes a greater disruption to perfusion than ventilation. Pulmonary circulation is also influenced by total blood volume.

3. While systemic hypoxia stimulates systemic vasodilation (to help offset oxygen lack in the tissues), pulmonary hypoxia stimulates pulmonary vasoconstriction, in order to enhance $\dot{V}_A/\dot{Q}$ matching, as described below.

1.8 VENTILATION/PERFUSION RELATIONSHIPS

It is no good having a well-ventilated alveolus if it is not supplied with blood, nor a well-perfused alveolus that is not ventilated. Fresh air and blood need to be in the same place at the same time for gas exchange to occur. The matching of these two essentials is expressed as the ratio of alveolar ventilation to perfusion ($\dot{V}_A/\dot{Q}$). Both ventilation and perfusion increase down the lung, but there is a steeper increase in perfusion, so that the $\dot{V}_A/\dot{Q}$ ratio decreases from an overventilated apex to an overperfused base.

When ventilation is reduced, an ingenious mechanism called **hypoxic vasoconstriction** limits $\dot{V}_A/\dot{Q}$ mismatch. Hypoxia, e.g. in the lung bases, causes local shutdown of vessels and forces blood to flow to better ventilated upper regions (upper lobe diversion). This becomes counterproductive when lung disease is severe and hypoxia is global, because generalized vasoconstriction increases pulmonary artery pressure.

1.9 ARTERIAL BLOOD GASES

PO_2 – partial pressure or tension of oxygen.
PaO_2 – partial pressure of oxygen in arterial blood, representing the oxygen dissolved in plasma (normal: 11–14 kPa or 80–100 mmHg).

SaO$_2$ – extent to which haemoglobin in arterial blood is saturated with oxygen, representing the capacity of blood to carry oxygen (normal: 95–98%).

Oxygen content – total amount of oxygen in blood, i.e. oxygen in both plasma and haemoglobin.

PaCO$_2$ – partial pressure of CO$_2$ in arterial blood, basis of respiratory acid-base balance (normal: 4.7–6.0 kPa or 35–45 mmHg).

HCO$_3$ – bicarbonate ion concentration, basis of metabolic acid-base balance (normal: 22–26 mmol/l).

pH – inverse of log of hydrogen ion concentration, which reflects acid-base balance and responds to metabolic or respiratory change but cannot differentiate between them. Low pH corresponds to acidosis, high pH to alkalosis (normal: 7.35–7.45).

Hypoxaemia – deficiency of oxygen in arterial blood, i.e. PaO$_2$ < 8 kPa (60 mmHg), SaO$_2$ < 90%.

Hypoxia – deficiency of oxygen at tissue level, the final common pathway for cardiorespiratory pathology (more important than hypoxaemia but more difficult to measure).

Hypocapnia/hypocarbia – deficiency of CO$_2$ in arterial blood.

Hypercapnia/hypercarbia – excess CO$_2$ in arterial blood.

Pulmonary shunt – blood that enters pulmonary veins and systemic arterial system without going through ventilated areas of lung.

1.9.1   Introduction

Arterial blood gas measurements give an indication of ventilation, gas exchange and acid-base status. Readings are relevant when related to previous values, the clinical state of the patient and the level of inspired oxygen. Resting PaO$_2$ does not reflect PaO$_2$ during exercise, nor predict accurately nocturnal PaO$_2$ (Hodgkin 1993, p. 66), nor does it necessarily correlate with airflow obstruction. A low PaO$_2$ is normal in people who smoke, have respiratory disease or are elderly.

Neither oxygen **tension** nor **saturation** tell exactly how much oxygen is being carried in blood. The PaO$_2$ describes only the 3% of oxygen dissolved in plasma. It determines the extent to which haemoglobin (Hb) can be saturated with oxygen and reflects the pressure needed to push oxygen from air to blood and blood to tissue cells. The SaO$_2$ describes the 97% of oxygen that is bound to Hb. An anaemic person may have a normal SaO$_2$ but deliver a subnormal load of oxygen. Only the oxygen **content** describes the total amount of oxygen that is carried in the blood, being related to PaO$_2$, SaO$_2$ and Hb, but in practice its value is assumed from the PaO$_2$ or SaO$_2$. None of these terms give a measure of oxygenation at tissue level.

1.9.2   Oxygen dissociation curve

The relationship between SaO$_2$ and PaO$_2$ is expressed by the oxygen dissociation curve, which represents the normal variation in the amount of oxygen that combines with Hb. Its peculiar shape represents the protective mechanisms that function in both health and disease (Fig. 1.7).

Upper flat portion of the curve

At the plateau of the curve, the combination of oxygen with Hb is favoured by a high PO$_2$, and its stability is not unduly disturbed by changes in arterial PO$_2$. In health, this encourages loading of oxygen in the high PO$_2$ environment of the lung, and discourages unloading of oxygen before blood reaches the capillary bed. In disease, a drop of PaO$_2$ to 10.7 kPa (80 mmHg) hardly affects the amount of oxygen in the blood.

Hb cannot be more than fully saturated, so that oxygen therapy is unhelpful for people with a high PaO$_2$, and hyperventilation of

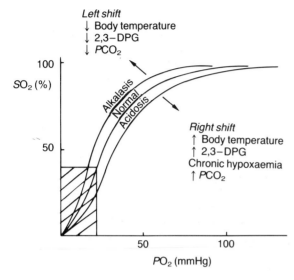

SO_2 (%)

Left shift
↓ Body temperature
↓ 2,3–DPG
↓ PCO_2

Right shift
↑ Body temperature
↑ 2,3–DPG
Chronic hypoxaemia
↑ PCO_2

100

50

50   100

PO_2 (mmHg)

Figure 1.7 Oxygen dissociation curve relating oxygen saturation to oxygen tension. Shaded area represents critical tissue hypoxia.

functioning alveoli cannot supersaturate arterial blood to compensate for hypoxaemia resulting from poorly functioning alveoli.

Steep portion of the curve

The dissociation of Hb becomes proportionately greater as PO_2 falls, so that small changes in PaO_2 greatly affect SaO_2. In health, this means that Hb can offload quantities of oxygen at the cellular level with maintenance of oxygen tension in the blood. In disease, large amounts of oxygen can be unloaded when tissues are hypoxic. A PaO_2 of 7.3 kPa (55 mmHg) marks the point where a significant reduction in oxygen delivery to the tissues begins, and further small drops in PaO_2 result in tissue hypoxia.

Shift of the curve

Another singular way in which the body responds to need is to adjust the affinity of Hb for oxygen, as reflected by a shift of the curve. A right shift means that Hb unloads oxygen more easily at a given PO_2. In health,

this occurs during exercise, when active muscle generates heat and makes blood hypercapnic and acidic. In disease, this shift occurs with fever and when tissues need extra oxygen.

A left shift means that Hb holds on to its oxygen tenaciously, as occurs in hyperventilation, hypometabolism or a cold environment. Pink ears and noses on frosty mornings are due to the reluctance of Hb to unload oxygen.

1.9.3 Hypoxia and hypoxaemia

Causes of hypoxia are:

- hypoxaemia,
- ↓ cardiac output, e.g. myocardial infarct,
- ↓ oxygen carrying capacity of the blood, e.g. anaemia,
- ↓ blood flow, e.g. circulatory shock or peripheral vascular disease,
- disrupted blood flow, e.g. multisystem failure,
- ↓ ability to extract oxygen, e.g. septic shock.

Causes of hypoxaemia are:

- low $\dot{V}_A/\dot{Q}$ ratio due to wasted perfusion (↑ shunt),
- high $\dot{V}_A/\dot{Q}$ ratio due to wasted ventilation (↑ dead space),
- hypoventilation,
- diffusion abnormality,
- ↓ F_IO_2, e.g. fire entrapment, high altitude, interrupted oxygen therapy.

Wasted perfusion occurs when blood is shunted through consolidated, collapsed or damaged areas of lung without picking up oxygen, leading to $\dot{V}_A/\dot{Q}$ mismatch (Fig. 1.8). Hypoxic vasoconstriction attenuates some of this effect, but is not well enough controlled to be localized only to non-ventilated regions. Hypoxaemia associated with shunt is refractory to oxygen therapy because added oxygen cannot reach the shunted blood. The mixing

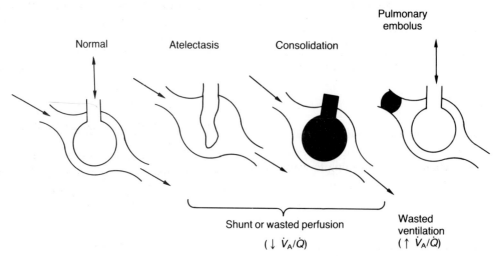

Figure 1.8 Alveoli and surrounding capillary network, showing how abnormal ventilation or perfusion can upset $\dot{V}_A/\dot{Q}$ balance.

of shunted venous blood with oxygenated blood is known as venous admixture. Some degree of shunt is normal due to part of the bronchial circulation mingling with pulmonary venous drainage. Extra-pulmonary shunt may also occur, e.g. congenital heart disease may cause right-to-left intracardiac shunting of unoxygenated blood.

Wasted ventilation occurs when a perfusion defect causes an increase in alveolar dead space, resulting in $\dot{V}_A/\dot{Q}$ mismatch in the other direction (Fig. 1.8). Pulmonary embolism is an example because fresh gas is delivered to non-perfused alveoli.

Hypoventilation leads to a fall in PaO_2 that is roughly equivalent to the increase in $PaCO_2$.

Diffusion abnormalities are rare, the hypoxaemia caused by disorders such as pulmonary oedema or fibrosing alveolitis being due to $\dot{V}_A/\dot{Q}$ mismatch more than impaired diffusion.

Normally, alveolar oxygen tension is slightly greater than arterial oxygen tension, the difference in tension being called the alveolar–arterial oxygen gradient (PA–aO_2). This can distinguish between hypoxaemia caused by hypoventilation and that caused by other alterations in gas exchange (Gray and Blalock 1991):

- hypo- or hyperventilation shows a normal PA–aO_2,
- diffusion defects cause a normal gradient at rest, a decrease on 100% oxygen but an increase on exercise,
- $\dot{V}_A/\dot{Q}$ abnormalities show an increased gradient.
- PA–aO_2 increases with age.

Clinical features

Table 1.1 shows how the body responds to hypoxia and hypercapnia. The brain is the organ that can least sustain oxygen deprivation, and normally responds to hypoxia by progressive signs:

PaO_2 < 7.3 kPa (55 mmHg) – memory defect, impaired judgement,
   < 5.3 kPa (40 mmHg) – tissue damage,
   < 4 kPa (30 mmHg) – unconsciousness,
   < 2.7 kPa (20 mmHg) – death.

The circulatory response to acute hypoxia is increased cardiac output and improved blood

Table 1.1 Clinical features of hypoxaemia and hypercapnia

Hypoxaemia	Hypercapnia
Cyanosis	Flapping tremor of hands
Tachypnoea	Tachypnoea
Tachycardia → arrhythmias/bradycardia	Tachycardia → bradycardia
Peripheral vasoconstriction	Peripheral vasodilation leading to warm hands
	Headache
Restlessness → confusion → coma	Drowsiness → hallucinations → coma
	Sweating

flow to the brain, respiratory muscles and liver, at the expense of reduced flow to gut, skin and bone (Kuwahira 1993). Worsening hypoxia leads to arrhythmias. Long-term sufferers compensate by developing polycythaemia (p. 53).

Hypercapnia reflects hypoventilation, which is due to respiratory depression, severe weakness, fatigue or an attempt to avoid fatigue by reducing ventilation and inspiratory muscle overload (Green and Moxham 1993). Both hypoxaemia and hypercapnia lead to reduced endurance of the diaphragm (Tobin 1988).

Blood gas patterns

PaO_2 is affected by one or a combination of the 'causes of hypoxaemia' mentioned on p. 11. $PaCO_2$ is affected only by ventilation because CO_2 is freely diffusible and is not altered by $\dot{V}_A/\dot{Q}$ changes. $PaCO_2$ is therefore used to assess ventilatory adequacy. Examples of blood gas abnormalities are:

- ↓ PaO_2 with ↑ $PaCO_2$ – hypercapnic respiratory failure, e.g. exacerbation of chronic lung disease,
- ↓ PaO_2 with ↓ $PaCO_2$ – hypocapnic res-

piratory failure in a patient who has maintained the ability to ventilate adequately,
- normal PaO_2 with ↓ $PaCO_2$ – hyperventilation, e.g. emotion, hyperventilation syndrome, painful arterial puncture.

The three above examples could, in reverse order, represent a developing asthma attack.

If we reduce our minute ventilation, $PaCO_2$ rises and PaO_2 falls, but the reverse is not true. Increased ventilation will blow off $PaCO_2$ but PaO_2 is maintained because Hb cannot be supersaturated.

1.9.4 Acid-base balance

Body cells and chemical reactions are acutely sensitive to the acidity or alkalinity of their environment, and any deviation from the normal slight alkalinity of body fluids is fiercely resisted, at whatever cost, by several homeostatic mechanisms. These work to dispose of the acids that are continually produced by the body's metabolic processes.

Regulation

The buffer system acts as a chemical sponge which neutralizes acids or bases by means of reactions that give up or absorb hydrogen ions, all within seconds. The base-buffer equation depends on the dissociation of carbonic acid in solution, which acts as a sink for hydrogen ions:

$$H^+ + HCO^-_3 \rightleftharpoons H_2CO_3 \rightleftharpoons H_2O + CO_2$$

The lungs then present an avenue for the escape of CO_2 that has been made available by this equation. Hyper- or hypoventilation can stabilize the acid-base balance within 1–15 minutes. The kidneys eliminate acid but take several days to normalize pH. When pH is restored to normal, the acidosis or alkalosis is known as fully compensated.

Acid-base balance is affected if the removal of CO_2 from the lungs is abnormal (respiratory acidosis or alkalosis) or production of

Table 1.2 Interpretation of acid-base readings

	Causes	Effects	Recognition
Acute respiratory acidosis	Hypoventilation e.g. oversedation, exhaustion	PCO_2 pH HCO_3^- ↑ ↑ ↓ Ⓝ (no time for renal compensation)	Shallow breathing, drowsiness
Chronic (compensated) respiratory acidosis	Airways obstruction, chronic hypoventilation e.g. COPD	PCO_2 pH HCO_3^- ↑ ↑ ↓ or Ⓝ ↑ ↑ (renal conservation of HCO_3^- in order to restore pH)	Signs of, e.g. COPD
Respiratory alkalosis	Acute hyperventilation, e.g. excess mechanical ventilation, anxiety or pain, early acute asthma, chronic hyperventilation	PCO_2 pH HCO_3^- ↓ ↓ ↑ ↓ ↓ (renal excretion of HCO_3^-)	Dizziness, tingling fingers, numbness around mouth
Metabolic acidosis	Ketoacidosis from diabetes, loss of alkali from, e.g. diarrhoea, chronic renal failure	PCO_2 pH HCO_3^- BE < −2 ↓ ↓ ↓ ↓ (respiratory compensation lowers PCO_2)	Hyperventilation, drowsiness, coma, arrhythmias if severe
Metabolic alkalosis	Volume depletion, diuretics, removal of acid, e.g. vomiting	PCO_2 pH HCO_3^- BE > +2 ↑ ↑ ↑ ↑	Delirium or tetany if severe

CO_2 from the tissues or elimination elsewhere is abnormal (metabolic acidosis or alkalosis).

Interpretation

It is best to look first at pH. Low pH means acidosis and high pH means alkalosis. Bicarbonate and base excess (BE) indicate the extent of renal compensation and quantify the metabolic component of acid-base disturbance. High bicarbonate or base excess means metabolic alkalosis and low bicarbonate or base excess means metabolic acidosis.

If pH and $PaCO_2$ change in opposite directions, it is usually a respiratory problem. A change in pH due to respiratory or metabolic disturbance is usually offset by a compensatory change in the other system so that pH normalizes. Respiratory and metabolic factors are often combined, and complex compensations can occur.

Cause, effect and recognition of acid-base imbalance are shown in Table 1.2. Examples are the following:

- pH 7.3, $PaCO_2$ 6.5 kPa (49 mmHg), HCO_3^- 30 mmol/l – compensated respiratory acidosis, since both $PaCO_2$ and HCO_3^- are increased but pH is low.
- pH 7.5, $PaCO_2$ 4 kPa (30 mmHg), HCO_3^- 18 mmol/l – compensated respiratory alkalosis, since both $PaCO_2$ and HCO_3^- are decreased but pH is high.
- pH 7.48, $PaCO_2$ 6.1 kPa (46 mmHg), HCO_3^- 30 mmol/l – compensated metabolic alkalosis, since both $PaCO_2$ and HCO_3^- are increased and pH is high.

Table 1.3 Examples of acid-base balance for common conditions (blood gases in kPa and mmHg)

	Normal	Acute asthma	COPD
PaO_2	12.7 (95)	9.3 (70)	7.3 (55)
$PaCO_2$	5.3 (40)	3.3 (25)	8 (60)
pH	7.4	7.5	7.4
HCO_3	24	24	29

- pH 7.3, $PaCO_2$ 4 kPa (30 mmHg), HCO^-_3 18 mmol/l – compensated metabolic acidosis, since both $PaCO_2$ and HCO^-_3 are decreased and pH is low.

Examples for common conditions are shown in Table 1.3.

1.10 OXYGEN DELIVERY, CONSUMPTION AND EXTRACTION

Even if ventilation, diffusion and perfusion are in order, gas exchange still has to take place at tissue level. Oxygen **delivery** (transport) to the tissues depends on the oxygen content of blood, cardiac output, haemoglobin levels and local perfusion. Oxygen **consumption** (uptake) by the tissues is roughly equivalent to oxygen demand, which is determined by the metabolic need of the tissues for oxygen.

Tissue oxygenation is determined by a balance between supply (oxygen delivery or DO_2) and demand (oxygen consumption or $\dot{V}O_2$). DO_2 is normally three or four times greater than $\dot{V}O_2$ (Epstein 1993) and an increase in $\dot{V}O_2$ is usually met without difficulty by higher DO_2 (through increased cardiac output and minute ventilation) and greater oxygen **extraction**. But $\dot{V}O_2$ varies with metabolic rate, and critically ill patients with sepsis can demand 50–60% extra oxygen, while patients with multiple trauma, septic shock or burns need 100% extra (Epstein 1993), so that oxygen requirements may not be met, thus causing sustained lactic acidosis. Measurement of tissue oxygenation is on p. 236.

1.11 EFFECT OF AGEING

A 90 year old has half the pulmonary function of a 30 year old. Changes due to ageing are related to the cumulative effect of the environment on the 'outdoor' lung. Changes with age that are relevant to the physiotherapist include the following:

- small airway narrowing, leading to ↑ closing volume (Fig. 1.9), airway closure during tidal breathing, $\dot{V}_A/\dot{Q}$ mismatch and transient hypoxaemia especially during REM sleep,
- ↓ respiratory muscle strength by 1% per year (Rochester and Arora 1983), due to factors such as a sedentary lifestyle, nutritional deficit, chronic illness and ageing itself,
- because of the above two factors, ↑ FEV_1 by 30 ml a year (Hodgkin 1993, p. 65),
- greater dependence on collateral ventilation due to airway closure in dependent lung regions,
- thinning of alveolar walls, which is similar to emphysema in increasing alveolar diameter and reducing gas exchange surface area, but is more evenly distributed and without alveolar destruction (Verbeken *et al* 1992),
- ↑ residual volume because closure of small airways prevents full expiration (this appears as hyperinflation on X-ray which can be misinterpreted as emphysema),
- ↓ chest wall compliance,
- ↓ exercise capacity, leading to ↓ function by 10% per decade (Hellman 1994),
- ↓ ventilatory response to both hypoxaemia and hypercapnia, leading to a risk of sleep-related disorders (Phillipson 1993),
- ↓ total blood volume, which impairs circulatory function (Davy and Seals 1994),
- postural hypotension,
- ↑ BP, especially systolic (Hellman 1994), which helps maintain tissue perfusion

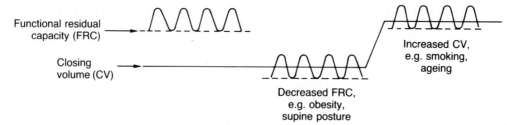

Functional residual capacity (FRC)

Closing volume (CV)

Increased CV, e.g. smoking, ageing

Decreased FRC, e.g. obesity, supine posture

Figure 1.9 Factors that shift tidal breathing into the closing volume range, leading to airway closure in lung bases during quiet breathing.

because a greater pressure is needed to overcome the resistance of hardening arteries.

Lung compliance does not alter with age, which accords with the concept that lung 'elasticity' is largely determined by surface tension (Nunn 1987, p. 34).

1.11.1   Clinical implications

During mobilization, time is needed when assisting elderly patients out of bed in case of postural hypotension. During deep breathing, collateral ventilation can be exploited with an end-inspiratory hold (p. 113). During exercise training, an ageing cardiovascular system is less able to adapt to the stress of exercise. During weaning from mechanical ventilation, extra help is needed because lung volume is especially compromised by the supine posture and low tidal volumes. When interpreting blood gas readings, a healthy 60-year-old has a PaO_2 of about 10.7 kPa (80 mmHg), thereafter losing 1 mmHg for each year of age.

1.12   EFFECT OF OBESITY

The obese and the elderly share a tendency towards poor basal ventilation. People who are overweight show lower lung volumes (especially expiratory reserve volume) and reduced lung and chest wall compliance (Jenkins and Moxham 1991). Hypercapnia is also a risk (Bégin 1991). In the lateral position, the normal downwards ventilation gradient is reversed because of lung compression from the abdomen (Hurewitz 1985), leading to less ventilation in the well-perfused bases, $\dot{V}_A/\dot{Q}$ mismatch and sometimes reduced PaO_2. Exercise demands high oxygen consumption. Breathing patterns tend to be rapid and shallow. Obesity increases the risk of cardiovascular disease, hypertension, diabetes, digestive diseases and some cancers (Chen *et al* 1993).

Obesity does not ensure adequate protein stores, and hospitalization can worsen the nutritional status of obese people. People with lung diseases may be obese from inactivity, and overweight from steroid medication.

1.12.1   Clinical implications

Head down postural drainage is inadvisable in obese people because of the extra load on the diaphragm and risk of atelectasis. After surgery, an obese patient should barely have emerged from anaesthesia before the physiotherapist becomes involved in pain control and positioning. Exercise tolerance is impaired by fat infiltration of muscle and a heavy work load.

1.13 EFFECT OF SMOKING

A custom loathsome to the eye, hateful to the nose, harmful to the brain and dangerous to the lungs.

King James I

Smoking is slow motion suicide. It is a form of drug addiction that is the leading preventable cause of premature death (Balfour 1993), killing one person every five minutes in the UK (Venables 1994). This comes as no surprise considering the 4000 chemicals in tobacco smoke, including cyanide, asbestos and 60 known carcinogens (HEA 1995). Apart from causing the well-known carnage to the respiratory and cardiovascular systems, including a 70% increased risk of heart disease (Brannon *et al* 1993), these chemicals wreak a litany of destruction, as described below.

1. Smoking increases low back pain (Ernst 1993), accelerates ageing (Kauffmann 1993), ulcerates the gut (Jones 1992), dislodges teeth (Jette 1993), causes cataract (Christen 1992) and glue ear (Couriel 1994a), depletes vitamin C by 30% (Strachan 1991), causes squint in children (Anon 1992), demineralizes bone (Ernst 1993), causes more bronchial hyperreactivity than cocaine (Tashkin *et al* 1993), increases the risk of subarachnoid haemorrhage sixfold (Partridge 1992) and risk of pneumothorax 16-fold (Light 1993), raises BP and reduces exercise tolerance (Gidding 1994).

2. Nicotine is the ingredient that imprisons smokers in the habit. It is more addictive than heroin, six to eight times as addictive as alcohol (Haas and Haas 1990, p. 67) and is delivered to the central nervous system within 7 seconds (Fisher *et al* 1990). It initially stimulates the brain, then acts as a sedative. The one redeeming feature of nicotine is that it ameliorates ulcerative colitis, for which nicotine patches have been advised (Pullan *et al* 1994).

3. Smokers show increased closing volumes

and greater $\dot{V}_A/\dot{Q}$ mismatch than non-smokers (Fig. 1.9). Premature closure of small airways occurs before the onset of symptoms or lung function abnormality, after which there is a doubling of the normal increase in airways obstruction (Zadai 1991).

4. Smoking weakens the immune system and damages surfactant (Pearce and Jones 1984).

5. Smoking doubles or triples female infertility (Partridge 1992). For those who pass this hurdle, smoking before and during pregnancy increases miscarriages, stillbirths and cot-deaths by one-third (Couriel 1994a), and creates children who are intellectually impaired (Olds 1994), smaller, slower growing and with increased respiratory and allergic disease throughout life (Partridge 1992). Even grandchildren do not escape – mothers born to women who smoked during pregnancy being more likely to have a miscarriage (Golding 1994).

6. Smoking is neither virile nor sexy. Male smokers have a high incidence of sperm abnormalities, and all smokers have breath that smells like an ashtray.

7. Smoking is the main risk factor for postoperative chest infection (Dilworth and White 1992).

8. Passive smoking increases infant mortality and the incidence of childhood respiratory diseases, impairs lung development (Gidding 1994) and forms lung carcinogens in the recipient within hours (Hecht 1993).

9. One tree is killed per fortnight to cure the tobacco for one average smoker (HEA 1995).

Marijuana smoking appears to be benign when the inhalation pattern is similar to tobacco smoking, but deep inhalation is common and causes bronchitic changes (Tashkin *et al* 1987), and additives are detrimental. Surprisingly, neonates of mothers who smoke marijuana have shown greater physiological stability than those who do not (Dreher *et al* 1994).

1.13.1   Clinical implications

Motivate, educate and cajole.

1.14   EFFECT OF EXERCISE

During exercise, oxygen delivery, consumption and extraction increase, extra oxygen being delivered to the heart and skeletal muscles by several mechanisms:

1. Ventilation can increase from 6 l/min to over 200 l/min (Salazar 1991). At low-intensity exercise, deeper breathing makes the largest contribution to minute ventilation, while at high intensity, rapid breathing is the main contributor.
2. Cardiac output can increase fourfold in an unconditioned young adult, and up to sixfold in a fit male (Epstein 1993), mostly due to rapid heart rate. Systolic blood pressure increases in proportion to oxygen consumption and may reach over 200 mmHg in a healthy man. Diastolic pressure increases slightly during isotonic exercise and significantly during isometric exercise (Salazar 1991).
3. Vascular resistance drops precipitately, and in the lungs, previously closed capillaries are recruited, primarily in the apices, and other capillaries become distended. Muscle blood flow increases 25-fold (Epstein 1993).
4. Oxygen extraction can increase 20-fold (Epstein 1993).
5. Bronchodilation occurs in normal lungs,
6. Mucus transport increases (Mier *et al* 1990).

Cardiovascular delivery of oxygen to the peripheral muscles imposes the primary limit to exercise in normal subjects (Hsia 1993). When blood flow becomes inadequate to maintain aerobic metabolism, the anaerobic threshold is reached, demand exceeds supply and lactic acidosis develops, with a disproportionate increase in minute ventilation relative to oxygen consumption.

PaO_2 changes little in people with normal lungs because of a matched increase in ventilation and perfusion. For people with obstructive lung disease, PaO_2 usually drops, and for those with restrictive disease, PaO_2 can fall dramatically due to diffusion limitation (Wagner 1992). Inspiratory muscle fatigue may develop in people with respiratory disease. Subjectively, exercise can be experienced as incapacitating, joyful or somewhere in between.

The effect of training is to reduce blood lactate levels for a given amount of exercise and lessen requirements for oxygen uptake, CO_2 output and ventilation. Training causes more complete oxygen extraction, a lower heart rate at rest and reduced BP on exercise (Casaburi 1992).

1.14.1   Clinical implications

When encouraging patients to exercise, accurate judgement is needed to achieve optimum activity without losing the patient's co-operation or causing oxygen desaturation.

1.15   EFFECT OF BED REST

Immobility reduces lung volumes and can lead to postural hypotension, constipation, urine retention, osteoporosis, depression and deconditioning (Mulley 1993). Saltin *et al* (1968) showed that 20 days' bed rest can reduce work capacity by 30%, returning to normal only after 3 weeks of intensive exercise. Muscles lose 20% strength per week (Sciaky 1994). Loss of gravitational stimulus to the cardiovascular system causes a negative fluid balance within 24 hours and is also a major cause of deconditioning. Reduced circulating blood volume and impaired vasoconstrictive ability cause postural hypotension, increased work of the heart and increased work of breathing (Dean and Ross 1992). Loss of plasma volume increases the risk of deep vein thrombosis (Sciaky 1994).

Deterioration occurs more rapidly in the respiratory and cardiovascular systems than the musculoskeletal systems, and recovery is slower than deterioration (Dean and Ross 1992). The more immobile the patient, the higher the risk of developing respiratory complications and pressure sores.

1.15.1 Clinical implications

If immobility is caused by pain, fatigue or depression, these should be addressed, e.g. by analgesia, rest or a listening ear, so that they do not prevent mobilization. If immobility is unavoidable for medical reasons, regular position change reduces some of the complications of bed rest. Passive and/or active exercise are necessary and encouragement of upright positions minimizes orthostatic intolerance.

1.16 EFFECT OF SLEEP

The sleeping patient is still a patient. His disease not only goes on while he sleeps, but may indeed progress in an entirely different fashion from its progression during the waking state.
Martin 1993

During sleep the brain is active, and significant alterations in the respiratory system occur. The rapid-eye-movement (REM) phase of the cycle occupies about 20% of total sleep time and is the restorative, dreaming and physiologically eventful phase. Changes during sleep include:

- ↓ mucociliary clearance (Agnew *et al* 1992),
- ↓ cough,
- ↓ PaO_2 and ↑ $PaCO_2$ (Piper *et al* 1992),
- ↓ muscle activity, including dissociation of diaphragmatic and intercostal activity during REM sleep (Mohsenin 1994), and ↓ tone in muscles which preserve

patency of the upper airway, leading to greater airflow resistance (Henke 1992),
- ↓ V_T by 25% during REM sleep (Nunn 1987, p. 304),
- for people whose respiratory system is already compromised, diaphragmatic fatigue and sometimes nocturnal respiratory failure. People at risk of sleep-disordered breathing are those with COPD (Fletcher 1992), and those who are elderly or obese. Sleep itself is disturbed by breathlessness and coughing.

1.16.1 Clinical implications

People on home oxygen should use it continuously during the night because the normal nocturnal drop in SaO_2 can be damaging for people who are already chronically hypoxaemic. Hospitalized patients on oxygen should maintain this at night, sometimes with a higher flow rate. Death from lung disease usually occurs at night.

RECOMMENDED READING

(*see also Further reading, p. 330*)

Halliwell, B. (1994) Free radicals, antioxidants, and human disease: curiosity, cause or consequence? *Lancet*, **344**, 721–4.

Higgins, T.L. and Yared, J.-P. (1993) Clinical effects of hypoxemia and tissue hypoxia. *Resp. Care*, **38**, 603–16.

Shapiro, C.M. and Flanigan, M.J. (1993) Function of sleep. *Br. Med. J.*, **306**, 383–5.

Stringfield, Y.N. (1993) Acidosis, alkalosis, and ABG's. *Am. J. Nurs.*, **93**, 43–4.

Tobin, M.J. (1988) Respiratory muscles in disease. *Clinics in Chest Med.*, **9**, 263–86.

Wagner, P.D. (1991) Clinical advances in pulmonary gas exchange. *Am. Rev. Resp. Dis.*, **143**, 883–8.

West, J.B. (1977) Ventilation-perfusion relationships. *Am. Rev. Res-ir. Dis.*, **116**, 919–42.

Westbrook, J.L. and Sykes, M.K. (1992) Peroperative arterial hypoxaemia. The interaction between intrapulmonary shunt and cardiac output. *Anaesthesia*, **47**, 307–10.

2. Assessment of the respiratory patient

2.1 INTRODUCTION

Accurate assessment is the linchpin of physiotherapy and forms the basis of rational practice. An inadequate assessment leads to reasoning such as: 'This is chronic bronchitis therefore I will turn the patient side-to-side and shake his chest.' A problem-based assessment leads to reasoning such as: 'This patient cannot cough up his sputum by himself. Why? Because it is thick. Why? Because he is dehydrated. Why? Because he feels too ill to drink.' A thoughtful assessment will lead to both effectiveness and efficiency because time will be saved by avoiding unnecessary intervention.

For the clinical assessment, a well-lit area is needed that is quiet, warm and private. A suggested approach is:

- assess the patient,
- identify problems,
- correlate these with the patient's expectations,
- formulate goals with the patient,
- agree on a management plan and time frame,
- treat the patient,

- re-assess,
- discuss and modify the management plan according to on-going assessment,
- check if goals are met.

Patients who cannot communicate or are on a ventilator can still be involved with decisions on the aims and methods of treatment. The more helpless the patient, the more important it is to ensure autonomy.

2.2 BACKGROUND

2.2.1 Ward reports and meetings

Referrals for physiotherapy come from medical staff and suggestions from nursing staff, but the initiative for requesting a referral often comes from the physiotherapist. It is the physiotherapist's job to clarify the indications for physiotherapy to other members of the health team, and to explain which changes in a patient's condition should be reported. If a patient is said to be 'too ill' to see the physiotherapist, this implies a lack of understanding of the scope of physiotherapy.

2.2.2 Notes and charts

Relevant details from the doctor's notes include:

- swallowing difficulty/tendency to aspirate,
- history of vertigo or light-headedness,
- bleeding disorder,
- social history, home situation, stairs,
- other conditions requiring physiotherapy such as arthritis,
- elevated white cell count ($> 10\,000/mm^3$ suggests infection),
- recent cardiopulmonary resuscitation (CPR),
- possibility of bony metastases,
- long-standing steroid therapy, leading to risk of osteoporosis,
- history of radiotherapy over the chest.

The last three findings would contraindicate percussion or vibrations over the ribs. Recent CPR necessitates close X-ray examination in case of aspiration or fracture.

The temperature chart should be checked at every visit because fever is the main harbinger of infection. Clinical examination will distinguish respiratory from other infection. Fever also occurs after surgery or if there is pulmonary embolism, connective tissue disease, blood transfusion, drug reaction or overdose.

Drug therapy, oxygen therapy and fluid balance are documented on the charts. The fluid chart should show a positive daily balance of approx 500–1000 ml due to insensible loss from the skin and respiratory tract. There are many normal reasons for a wide variation in this, including major fluid shifts after surgery, but a trend towards a negative balance suggests the possibility of dehydration and sputum retention, while a trend towards fluid overload might be associated with pulmonary oedema.

The charts should show a BP that is stable and near the norm of 120/80. Patients with a diastolic pressure above 95 mmHg should not normally be tipped head down. Those with a systolic pressure below 90 mmHg should be mobilized only with close observation for light-headedness. The relevance of BP to exercise training, heart surgery and bag-squeezing are discussed in Chapters 6, 7 and 10. Heart rate ranges from 60–100 bpm in adults. A high value suggests hypoxaemia, hypotension, anxiety, pain, fever or sympathomimetic drugs. A low value might also reflect hypoxaemia, as well as arrhythmias, heart block, the effect of drugs, vagal stimulation from suctioning or athletic conditioning.

2.3 SUBJECTIVE ASSESSMENT

The subjective assessment is what matters to the patient. Subjective problems, such as breathlessness, are more closely related to general health and quality of life than physiological measurements (Mahler 1995). Before questioning the patient, introductions and explanations are needed because the public perception of physiotherapy is often limited to football and backache. Patients need to be given the opportunity to define their problems and how these influence their lifestyle. It is worth building up rapport at this stage to encourage accuracy and set the foundations for a co-operative relationship. Respect for a patient's opinions is a potent motivating factor.

2.3.1   Symptoms

How long have symptoms been troublesome? What is their frequency and duration? Are they getting better or worse? What are aggravating or relieving factors?

The four cardinal symptoms of chest disease are wheeze, pain, breathlessness and cough with or without sputum.

A **wheeze** increases the work of breathing. The feeling should be explained to patients as tightness of the chest on breathing out, not just noisy, laboured or rattly breathing. Is the wheeze aggravated by exertion or allergic factors, suggesting asthma? It is confirmed objectively with the stethoscope.

Is there **pain**? Chest pain can be musculoskeletal, cardiac, alimentary or respiratory in origin. Many patients associate chest pain with heart attacks, and anxiety may modify their perception and description of it. Chest pains that are relevant to the physiotherapist are:

- pleuritic pain which is sharp, stabbing and worse on deep breathing and coughing; it is caused by pleurisy, some pneumonias, spontaneous pneumothorax or pulmonary embolism,
- angina pectoris which is a paroxysmal suffocating pain due to myocardial ischaemia,
- raw central chest pain, worse on coughing, which is caused by tracheitis and associated with upper respiratory tract infection.

Breathlessness signifies increased work of breathing. It is abnormal if inappropriate to the level of activity. Causes can be pulmonary, cardiovascular, metabolic or neuromuscular. It may be related to posture. Patients often deny breathlessness if it has developed gradually, but it is significant if they need to pause during undressing or talking, or if they cannot walk and talk at the same time. A key question at each visit can be a comparative measurement for that individual, e.g. how much can you do at your best/worst? What are you unable to do now because of your breathing?

Subjectively, questions on breathlessness could include: What does your breathing feel like? What makes it better or worse? How does it affect your life? Patients describe their breathlessness with expressions such as tightness, smothering, gasping or hunger for air. They can usually identify the quality as well as the intensity of breathlessness (Wilson and Jones 1991). Details of breathlessness measurement are in Chapter 6.

Breathlessness that increases in supine can be caused by lung or heart problems. In lung disease, pressure on the diaphragm from the abdominal viscera compromises breathing. In heart disease, breathlessness on lying down is called **orthopnoea** and is caused by the inability of a poorly-functioning left ventricle to tolerate the increased volume of blood returning to the heart. **Paroxysmal nocturnal dyspnoea** is breathlessness at night caused by orthopnoeic patients sliding off their pillows during sleep, leading them to seek relief by sitting up over the edge of the bed. Breathlessness due to lung or heart disorders can be distinguished by peak flow readings (McNamara 1992), auscultation, X-ray signs or exercise testing.

Cough is abnormal if it is persistent, painful or productive of sputum. It may be related to inflammation, irritation, habit or serious disease, but is often underestimated by smokers and people who swallow their sputum. Suggested questions are:

- What started off the cough?
- Is there sputum?
- If so, what is the sputum like?
- Has it changed in quality or quantity?
- Is there sometimes blood?
- Does the cough occur at night (suggesting asthma and/or gastro-oesophageal reflux)?
- Does it cause pleuritic pain?

A cough that is associated with eating or drinking may be a sign of repeated minor aspiration of stomach contents, especially in people who are weak or elderly. Chronic persistent cough may be associated with postnasal drip or gastro-oesophageal reflux (Ing *et al* 1992), and a dry cough can be caused by asthma, interstitial lung disease, recent viral infection, hyperventilation syndrome, ACE inhibitor drugs or mucosal irritation following removal of an endotracheal tube. The patient can be asked to cough in order to check for weakness or pick up sounds that may be missed by the stethoscope but stimulated by a cough.

Other relevant symptoms are fatigue and weakness, one or both of which may be present. It is useful to adopt the practice of asking patients the cause of their symptoms because their perceptions are often surprisingly accurate.

2.3.2 Functional limitations

Problems with activities of daily living, finance, employment and housing loom large for people with respiratory disease. What is the level of daily exercise? Is the patient employed? How many stairs are there at work or home? Is the environment well-heated, smoky, dusty? Does the patient live alone, eat well, smoke? Is it difficult to shop, bathe, dress? What support is available? Limitation of activity is not in itself an accurate indicator of respiratory disease because of many variables, but a change in activity level is noteworthy.

Fatigue is closely associated with breathlessness (Kellner, *et al* 1992) and depression (Small and Graydon, 1992), which can reduce motivation and the ability to co-operate. How does the patient feel about the disease? This question provides the opportunity for patients to describe their feelings. Anxiety is common if symptoms are unpredictable. Other distressing factors are frustration, embarrassment, restricted social function and a feeling of loss of control. If the patient spends the day flopped in front of the TV, is this because of preference, exercise limitation or depression?

Details of previous experience with physiotherapy will give an indication of which interventions have been beneficial. If the patient is unable to give a history, relatives can be questioned, bearing in mind that they may identify fewer problems and see them from a different perspective. A questionnaire is an efficient way of gaining more detail about symptom-related problems, functional activity and the patient's emotional reaction to the disease (Table 6.1, p. 151).

Details of assessment specifically for chronic problems are given in Chapter 6.

2.4 OBSERVATION

Preliminary observation of the breathing rate and breathing pattern should be made before the patient is aware of the physiotherapist's presence. Detailed observation can then be undertaken.

2.4.1 Apparatus

Is the patient using oxygen? Is it being used as prescribed? Is the humidifier working effectively? Are drips, drains and chest drains in order?

2.4.2 Sputum

Sputum production is always abnormal because daily secretions are swallowed in healthy people. **Serous** secretions are produced in pulmonary oedema. They are frothy because of a mixture of air and liquid, and sometimes pink if blood has squeezed into the alveoli. Chronic bronchitis is characterized by sticky grey **mucoid** sputum, which is like raw egg white. Asthmatic people may produce tenacious mucoid sputum, sometimes containing thick plugs. **Purulent** sputum is thick, usually coloured and often infected; if yellow, it signifies infection or the excess eosinophils seen in asthma; if green, it signifies infection or may have lingered in the airways awhile as in bronchiectasis. Foul-smelling green sputum occurs with *pseudomonas* infection.

Haemoptysis is expectoration of sputum containing blood, which can be an alarming experience for the patient. It varies in severity from slight streaking to frank bleeding. It is bright red if fresh, pink if mixed with sputum, or rusty brown if it is old blood. Causes are:

- pulmonary carcinoma,
- pulmonary tuberculosis,
- bronchiectasis,
- pulmonary embolus,
- lung abscess,
- pulmonary oedema or mitral stenosis,
- pneumococcal pneumonia,
- blood clotting abnormality,
- trauma such as intubation, tracheostomy, lung contusion or frequent tracheal suction.

Haematemesis occurs when blood is vomited, and may be confused with haemoptysis. It is characterized by acidity and dark red blood which resembles coffee grounds, and it may be accompanied by melaena (digested blood passed per rectum) or nausea.

2.4.3 General appearance

Does the posture suggest fatigue, pain, altered consciousness or respiratory distress? Breathless people characteristically brace their arms so that their shoulder girdle muscles can work as accessory muscles of respiration. Is the patient obese, thus compromising diaphragmatic function, or cachectic, indicating poor nutrition and weakness? If the patient is unkempt, does this reflect difficulty with self-care or a measure of how the disease has affected self-esteem? Is the patient restless or incoherent, possibly due to hypoxaemia?

For mobile patients, the gait gives an indication of mood, breathlessness, co-ordination, fatigue, shoulder girdle tension or a tense rigid posture with lack of arm swinging during walking.

2.4.4 Colour

Pallor is associated with anaemia, reduced cardiac output or hypovolaemic shock. A plethoric appearance is due to the excess red blood cells of polycythaemia. Cyanosis is blue colouration due to unsaturated haemoglobin in the blood, caused by lung or cardiovascular disease.

Central cyanosis is evident at the mouth, lips and tip of the tongue, but it is an unreliable guide to hypoxaemia and can be identified at SaO_2 levels that vary between 72% and 95% (Martin 1990). Its detection depends on skin pigmentation, patency of vessels, ambient lighting, keeness of the observer's eye and the level of haemoglobin in the blood. It may be masked by anaemia or exaggerated in polycythaemia. Cyanosis should be viewed as a warning rather than a measurement, and its absence should not lead to a false sense of security.

Peripheral cyanosis shows at the fingers, toes and ear lobes, and signifies a problem with circulation rather than gas exchange. Stagnant blood gives up its available oxygen and the peripheries appear blue as a result of a cold environment or pathology, such as peripheral vascular disease.

2.4.5 Hands

The hands are a rich source of information. Cold hands could be caused by poor cardiac output. CO_2 retention is indicated by warm hands due to peripheral vasodilation, and a flapping parkinsonian-like tremor of the outstretched hands (asterixis). A fine tremor may be a side-effect of bronchodilator drugs. For patients who are unable to give a smoking history, nicotine stains provide irrefutable evidence of the deadly habit.

Clubbing is recognized by loss of the angle between nail and nail bed, and in later stages by bulbous ends to the fingers which look like drumsticks. It is associated with an array of heart, lung, liver and bowel disorders. Pulmonary causes include sepsis and fibrosing alveolitis. Recent-onset clubbing may be the first sign of bronchial carcinoma. The exact mechanism of clubbing is unknown, but it is associated with increased local perfusion due to fluid accumulation (Currie and Gallagher 1988). Clubbing is of supreme unimportance to the physiotherapist because it is not affected by physiotherapy. It is only known to be reversed by lung transplantation.

2.4.6 Oedema

Oedema accumulates at the ankles or sacral area, depending on posture. In the respiratory patient, it is associated with chronic hypoxaemia and heart failure. More details are on p. 54.

2.4.7 Chest shape

Patients should be asked to undress, if they feel comfortable with this, so that the chest and abdomen are visible. A normal chest shape is shown in Fig. 2.1. Chronic lung disease can lead to a rigid barrel-shaped hyperinflated chest, with horizontal ribs and increased antero-posterior diameter relative to transverse diameter (p. 56).

Abnormalities of the chest wall may increase the work of breathing, e.g. a restrictive defect can be caused by kyphosis, kyphoscoliosis or scoliosis. A kyphotic curvature exceeding 70° increases the risk of respiratory failure, and a curvature exceeding 100° is associated with hypoxaemia and cor pulmonale (Ras *et al* 1994). Rarer conditions are pigeon chest (pectus carinatum) which protrudes the sternum, and funnel chest (pectus excavatum) which depresses the sternum; these do not usually restrict lung function, but may require cosmetic surgery.

2.4.8 Breathing rate

The normal respiratory rate (RR) is 10–20/min. A rate over 40/min increases the work of breathing, is inefficient and leads to respiratory alkalosis. A rate below 8/min pushes up the $PaCO_2$ to unacceptable levels. Causes for deviations from the norm are indicated below:

↑ RR	↓ RR
lung or heart disease	drug overdose
pain or anxiety	brain damage
anaemia	diabetic coma
inspiratory muscle fatigue	
or weakness	exhaustion
pulmonary oedema	
pulmonary embolus	
spontaneous pneumothorax	
fever.	

2.4.9 Breathing pattern

Normal breathing is rhythmic, with active inspiration, passive expiration and an inspiratory to expiratory (I:E) ratio of about 1:2. Many individual variations are normal, the same ventilation being achieved by different combinations of rate and depth or different combinations of chest and abdominal movement. Other patterns suggest increased work of breathing and/or neurological defect. Laboured breathing is shown by the following:

1. Obvious accessory muscle contraction (Fig. 2.2), which reflects the effort of

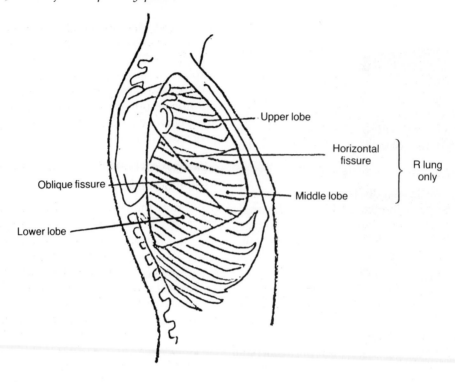

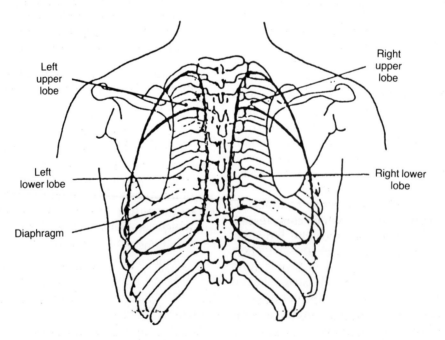

Figure 2.1 Lateral and posterior views of the lobes and fissures of the lung.

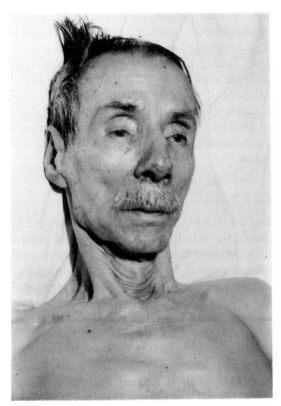

Figure 2.2 Patient with hypertrophied accessory muscles and soft-tissue recession.

age (Ingram 1967) and disrupts pulmonary blood flow and cardiac output (Cameron and Bateman, 1990). Pursed lip breathing may improve SaO_2, but does not improve oxygen uptake (Breslin 1992), probably because of impaired cardiac output. More details are in Chapter 6.

Paradoxical breathing increases the work of breathing, e.g.:

1. If more than one rib has been fractured in more than one place, a flail segment of chest is sucked in during inspiration and pushed out on expiration (Fig. 11.1).
2. The flattened diaphragm that occurs in hyperinflation can become in effect an expiratory muscle, pulling in the lower ribs on inspiration (Hoover's sign, p. 56).
3. If there is increased inspiratory load, or diaphragmatic weakness or paralysis, abdominal paradox may be observed. On inspiration, the inadequate diaphragm is pulled up by negative pressure generated in the chest and the abdomen is sucked in. Palpation distinguishes this from active contraction of the abdominal muscles.

The following three signs indicate inspiratory muscle fatigue, weakness and/or overload (Mador 1991):

- abdominal paradox, as described above,
- rapid shallow breathing, which reduces elastic loading (Mador 1991),
- less commonly, alternation between abdominal and rib cage movement so that each muscle group can rest in turn, which is similar to shifting a heavy suitcase from hand to hand.

Exhaustion is presaged by ↓ RR with ↑ $PaCO_2$. This is a danger sign which indicates that the patient may need some form of mechanical assistance.

Periods of apnoea with waxing and waning of the rate and depth of breathing is called Cheyne–Stokes breathing when regular, and

overcoming the resistance of obstructed airways and the mechanical disadvantage of a hyperinflated chest.
2. Indrawing or recession of soft tissues of the chest wall on inspiration, caused by excessive negative pressure in the chest, which sucks in supraclavicular, suprasternal and intercostal spaces.
3. Forced expiration with active contraction of abdominal muscles, which compresses the airways and increases the work of breathing yet further (Ninane *et al* 1992). It does not speed expiratory flow (Tobin 1988).
4. Pursed lip breathing, which is adopted to stabilize the airways internally and delay expiratory collapse. However, it increases the overall work of breathing (Roa 1991), offers no mechanical advant-

from the bath with ears just above the water. Low pitched bronchial breathing may be heard over fibrotic lung tissue.

Diminished breath sounds are heard if:

- the patient is obese, in a poor position or not breathing deeply,
- there is no air entry to generate the sound, e.g. atelectasis with occluded airway,
- there is air entry but insufficient airflow to generate sound, e.g. acute asthma, emphysema (Schreur *et al* 1992).
- there is air entry but transmission of sound is deflected by an acoustic barrier, such as the air/solid or air/fluid interface of a pneumothorax or pleural effusion (Fig. 2.3).

Both diminished and bronchial breath sounds indicate loss of functioning lung volume.

If breath sounds are inaudible over the chest of a person with acute asthma, he or she should be transferred to an intensive care unit where mechanical ventilation is available if needed. This 'silent chest' is a danger sign because airflow is reduced to the point of ventilatory failure.

2.5.3 Added sounds

Added sounds are superimposed on the intensity of breath sounds and are more obvious, and so can mask the breath sounds. If added sounds are louder on one side of the chest than the other, this may be due to ↑ added sounds on the same side, or ↓ breath sounds on the other side. Non-respiratory sounds occur independently of the breathing cycle and may be transmitted from the abdomen, voice or water in humidifier tubing.

Crackles

Crackles indicate secretions or parenchymal disease (Piirilä *et al* 1991) and are created when air is forced through airways which have been narrowed by oedema, inflamma-

tion or secretions, or when a group of airless alveoli spring open. They are principally heard on inspiration, and their timing depends on the source. Early-inspiratory crackles arise in the large airways and are heard in COPD. Mid-inspiratory crackles are characteristic of bronchiectasis. Late-inspiratory crackles originate in peripheral airways as they open at the end of inspiration, and are associated with pneumonia, fibrosis or pulmonary oedema. The weight of the lung itself causes a degree of airway closure so that late-inspiratory crackles may be heard in dependent regions, especially in elderly obese people who have been recumbent for some time. Late-inspiratory crackles are sometimes called fine crackles, Velcro crackles or crepitations. Both inspiratory and expiratory crackles are heard in bronchiectasis (coarse) and fibrosing alveolitis (fine).

Wheeze

Wheezes are generated by vibration of the wall of a narrowed airway as air rushes through. Expiratory wheeze, combined with prolonged expiration, is usually caused by bronchospasm. Wheeze on both inspiration and expiration can be caused by other forms of airways obstruction such as mucosal oedema, pulmonary oedema, sputum, tumours and foreign bodies. Understanding the timing is relevant because bronchospasm might be exacerbated by certain interventions, while sputum clearance might benefit from these same interventions. A monophonic wheeze can mean local airway obstruction from a foreign body or tumour.

Pleural rub

Inflammation with roughening of the pleural surface occurs in pleurisy, producing a pleural rub which sounds like boots crunching on snow, stronger on inspiration than expiration. The sound is localized, but is best heard over the lower lobes because excursion of the pleura is greater basally.

2.5.4 Voice sounds

The vibrations of the spoken word can be felt by the hands (tactile vocal fremitus), or heard through the stethoscope (vocal resonance). The patient is asked to say '99' or is engaged in conversation.

Voice sounds are normally an unintelligible mumble because the vowels are filtered out through air-containing lung. Sensible speech can be heard when the voice is transmitted through the solid medium of consolidated lung or collapsed lung with a patent airway. This is known as increased vocal resonance or **bronchophony** and is associated with bronchial breathing. Voice sounds transmitted through the fluid/air interface at the top of a pleural effusion have a characteristic nasal bleating quality, a slightly different form of increased vocal resonance called **aegophony**.

Another confirmatory test is to ask the patient to whisper '99'. Over normal lung tissue, whispered words are barely audible, but through a solid medium, such as consolidation, individual syllables are recognizable. This is known as **whispering pectoriloquy**.

Table 2.1 relates physical signs to different disorders, and Table 2.2 differentiates the signs of excess sputum and of pulmonary oedema.

2.6 PALPATION

2.6.1. Abdomen

The abdomen enjoys an intimate relationship with the diaphragm and should be gently palpated at every assessment. A mildly distended abdomen restricts lung volume, while an acute abdomen splints the diaphragm rigidly. Causes of a distended abdomen include pain and guarding spasm, paralytic ileus, constipation, enlarged liver, ascites, obesity and flatulence.

2.6.2 Chest expansion

Chest movement gives an indication of lung expansion. It can be evaluated by inspection or palpation. Apical expansion is best assessed by observing the supine patient from the foot of the bed. To assess the rest of the chest, the patient sits with legs over the edge of the bed if possible, and the clinician stands behind and grips the sides of the chest with the fingers, resting the thumbs lightly on the skin on each side of the spine. On inspiration, separation of the thumb tips should be symmetrical. Lower lobe movement is wholly lateral in the sitting-up position, but both lateral and antero-posterior in side-lying. If expansion needs to be assessed from the front, symmetry of thumb movement from the xiphisternum is used.

While palpating for expansion, other signs may be felt, such as the crackling of sputum or, around the neck and upper chest, the puffing skin of subcutaneous emphysema (air in subcutaneous tissues).

2.6.3 Percussion note

A percussion note is elicited by tapping the chest wall to determine whether underlying tissue contains air, fluid or solid. It is a simple test that evaluates the lung to a depth of 5–7 cm below the chest wall (Wilkins *et al* 1990). It sometimes reveals what the stethoscope cannot, especially in patients who are unable to take a deep breath or when added sounds obscure underlying breath sounds.

One finger is placed firmly on an intercostal space and struck sharply by the middle finger of the opposite hand. To avoid damping the vibrations, immediate recoil is necessary as when a woodpecker strikes a tree. Each side of the chest should be percussed alternately for comparison.

The percussion note is resonant over normal lung tissue. A booming sound suggests hyperresonance and indicates excess air, as in hyperinflation or pneumothorax, but is an inexact guide to these conditions which are more easily detected by X-ray. A dull note is heard when lung volume is

Table 2.1 The relation of respiratory conditions to clinical signs

	Observation	Percussion note	Breath sounds (BS)	Added sounds	Vocal resonance/tactile vocal fremitus
Consolidation	Normal	Dull	Bronchial breathing	–	Increased
Atelectasis with patent airway	Expansion sometimes decreased over affected area Tracheal deviation	Dull	Bronchial breathing	–	Increased
Atelectasis with occluded airway	As above	Dull	BS decreased	–	Decreased
Pneumothorax	Expansion normal or decreased	Hyperresonant	Normal or decreased or absent on affected side	–	Normal or decreased or absent on affected side
Pleural effusion	Expansion normal or decreased	Stony dull	BS decreased Aegophony at upper level of effusion	–	As above Increased at upper level of effusion
Acute asthma	Hyperinflated chest	Hyperresonant	?'Silent chest'	Expiratory wheeze	Normal
Emphysema	Prolonged expiration Pursed lip breathing Hyperinflated chest Barrel chest	Hyperresonant	BS decreased	–	Normal or decreased
Chronic bronchitis	Normal	Resonant, i.e. normal	Normal	Early inspiratory crackles ± wheeze	Normal
Bronchiectasis	Normal	Resonant	Normal	Inspiratory and expiratory crackles	Normal
Pulmonary oedema	Normal	Resonant	Normal	Crackles at bases ± wheeze	Normal
Interstitial lung disease	Expansion symmetrically decreased	Resonant	Normal or decreased	End-inspiratory crackles	Normal
Localized fibrosis	?Expansion decreased over affected area ?Tracheal deviation	Dull over affected area	Normal	Localized end-inspiratory crackles	Normal

Table 2.2 Comparative signs of excess sputum and pulmonary oedema

History	Lung disease	Heart disease (may be secondary to lung disease)
Temperature	↑ if chest infection	Normal
Fluid balance chart	Normal	Fluid retention usually
Crackles	Patchy	Bilateral, usually late-inspiratory, in dependent areas
Secretions	Mucoid or purulent	Frothy, white or pink
Clearance of secretions	By cough or suction	By diuretics
Chest X-ray	Normal, or related to lung disease	Bilateral hilar flare, often enlarged heart, sometimes pleural effusion

reduced by solid tissue replacing air-filled lung, as in consolidation or atelectasis. A stony dull note is an unmistakable sound heard over a pleural effusion.

2.6.4 Hydration

Patients need 1500 ml of fluid a day, which is commonly not achieved. Respiratory patients should always be tested for dehydration. Patients at risk are:

- the elderly, who often have reduced total body water, altered perception of thirst, impaired renal function and reduced mobility which inhibits self-regulation of fluids and increases fear of incontinence,
- patients who are not on a drip,
- people in heart failure, who retain fluid in the interstitial compartment of the body rather than the plasma, and are often on diuretics and so pass excess urine.

Dehydration causes inelastic skin, but so does ageing; it produces dry lips, but so does mouth breathing or oxygen therapy. Clinical assessment for dehydration is imperfect, but the following are adequate:

- the skin over the sternum shows little loss of elasticity in the elderly, so this can be pinched gently, and if it does not bounce back, dehydration is suspected,
- the axilla has a dry, velvety feel in most dehydrated people (Eaton *et al* 1994).

Dehydration is also suspected in a patient with dark urine, postural hypotension with increased heart rate, or electrolyte imbalance, such as increased urea, creatinine, sodium and potassium levels. A patient who has cor pulmonale and does not have swollen ankles should be closely examined for dehydration. Weakness, malaise, headache, nausea, vomiting, cramps and low-grade fever are indicative of, but not specific to, dehydration.

2.6.5 Trachea

Tracheal deviation is detected by palpating with one finger each side of the trachea. In the absence of thyroid enlargement, deviation is due to shift of the mediastinum away from a large pleural effusion, tumour or tension pneumothorax, or a shift towards atelectasis or fibrosis.

A hyperinflated chest means that the low diaphragm shortens the cricosternal distance to less than the normal two to three fingers' breadth, and causes a tracheal tug in which the thyroid cartilage is pulled down on inspiration.

2.7 EXERCISE TESTING

Exercise limitation is directly related to quality of life and is better assessed by exercise testing than laboratory tests (Palange 1994). The patient's own estimate of exercise tolerance accommodates to a slowly deteriorating capacity, so it is best measured objectively by walking or stair climbing. This gives an accurate indication of an individual's progress, but is not a good comparison between patients. Observation of the patient during walking also provides information on the quality of movement and degree of fatigue.

2.7.1 Tests by the physiotherapist

Six-minute distance

Patients are asked to walk for six minutes as fast as reasonably possible along a measured flat corridor. Stopping to rest is allowed, but patients should feel at the end that they have performed to their maximum capacity. The physiotherapist can tell the patient when each minute is completed, but should not walk alongside because this might influence their speed. If an oximeter is necessary, the physiotherapist carries it while walking just behind. Oximetry is useful because resting SaO_2 is not a predictor of exercise desaturation or breathlessness (Mak *et al* 1993).

The data to record are the six-minute distance, time taken to rest, symptoms and SaO_2. If desaturation occurs, the heart rate is noted at that point so that desaturation can be avoided in future. Limitations such as orthopaedic or neurological problems are noted so that exercise programmes can be individualized.

Several practice walks are needed, followed by a 20-minute rest before the test walk. Repeat tests should be performed at the same time in relation to any bronchodilator drugs.

Stair climbing

The stair climbing test is done under the same conditions, and involves counting the number of stairs that can be climbed up and down in two minutes. Stair climbing is also used to assess cardiopulmonary reserve, a climb of at least five flights indicating that the patient is suitable for lung surgery (Pollock *et al* 1993).

Shuttle test

For a more accurate and reproducible walking test, the shuttle test is used. This is incremental, externally paced, needs only one practice walk and is less dependent on motivation and encouragement. Patients are asked to walk around a 10 m oval circuit with two cones at each end to prevent an abrupt turn. The speed of walking is dictated by a taped bleep which is increased each minute. The tape (see Appendix C) also gives standardized instructions. The physiotherapist walks alongside for the first minute to help the patient establish the initial speed. The end point of the test is decided by the patient when symptoms are too great, or by the physiotherapist if the patient fails to complete a circuit in the time allowed (Singh 1992).

2.7.2 Tests in the laboratory

Exercise testing based on treadmill walking or cycle ergometry is unfamiliar to patients, unreliable in relation to everyday activity (Mak *et al* 1993), and less related to exercise capacity than breathlessness (Wijkstra 1994). However, measurable workloads can be imposed in the laboratory while monitoring minute ventilation, CO_2 output, heart rate, BP, SaO_2, blood gases and oxygen consumption ($\dot{V}O_2$). This helps to highlight the interaction between various systems involved in oxygen delivery to the tissues.

Maximum oxygen consumption ($\dot{V}O_{2max}$) indicates the anaerobic threshold, i.e. the oxygen consumption before the start of lactic acid production. It reflects the ability of the cardiopulmonary system to deliver oxygen to muscles and the ability of the muscles to use it. It is an exhausting test that entails increasing the work load until a plateau $\dot{V}O_2$ is reached. $\dot{V}O_{2max}$ is a reliable guide to aerobic capacity in normal subjects, but of limited use

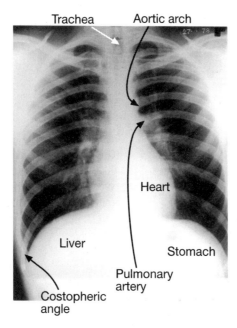

Trachea Aortic arch

Heart

Liver

Stomach

Pulmonary
artery

Costopheric
angle

Figure 2.4 Normal PA film.

in patients with respiratory disease if their peak exercise levels are limited by breathlessness.

Exercise testing can help determine the cause of exercise limitation. If breathlessness is the limiting factor, there is probably respiratory impairment. If a person reaches the anaerobic threshold early, i.e. at less than 40% predicted $\dot{V}O_{2max}$, or if maximum predicted heart rate is reached early, limitation is probably due to cardiovascular disease. Many respiratory patients have cardiovascular involvement, and both respiratory and cardiac patients are often unfit.

2.8 CHEST X-RAY

The X-ray provides a unique insight into the state of the lungs and chest wall, but physiotherapists should not fall into the trap of 'treating the X-ray' because there are several limitations:

1. X-ray findings lag behind other measurements, e.g. they are a later indication of chest infection than pyrexia, and pneumonia may have been resolved for weeks or even months while X-ray signs still linger.

2. A normal X-ray does not rule out disease. Its contribution is anatomical and interpretation is often by inference, e.g. the structural changes of emphysema are more apparent than the hypersecretion of chronic bronchitis, and postoperative patients with reduced lung volume and oxygenation may have normal X-rays (Weiner 1992).

3. The two-dimensional representation of a Three-dimensional object can obscure the relationship between certain structures and limit the accurate location of lesions. It is customary to refer to zones rather than lobes unless a lateral film is available to pinpoint the site.

If possible, a postero-anterior (PA) view is taken, in which the source of rays is behind the patient (Fig. 2.4). This makes for an optimum view of the lungs, the patient taking a deep breath in the standing position with shoulders abducted and scapulae held clear of the film. For less mobile patients, a portable film is taken, with the rays passing anteroposteriorly (AP). The lung fields in an AP view are partly obscured by the scapulae, raised diaphragm, magnified heart, and accentuated lung markings if the patient is unable to take a deep breath.

Dense structures absorb most rays and appear white or opaque, while air has low density and appears black. Allowance should be made for normal variations between individuals, such as different-shaped diaphragms. Comparison with previous films is useful. Chest films show bilateral symmetry, i.e. paired structures look alike, so that opposite sides should be compared.

2.8.1   Systematic analysis

It is worth using a systematic approach to examine the film. This may feel cumbersome at first, but will become second nature and lead to quick and accurate identification of problems.

Preliminary checks

The patient's **name** and the **date** should be checked. Then the **projection** is checked to see whether it is a PA or AP film. This avoids misinterpretation about the heart or diaphragm.

The **exposure** is then checked, an underexposed film appearing too white and an over-exposed film too black. Correct exposure means that it is just possible to distinguish the space between vertebrae through the heart shadow. This avoids misinterpretation about the density of tissues.

The **symmetry** is correct if the medial ends of the clavicles are equidistant from the spinous processes, which appear as tear-drop shapes down the spine. If the patient is rotated towards either side of the plate, the heart shadow is shifted towards that side because the heart is near the front of the

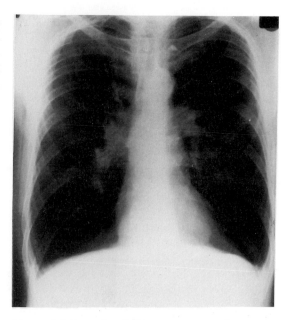

Figure 2.5 Low flat diaphragm, narrow heart and dark lung fields of emphysema.

chest. This check avoids misinterpretation about displacement of the heart.

Trachea

The dark column of air overlying the upper vertebrae represents the trachea, which is in the midline down to the clavicles and then displaced slightly to the right by the aortic arch before branching into the main stem bronchi. It is displaced for similar reasons as displacement of the heart.

Heart

The size, position and borders of the heart are observed. The transverse diameter is normally less than half the internal diameter of the chest in the PA film. An apparently big heart could be due to ventricular enlargement, pulmonary hypertension or poor inspiratory effort. A narrow heart is caused by hyperinflation, in which the diaphragm pulls down the mediastinum (Fig. 2.5), or it may be normal in tall thin people.

The heart normally lies slightly to the left of

midline. It is displaced away from a large pleural effusion or tension pneumothorax, and towards unilateral loss of lung volume, such as atelectasis, resection or fibrosis. The right or left heart borders are blurred if there is consolidation of the right middle lobe or lingula, which are on the same plane as the heart. If there is blurring but the border is still visible, this 'silhouette sign' indicates consolidation of the lower lobe, which is on a different plane to the heart. Lower lobe atelectasis may be concealed behind the heart, or a flattening of the normally-curved border might be the only sign of lower lobe collapse or previous resection.

Hila

Pulmonary vessels and lymph nodes make up the hilar shadows, the left hilum being slightly higher than the right. Hila are elevated by fibrosis, atelectasis or lobectomy of the upper lobe, and depressed by lower lobe atelectasis. Ring shadows near the hilum are normal large airways seen end-on. Bilateral enlargement is associated with pulmonary hypertension, and unilateral enlargement raises suspicions of malignancy.

Diaphragm

On full inspiration, the height of the diaphragm should be level with the 6th rib anteriorly, 8th laterally and 10th posteriorly (Fig. 2.1), with the left side slightly lower than the right because it is pushed down by the heart. A low, flat diaphragm suggests emphysema (Fig. 2.5). An elevated diaphragm could be (1) positional as in an AP film, (2) physiological due to lack of a full inspiration, or (3) pathological due to abdominal distension or generalized lung fibrosis. If one side of the diaphragm is raised, this could be due to atelectasis (Fig. 2.6), a paralysed hemidiaphragm or excess gas in the stomach.

The shape of the diaphragm should be rounded and smooth. Flattening is caused

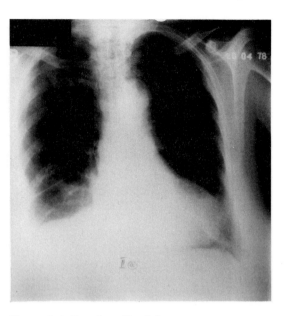

Figure 2.6 Opacity of both lower zones suggests consolidation. The right side also shows the hemidiaphragm shifted upwards and horizontal fissure shifted downwards, consistent with right lower lobe atelectasis.

by hyperinflation, excess doming caused by fibrosis and blurring of the smooth surface caused by lung or pleural abnormality.

The costophrenic angle provides the first clue to problems that hide behind the dome of the diaphragm. The normally acute angle may be obliterated by the meniscus of a small pleural effusion, or the patchy shadow of consolidation.

Air under the left hemidiaphragm is in the stomach and therefore normal. Air under the right is only normal following abdominal surgery or if the colon is displaced above the liver, otherwise it may indicate a subphrenic abscess or perforated gut.

Lung fields

Normal lung contains air and is dark. A film that is too dark suggests hyperinflation (Fig. 2.5). A localized dark area bounded laterally by the chest wall and medially by the thin line of the visceral pleura, and containing no

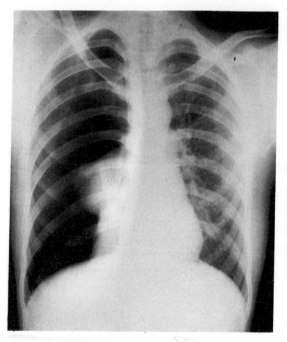

Figure 2.7 Pneumothorax, as shown by the right lung shrivelled down towards the hilum and replaced by a darkened area representing air in the pleural space.

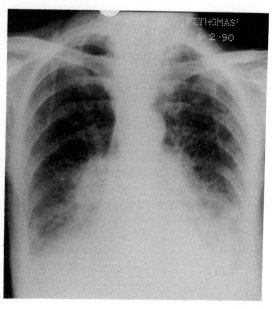

Figure 2.8 Pulmonary oedema, showing bilateral shadowing spreading from the hila, upper lobe diversion and enlarged heart.

vascular markings, suggests a pneumothorax (Fig. 2.7).

Opaque lung fields suggest generalized infiltration, e.g. pulmonary oedema (Fig. 2.8) or interstitial lung disease (Fig. 2.9). Localized opacity suggests consolidation or malignancy. Consolidation is often seen with pneumonia or after surgery, and usually occupies a lobe or segment (Fig. 2.6). If a patient has had a recent cardiac arrest or unexpected loss of consciousness, the right mid-zone should be inspected for consolidation because in the supine position the apical segment of the right lower lobe is dependent and, therefore, the target of any aspirated substances. Complete opacity on one side of the chest, or white-out, is due to lung collapse, pneumonectomy or large pleural effusion. The mediastinum is shifted towards a collapse or pneumonectomy and away from

a large pleural effusion or tension pneumothorax.

The fine white lines fanning out from the hila are vascular markings, which should be:

- symmetrical right and left,
- larger in the lower zones to reflect the greater perfusion,
- visible up to 2 cm from the lung margin,
- more prominent if there is poor inspiration.

In conditions that reduce ventilation to the bases, such as COPD or pulmonary oedema, hypoxic vasoconstriction causes upper lobe diversion (p. 9) by squeezing blood from the bases to match the better ventilated upper lobes (Fig. 2.8).

Airways do not normally show up on X-ray, nor the sputum contained in them. However, they are visible if their walls are thickened as in bronchiectasis, or if they are surrounded by consolidation or generalized white-out, so that the air within them is contrasted against

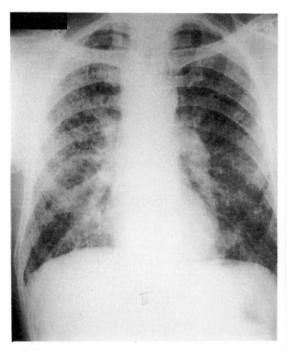

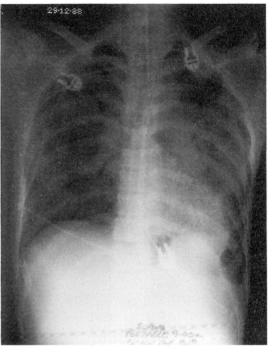

Figure 2.9 Interstitial lung disease, showing reticular shadowing of lung fields.

Figure 2.10 Diffuse shadowing of lung fields indicates generalized pneumonia (*Pneumocystis carinii* pneumonia). Ring shadow at left costophrenic angle is a bulla. Endotracheal tube and ECG leads are present.

a white background, creating an 'air bronchogram' (Fig. 2.10).

Ring shadows may represent (1) an abscess, shown as a thick-walled lesion often containing fluid, (2) a cyst, which is thick-walled, comes in clusters and is often associated with bronchiectasis or cystic fibrosis, or (3) a bulla (Fig. 2.10), which is thin-walled, air-filled and associated with emphysema or barotrauma.

A fluid line spans the width of the lung in a pleural effusion (Fig. 2.11), but is localized in an abscess (Fig. 2.12). Streaky shadowing with some traction on moveable structures suggests fibrosis.

Bones

The bones are examined with particular care following cardiopulmonary resuscitation or other trauma, or if the patient is suspected of

having osteoporosis or malignant secondary deposits. Bony secondaries are commonest with cancer of the lung, breast, prostate, thyroid and kidney.

If a patient has fractured ribs, it is advisable to ask a radiologist to check the film before contemplating any positive pressure treatments because a hidden pneumothorax may be lurking behind the cluster of rib shadows at the apex.

Soft tissues

Extrathoracic tissues cause shadows that project on to the lung fields and can cause confusion unless the origin is identified. Breast shadows may obscure the costophrenic angles in obese people, and prominent

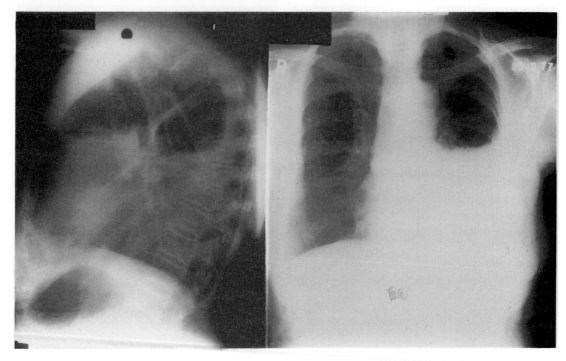

Figure 2.11 Lateral and PA films showing pleural effusion. Lateral film shows fluid seeping into the oblique fissure.

nipple shadows can produce an apparent opacity. Rolls of fat pressed against the plate may be visible. Subcutaneous emphysema shows up along the fibres of chest wall muscles.

2.8.2   Lateral film

A lateral film is needed if accurate postural drainage is required, e.g. for bronchiectasis or an abscess, or to show up lesions that are concealed behind the diaphragm or heart. The lateral film shows the lungs superimposed so that some structures are not easily distinguishable, but other structures can be identified which cannot be seen on the straight film (Fig. 2.13). The hilum is at the centre of the film, and the aorta is seen arching above and behind the heart. The white borders of the scapulae and the dark outline of the trachea can be seen, and the

oblique fissure may be visible. Clear spaces indicate where the lungs touch.

2.8.3   Other tests

Fluoroscopy

Visualization of moving structures is achieved by fluoroscopy, which projects the image on to a monitor. Diaphragmatic paralysis can be identified in this way.

Radionuclide imaging

A $\dot{V}/\dot{Q}$ scan is a map of the distribution of ventilation and perfusion in the lung. The patient first inhales a radioactive gas, and is then injected with radioactive material. The distribution of each is traced by radiation detectors on the chest, and the two images projected and compared. Areas of poor perfusion but good ventilation are diagnostic of pulmonary emboli (Fig. 2.14) or thrombosis.

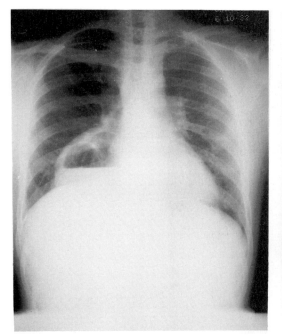 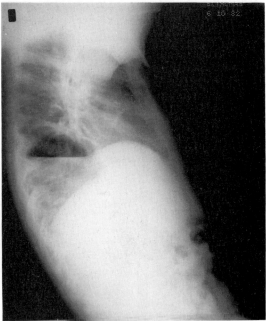

Figure 2.12 PA and lateral films showing a lung abscess in the posterior basal segment of the right lower lobe.

Angiography and bronchography

A pulmonary angiogram is obtained by injecting contrast medium into the pulmonary artery, causing the pulmonary vascular tree to become opaque on X-ray. This shows up pulmonary emboli and vessel malformation. A bronchogram is created by passing a bronchoscope into the airway, where contrast medium is injected into the airways. This shows, for example, the dilated airways of bronchiectasis. Angiography and bronchography are invasive procedures and have been largely superseded by the $\dot{V}/\dot{Q}$ scan.

Computed tomography (CT)

CT scans provide a display of the chest in cross-section, viewed as if from the patient's feet. Computer manipulation of the data produces images in any plane, creating greater sensitivity to different soft tissues than conventional X-rays and overcoming the interference of chest wall structures. CT scans identify consolidation, atelectasis, abscesses, pleural effusions, bullae, the thick-walled dilated airways of bronchiectasis and the distinction between different causes of white-out. It enhances diagnosis in emphysema (Morgan 1992), pneumothorax (Engdahl 1993) and air trapping in hyperinflation conditions (Newman *et al* 1994).

2.8.4 Checklist

The conditions below will show one or more of the signs indicated:

Consolidation (Fig. 2.6)

- patchy opacity with ill-defined margins due to piecemeal alveolar involvement,
- no loss of physical volume (compared with atelectasis),
- air bronchogram,
- silhouette sign.

Anterior ⟶

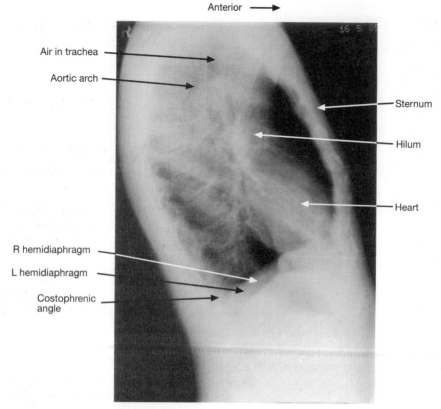

Air in trachea

Aortic arch

Sternum

Hilum

Heart

R hemidiaphragm

L hemidiaphragm

Costophrenic angle

Figure 2.13 Lateral film of a normal lung (patient has a tracheostomy bib).

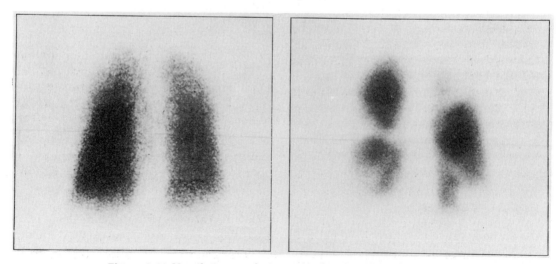

Figure 2.14 Ventilation–perfusion scan showing normal ventilation (left) and patchy abnormal perfusion (right), suggesting multiple pulmonary emboli.

Atelectasis (Fig. 2.6)

- often associated with consolidation,
- ↓ lung volume, as shown by shift of an adjacent structure, e.g. diaphragm or fissure, towards collapsed area,
- ↑ density of collapsed area,
- other lobes appear translucent (darker) because they distend to compensate,
- if the entire lung is collapsed, the hemithorax is opaque, the mediastinum shifts towards the affected side and the ribs crowd together.

Pleural effusion (Fig. 2.11)

- dense opacity across the hemithorax with a horizontal or concave fluid line as the upper border,
- obliterated costophrenic angle or hemidiaphragm.

Pulmonary oedema (Fig. 2.8)

- at first, upper lobe diversion,
- secondly, short horizontal peripheral 'Kerley B' lines at the bases which become visible when the pulmonary artery wedge pressure is more that 25 mmHg (Hodgkinson *et al* 1993); these represent engorged lymphatics, i.e. interstitial oedema,
- then bilateral fleecy mottling spreading from the hila, known as batswing or butterfly shadows, progressing to generalized haziness i.e. alveolar oedema,
- later, pleural effusion as fluid seeps into the pleural space,
- often an enlarged heart.

Pneumothorax (Fig. 2.7)

- black, non-vascular area demarcated medially by the white line of the visceral pleura, often irregular.
- for a large pneumothorax: the lung is shrivelled around the hilum, and sometimes the mediastinum is shifted away from the affected side, especially if under tension.

  A film taken on expiration shows up a

pneumothorax more clearly than a normal inspiratory film.

Hyperinflation (Fig. 2.5)

- dark lung fields, flat diaphragm, narrow heart.

2.9 RESPIRATORY FUNCTION TESTS

The aims of respiratory function tests (RFTs) are to:

- define an abnormality, e.g. distinguish restrictive from obstructive disorders,
- indicate the progress of a disease or response to treatment,
- provide preoperative assessment.

Certain RFTs can be life saving when used for detecting an impending asthma attack in a symptomless patient.

2.9.1 Working definitions

Measurements vary with posture, sex, stature and age. Some depend on fitness and the time of day or year. If two or more subdivisions of the total lung capacity are taken together, the sum of their volumes is called a capacity.

Peak expiratory flow or peak flow

This is the highest flow that can be achieved during a forced expiration from a full inspiration. Peak flow reflects the ease with which the lungs can be ventilated and relates to airflow resistance, elasticity of lung parenchyma and effort.

Normal value: 300–600 l/min.
Less than 1 l/min indicates severe airflow obstruction.

Vital capacity (VC) (Fig. 2.15)

The volume of gas that can be exhaled after a full inspiration, i.e. the three volumes that are under volitional control (IRV, V_T, ERV, see definitions below or in glossary). It is sometimes reduced in obstructive disorders, and always in restrictive disorders. It reflects the ability to breathe deeply and cough, indicating inspiratory and expiratory muscle strength. Less than 1 l suggests an ineffective cough. It is subject to day-to-day fluctuations.

Normal value: 3–6 l, or approx 80% of TLC.

Forced vital capacity (FVC)

As above but with forced exhalation.

Normal: equal to VC.
COPD: FVC < VC because the manoeuvre causes airway collapse.

Forced expiratory volume in one second (FEV$_1$)

This is the volume of gas expelled in the first second by a forced exhalation from a full inhalation. It is a similar measurement to peak flow, but more accurate and closely related to the development of obstructive lung disease. As with any forced manoeuvre, it is difficult for breathless patients and may bring on bronchospasm in susceptible patients. It is subject to day-to-day fluctuations.

Normal: 70–80% of VC, or approx 2–4 l.
Severe airways obstruction (e.g. hypercapnic patients): < 60% predicted.

FEV$_1$/FVC

This expresses FEV$_1$ in relation to vital capacity, and is more accurate for diagnosis than FEV$_1$ alone.

Normal: 70–80, i.e. FEV$_1$ = 70–80% of FVC.
Moderate airflow obstruction: 50–60%.
Severe airflow obstruction: 30% (both values reduced but greater drop in FEV$_1$)
Restrictive disease: up to 100% (both values reduced but greater drop in FVC).

Total lung capacity (TLC) (Figs. 2.15 and 2.16)

This is the total volume of gas in the lungs after maximum inspiration, i.e. the sum of the four primary lung volumes (V_T, IRV, ERV, RV).
Normal: 3–8 l.

Functional residual capacity (FRC) (Fig. 2.16)

This is the volume of gas remaining at the end of a tidal exhalation. It is a useful indicator of lung volume because it does not depend on effort. It reflects the resting position when the inward pull of lung elastic recoil is balanced by the outward pull of chest wall recoil – a comfortable place to be. Active exhalation is necessary if further reduction in lung volume is required.

FRC decreases with restrictive disorders and increases with air trapping or hyperinflation, the ratio of FRC to TLC being an index of hyperinflation. The normal large capacity is needed to dilute extreme changes in alveolar oxygen tension with each breath.

Normal in standing: 40% of TLC, i.e. approx 1–3 l.
Normal in supine: up to 2.2 l.
COPD: up to 80% of TLC.

Tidal volume (V$_r$)

This is the volume of air inhaled and exhaled during one respiratory cycle.

Normal: 10% of TLC, i.e. approx 300–800 ml.

Inspiratory reserve volume (IRV) (Fig. 2.15)

This is usually kept in reserve; IRV is the extra volume of gas that can be inhaled voluntarily from end-inspiratory tidal volume. It is increased during deep breathing exercises.

Expiratory reserve volume (ERV) (Fig. 2.15)

This is the extra volume of gas that can be exhaled voluntarily from end-expiratory tidal volume. It is decreased with obesity, ascites or after upper abdominal surgery.

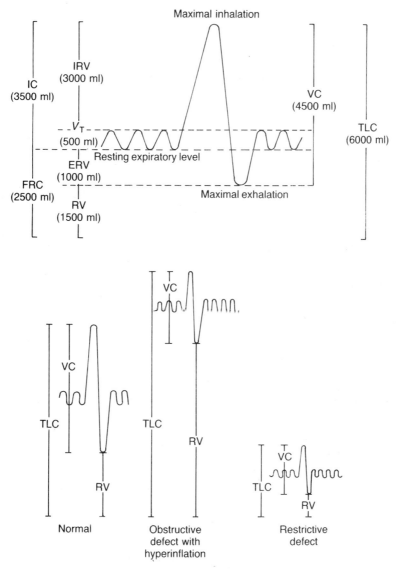

Figure 2.15 Subdivisions of total lung capacity, with variations for different disorders. Hyperinflated lungs show increased TLC, RV and FRC. Restricted disorders show a decrease in all volumes.

Residual volume (RV) (Figs. 2.15 and 2.16)

This is the volume of gas remaining in the lungs after maximum exhalation. It cannot be measured directly. It is inhaled with the first breath at birth and not exhaled until death because the chest wall prevents total lung collapse, i.e. the lungs never empty completely. RV increases with air trapping and age. The ratio of RV to TLC is an index of hyperinflation.

Normal: 20–30% of TLC.
Airways obstruction: approx. 75% of TLC.

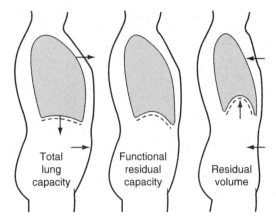

Figure 2.16 Volumes and capacities and the effect of a deep inspiration and expiration. Arrows represent the direction of movement. (From Luce, J.M. and Carver, B.H. (1982) Respiratory muscle function in health and disease, *Chest*, **81**(1), 82–90, with permission.)

Minute volume/ventilation

This is the volume of gas breathed in or out per minute, i.e. $V_T \times RR$.

Normal: approx 7 l/min.
COPD: approx 9 l/min.

Maximum voluntary ventilation (MVV)

This is the volume of air inhaled and exhaled with maximum effort over 15 seconds. It correlates with FEV_1, but particularly relates to maximum ventilation on exercise.

Normal: 50–200 l/min.

2.9.2   Airways obstruction

Serial measurements should be taken on well-rested patients in a uniform posture at the same time each day. This minimizes the normal daily variation which can be greater than the improvement with bronchodilator drugs (Burge 1992). In asthma, peak flow and FEV_1 are lowest in the early morning.

Peak flow

A peak flow meter provides a quick and simple indication of airways obstruction. Three tests are performed, with a rest in between, and the best recorded. Subsequent tests should be at the same time in relation to any drugs. Suggested guidelines are:

- ask the patient to avoid tight clothes, vigorous exercise within the last 30 minutes, a heavy meal within two hours or smoking within 24 hours (BTS 1994),
- explain the purpose and technique of the test (the meter is effort-dependent and reliability depends on the patient understanding and not feeling hurried),
- have the patient seated upright, avoid occluding the exhaust holes and check the pointer is at zero,
- demonstrate the technique with a separate mouthpiece,
- have the patient hold the meter horizontally,
- ask the patient to take a deep breath until the lungs are full, then take a firm seal on the mouthpiece and blow 'short, sharp and as hard as possible'.

The limitations of peak flow measurements are that they are effort-dependent, inaccurate for children under four years, sensitive only to resistance in the large airways and their reliability is variable (Frischer 1995). Peak flow meters should be tested regularly, the portable models replaced annually and the same device used for the same patient.

Peak flow meters are available on prescription in the UK. Regular home measurement is a necessity for people with unstable asthma because lung function can decline to 50–60% of normal before symptoms are noticeable, and subsequent deterioration can be rapid. Less dramatically, peak flow reveals untreated chronic asthma and determines accurate drug therapy.

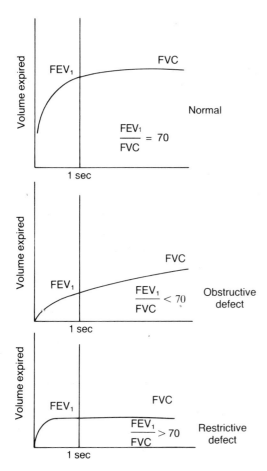

Figure 2.17 Spirograms. **Normal** trace shows most FVC expelled within 3 seconds (the decreasing slope of the curve is due to progressive airway compression and lower elastic recoil as the subject exhales). **Obstructive** pattern shows prolonged expiration. **Restrictive** pattern shows reduced FVC, all of which is expelled within 1 second due to augmented elastic recoil.

Spirometry

Spirometry is an effort-dependent test which uses a spirometer such as the Vitalograph to assess ventilatory function by measuring FEV_1 and FVC (Fig. 2.17). Using the Vitalograph is more tiring than the peak flow meter. Instructions are similar, but instead of a short, sharp blow, patients are exhorted to 'blow the living daylights out of the machine, and keep blowing until your lungs are empty'. Much uninhibited encouragement is required, repeated on subsequent measurements. It may be necessary for some patients to wear a noseclip, so long as they are not breathless.

If a relaxed, not forced, vital capacity is required, the patient blows out from maximal inspiration, but blows at a comfortable and sustained speed until no more can be exhaled (BTS 1994).

Further measurement of large airways resistance

More sophisticated measurements of airway calibre are available. Airways resistance in the large airways depends on flow rate at the mouth and the pressure difference between mouth and alveoli. Flow at the mouth is measured by a pneumotachograph, in which a manometer detects the pressure drop across a slight resistance placed in the airstream. Pressure difference is measured in an airtight body box called the plethysmograph.

Further measurement of small airways resistance

Early detection of resistance in the small airways, where changes occur in the early stages of obstructive disease, improves the success of treatment before changes are irreversible. The small airways contribute only 10–20% of total airflow resistance, and patients with changes in this 'silent zone' may have otherwise normal lung function tests and be symptomless.

The **flow volume loop** records flow and volume during forced inspiration and expiration (Fig. 2.18). During inspiration, flow is dependent on effort throughout. During expiration, the highest flow occurs initially, where it is dependent on effort and represents large airways function, but after only a

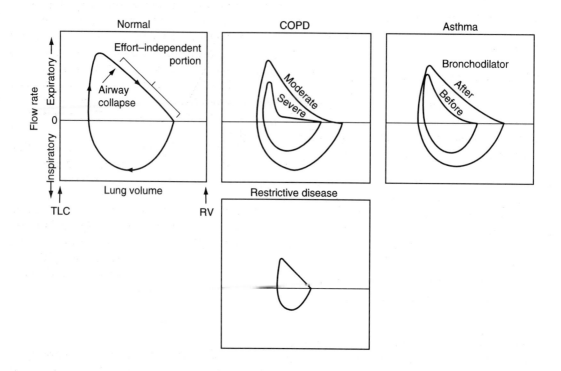

Figure 2.18 Flow-volume loops. Increasing severity of obstructive lung disease is reflected by the increasing concavity of the effort-independent portion of the expiratory curve. Restrictive pattern is represented by a small loop and rapid expiration.

small proportion of VC has been expired, flow is independent of effort and depends solely on elastic recoil and small airways resistance. In obstructive disease, expiratory flow shows a scooped-out appearance representing sudden attenuation of expiration as floppy airways collapse or narrowed airways obstruct. Restrictive disease shows rapid flow during exhalation due to exaggerated elastic recoil.

Maximum mid-expiratory flow (MMEF, MEF_{50} or FEF_{25-75}), is the mean forced mid-expiratory flow during the middle half of FVC. It is independent of effort and reflects small airways resistance.

2.9.3 Lung volumes

FRC is estimated in one of the following ways:

- by plethysmography: air in the chest is compressed and lung volume calculated from the change in pressure,
- by the gas dilution technique: air in the lungs is mixed with an inert gas such as helium, the dilution of which gives an indication of lung volume,
- by the nitrogen washout method: the nitrogen content of air is known to be about 80%, and lung volume can be calculated by having the patient breathe

nitrogen-free oxygen and measuring the expired nitrogen.

TLC and RV can be measured by using one of these measurements plus spirometry.

2.9.4 Respiratory muscle function

Increased strength – ability to generate greater force.

Increased endurance – ability to generate the same work for a longer time.

Respiratory muscle strength is related to exercise capacity (Wijkstra 1994). The technique used to test muscle strength must be meticulous and the patient position standardized because normal values vary 10-fold due to variability between subjects, different diaphragmatic lengths and different test procedures (McKenzie 1994). The following tests are available:

1. Vital capacity is a simple measurement, but insensitive and non-specific. Small pressures are required to inflate the lung, therefore a fall in VC only occurs with severe muscle weakness. The outcome is influenced by effort, fitness and compliance of the lung and chest wall.
2. Maximum static mouth pressure (Chatham *et al* 1994) is also simple to measure. Maximal inspiratory pressure (MIP), indicating diaphragmatic strength, is measured from RV or FRC. Maximal expiratory pressure (MEP), indicating the strength of the abdominals and intercostals, is measured from TLC. A pressure gauge or transducer is connected to a mouthpiece, the patient inhales or exhales sharply, keeping a firm lip seal and taut cheeks, and the best of three efforts is recorded. For non-paralysed ventilated patients, MIP can be measured by briefly occluding the airway with a one-way valve (Truwit 1992). Intrinsic

PEEP (p. 55) causes an underestimation of MIP (Aldrich 1993).

3. Transdiaphragmatic pressure is a more accurate measurement obtained by comparing oesophageal (pleural) and gastric (abdominal) pressures, using swallowed balloons (Green and Moxham 1993).
4. Phrenic nerve stimulation or reduced relaxation rate of muscle are relatively accurate measurements (Green and Moxham 1993).
5. Nocturnal hypercapnia indicate that inspiratory muscle strength is below 30% of normal (Green and Moxham 1993).

Respiratory muscle endurance is difficult to measure and cannot necessarily be inferred from strength. It is assessed by MVV, which is also influenced by co-ordination, pulmonary mechanics and effort (Bardsley *et al* 1993).

2.9.5 Gas transfer

Gas transfer (transfer factor), is the ability of the lungs to transfer gas from alveoli to capillary blood, and is measured by the total lung transfer capacity for carbon monoxide (TLCO). The patient takes a single deep breath of a gas that includes carbon monoxide, breath-holds for 10 seconds, then exhales. The amount of expired carbon monoxide indicates its passage across the alveolar–capillary membrane.

Reduced TLCO indicates $\dot{V}_A/\dot{Q}$ abnormality, low haemoglobin, or diffusion that is impaired by damage to the pulmonary capillaries, lung tissue or alveolar–capillary membrane. TLCO is closely correlated with exercise limitation (Wijkstra 1994) and breathlessness due to emphysema or lung fibrosis (O'Donnell and Webb 1992). In emphysema it may be 50% of normal (Brannon *et al* 1993). It is reduced in anaemia and increased in polycythaemia.

Diffusion of oxygen is influenced by factors other than diffusion *per se*, which is why the

Table 2.3 Checklist of major points of pulmonary assessment

Patient's notes
   history (past, present, family, social)
   investigations
Charts
   temperature
   arterial blood gases
   medication
   oxygen prescription
   peak flow
   fluid balance
   BP
Subjective assessment
   symptoms
   functional limitations
Apparatus
   oxygen
   humidification
   oximeter
   drips
   chest drains
Sputum
Observation
   posture
   colour
   hands
   oedema
   chest shape
   breathing rate
   breathing pattern
Palpation
   abdomen
   expansion
   percussion note
   hydration
Auscultation
   breath sounds
   added sounds
   voice sounds
Exercise tolerance
Chest X-ray

---

terms 'gas transfer' or 'transfer factor' are used. These are broad measures incorporating not just diffusion properties, but also the influence of alveolar volume and capillary blood. The old term 'diffusing capacity' is less accurate because it encompasses only the passage of gas from blood to alveoli.

2.9.6 Oxygen consumption and carbon dioxide production

$\dot{V}O_2$ and $\dot{V}CO_2$ are measured by analysis of inhaled and exhaled gas volumes. When compared with predicted values for age and sex, aerobic and anaerobic contributions to metabolic activity can be assessed.

Table 2.3 summarizes the main aspects of assessment.

RECOMMENDED READING

Curtis, J.R, Deyo, R.A. and Hudson, L.D. (1994) Health-related quality of life among patients with COPD. *Thorax*, **49**, 162–70.

Earis, J. (1992) Lung sounds. *Thorax*, **47**, 671–2.

Hodgkinson, D.W, O'Driscoll, B.R, Driscoll, P.A. *et al.* (1993) Chest radiographs. *Br. Med. J.*, **307**, 1202–6, 1417.

Holleman, D.R. (1995) Does the clinical examination predict airflow limitation? *JAMA*, 273, 313–19.

McCord, M. and Cronin, D. (1992) Operationalizing dyspnea: focus on measurement. *Heart Lung*, **21**, 167–79.

Mootoosamy, I.M. (1993) Computed tomography scanning of the thorax. *Br. J. Hosp. Med.*, **50** (2/3), 95–105.

Quanjer, P.H. (1993) Lung volumes and forced ventilatory flows. *Eur. Respir. J.*, **6**(suppl.), 5–40.

Stiesmeyer, J.K. (1993) A four-step approach to pulmonary assessment. *Am. J. Nurs.*, **93**(8), 22–8.

3. *Respiratory disorders*

3.1 INTRODUCTION

It would be convenient to divide lung diseases into those of airways and those of alveoli, thus identifying them according to the functions of ventilation and gas exchange, but the body refuses to be neatly classified, and conditions such as COPD straddle the fence. Lung disorders are usually divided into obstructive and restrictive disease, plus those that fit neither or both categories.

Airways obstruction is due to:

- reversible factors, e.g. inflammation, bronchospasm or mucus plugging,
- irreversible factors, e.g. fibrotic airway walls or damaged alveoli leading to loss of elastic recoil that supports the airways (Fig. 3.1),
- localized lesions, e.g. tumour or foreign body.

Restrictive disorders are characterized by reduced lung volume and reduced compliance due to impaired lung, pleura, chest wall or neuromuscular mechanisms.

3.2 OBSTRUCTIVE DISORDERS

The common disease entity of chronic bronchitis and emphysema is known as chronic obstructive pulmonary disease (COPD) or chronic obstructive airways disease. Asthma can overlap with COPD (Fig. 3.2). This convenient lumping together occurs because it is not easy to determine the relative proportions of each disorder.

3.2.1 Chronic bronchitis

Chronic bronchitis is a disease of the airways. It is characterized by excess mucus secretion and productive cough. The cough is called a

(a)

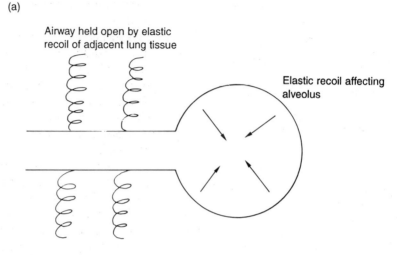

Airway held open by elastic
recoil of adjacent lung tissue

Elastic recoil affecting
alveolus

(b)

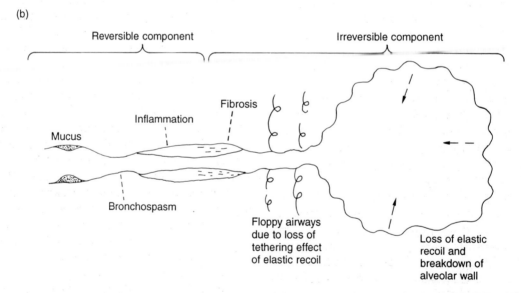

Reversible component

Irreversible component

Fibrosis

Inflammation

Mucus

Bronchospasm

Floppy airways
due to loss of
tethering effect
of elastic recoil

Loss of elastic
recoil and
breakdown of
alveolar wall

Figure 3.1 Mechanism of airways obstruction: (a) normal,
(b) COPD.

smokers' cough in the early stages, but once it has occurred for three months per year for two years, it becomes the inadequate, but traditional, definition of chronic bronchitis.

Causes

Smoking is the major cause of chronic bronchitis, although other pollutants contribute.

Risk factors are male sex and poverty (both associated with smoking), occupation, housing, climate and childhood respiratory illness (Clarke 1991).

Pathophysiology

Repeated inhalation of pollutants causes irritation of the sensitive lining of the airways,

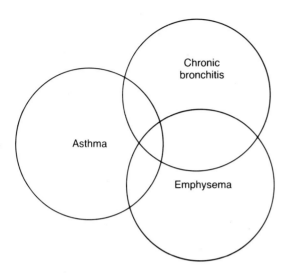

Figure 3.2 Relationship between the common forms of obstructive lung disease.

inflammation, mucus hypersecretion and sometimes bronchospasm.

Inflammation is the key process in chronic bronchitis. It causes narrowing first in the small and then the large airways. Acute inflammation resolves, but chronic inflammation leads to fibrotic changes, scarring and permanent damage.

Mucus hypersecretion is caused by rampant increase in the size and number of mucus-secreting goblet cells. Excess mucus has traditionally engaged the attention of physiotherapists, but causes little overall airways obstruction, correlates little with physiological disturbances (Faling 1986) and does not relate to mortality (Wiles and Hnizdo 1991). Breathlessness is more significant to the patient and more related to inflammatory damage and airway narrowing (Peto *et al* 1983). However, excess mucus predisposes to infection and clearance is hampered by cilia rendered inefficient by damaged epithelium, airway collapse and abnormal hydration (Smalldone 1993).

Bronchospasm is thought to be caused by acetylcholine release due to inflammatory stimulation of the parasympathetic nervous system.

Gradual patchy airway narrowing, often augmented by the floppy airways of emphysema (Gelb *et al* 1993), leads to uneven distribution of ventilation and hypoxaemia. The inexorable downhill path of advanced chronic bronchitis is shown in Fig. 3.3. Polycythaemia is red cell proliferation and represents an attempt to compensate for hypoxaemia by boosting arterial oxygen capacity. It manifests as increased red cell count, haemoglobin concentration and packed cell volume. The associated rise in blood viscosity can reduce cardiac output, hinder oxygen delivery, increase pulmonary hypertension and cause headaches. If the disadvantages of polycythaemia are greater than the advantages, venesection (blood-letting), with reinfusion of the plasma, brings temporary relief.

Capillary destruction and widespread hypoxic pulmonary vasoconstriction increases pulmonary vascular resistance (Vender 1994). Pulmonary hypertension increases the load against which the right ventricle must pump, leading to hypertrophy and dilation, a condition known as cor pulmonale. This reduces the efficiency of the heart and further impairs oxygen delivery. Right heart failure then supervenes, followed by a rise in systemic BP in order to overcome the increased right atrial pressure and maintain cardiac output. This process eventually strains the left ventricle and leads to left heart failure, but death is ultimately due to inadequate gas exchange rather than cardiac involvement (Harris 1989).

Clinical features

The natural history of chronic bronchitis spans 20–50 years, but the disease is asymptomatic at first because changes in the small airways barely affect total airways resistance. Onset of symptoms is then insidious, and a morning cough is tolerable and considered

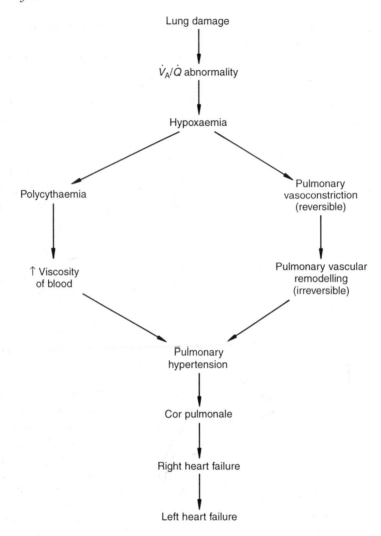

Figure 3.3 Sequence of events in COPD.

normal among smokers, who may not seek medical advice until the lungs are considerably damaged.

Patients then gradually develop breathlessness, which should be routinely measured in COPD patients (Mahler 1995), reduced exercise tolerance and fatigue. Sleep is no longer recuperative but is disturbed by breathlessness, while nocturnal oxygen desaturation plays a role in progression of the disease. Objectively, there is a rich tapestry of signs, such as laboured breathing, a plethoric or cyanotic appearance and crackles on auscultation (Piirilä *et al* 1991). FEV_1 declines by 60–120 ml a year (Hodgkin 1993, p. 65) and is a useful indicator of obstruction but relates weakly to functional impairment (Mahler 1995). X-ray signs may be insignificant or may show a feathery appearance, upper lobe diversion and later the enlarged heart of cor pulmonale.

The appearance of peripheral oedema is a turning point in the disease process, indicating a $PaO_2 < 7.3\,kPa$ (55 mmHg) (Stewart and Howard 1992). Although often associated with cor pulmonale, oedema is not caused by right heart failure, but reflects impaired water handling by the kidneys due to hypoxaemia and hypercapnia (Henderson 1994) and the release of intracellular water during hypoxic dissolution of tissue matrix. Oedema is reduced by oxygen therapy (Howes *et al* 1995). Other systems affected by hypoxia include the gut, leading to the association of COPD with peptic ulcers.

3.2.2 Emphysema

Sometimes when exhausted by breathless
  endeavor
I wish I could sleep forever and ever.
But then this thought my longing allays:
I shall be doing it one of these days.

                    Carroll O'Carroll, Chicago

Emphysema usually coexists with chronic bronchitis and shares a similar aetiology, but is primarily a disease of alveoli with secondary effects on the airways. It is commonly caused by smoking. Rarely, primary emphysema is caused by congenital lack of alpha$_1$-antitrypsin.

Pathophysiology

Protein breakdown is the villain of emphysema, causing erosion of alveolar septa, dilatation of distal airspaces and destruction of elastic fibres. This leads to a hyperinflated chest by three mechanisms:

1. The walls of the terminal bronchi are normally supported by radial traction exerted by alveolar septa. Loss of elastic tissue means that during expiration compressive forces are not opposed by radial traction, and the floppy airways tend to collapse (Fig. 3.1), a phenomenon known as dynamic compression of the airways. This leads to air trapping distally and **passive hyperinflation**.
2. The patient has to maintain hyperinflation actively by sustained inspiratory

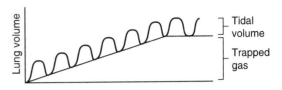

Figure 3.4 Development of intrinsic PEEP.

muscle contraction in order to hold the airways open, a mechanism known as **dynamic hyperinflation** (McCarren 1992). This unfortunate but necessary process is achieved at the cost of excess work of breathing, barrel chest and a lung volume that can actually exceed the predicted TLC (Decramer 1989).

3. Obstructed airways mean that air from the previous breath may not be fully expelled before the next inspiration starts, creating positive pressure in the chest known as **intrinsic PEEP** (Fig. 3.4).

The latter was first described during mechanical ventilation but occurs spontaneously in some COPD patients, especially during exacerbations or when breathing rapidly, e.g. during exercise. The lungs are prevented from emptying to their usual relaxed volume between inflations by an average positive pressure of 2 cmH$_2$O (Ninane *et al* 1993), imposing an extra load at the start of inspiration, hindering cardiac output and impairing perfusion to the labouring inspiratory muscles (Kawagoe 1994). Stabilization occurs at volumes and pressures that are higher than normal, which reduces lung compliance. The distended alveoli require greater than normal pressure for inflation, thus overturning the old concept that emphysematous lungs are hypercompliant (Macklem and Eidelman 1990).

The flat diaphragm of a hyperinflated chest is inefficient and susceptible to fatigue, as with any muscle which deviates from its resting length (Yan 1992). Extra energy is required to:

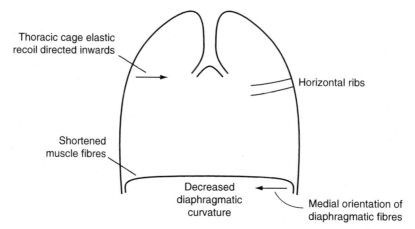

Figure 3.5 The detrimental effects of hyperinflation on the mechanics of breathing. (From Tobin, M. (1988) Respiratory muscles in disease. *Clinics in Chest Medicine*, **9**, 264, with permission.)

- compensate for this inefficient muscle contraction,
- compensate for loss of the 'bucket handle' action of the ribs (Fig. 3.5),
- compensate for reversed action of rib cage elastic recoil, which in the hyperinflated chest is directed inwards rather than outwards, thus resisting instead of assisting inspiration (Fig. 3.5),
- sustain inspiratory muscle action so that high lung volumes are maintained, alveoli being opened at a high point on the pressure–volume curve (Fig. 1.3),
- assist expiration, which has become active in an attempt to squeeze air out through floppy airways on expiration.

People with emphysema are doubly burdened because airways resistance makes it harder to breathe, while hyperinflation impairs the capacity of the inspiratory muscles to handle the added load. The flat diaphragm works paradoxically and becomes expiratory in action, the lower ribs being drawn in on inspiration (Hoover's sign). Some patients can only inhale by lifting up their entire rigid rib cage with their accessory muscles.

Normal muscle is able to respond to increased load by hypertrophy, but an emphysematous diaphragm often labours under further handicaps, such as malnutrition, so diaphragmatic weakness is common (Duranti 1995). Malnourishment is caused by excess energy demand due to the work of breathing, and impaired energy supply due to difficulty in eating when breathless. It leads to cannibalization of the respiratory muscles for their protein, further impairing ventilation. Malnutrition also accelerates the process of emphysema itself (Schlichtig and Sargent 1990).

Two types of emphysema are described, although they may coexist. Centrilobular emphysema affects the respiratory bronchioles, leaving the alveoli relatively unscathed. Panlobular/panacinar emphysema is associated with severe $alpha_1$-antitrypsin deficiency and affects the alveoli themselves, causing more extensive destruction. Breakdown of lung tissue may lead to the formation of bullae (see Glossary), which occasionally require laser ablation (Barker *et al* 1993) or surgery (Nickoladze 1992).

Clinical features

Emphysema shares many of the features of chronic bronchitis. Its hallmarks are breath-

(a)

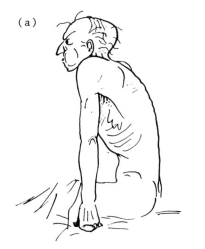

(b)

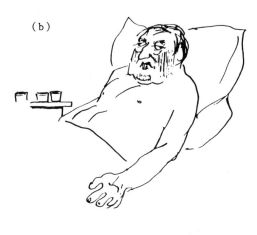

Figure 3.6 Patients with (a) pink puffer and (b) blue bloater characteristics of COPD. (From Brewis, R.A.L. (1977) *Lecture Notes in Respiratory Disease*, Blackwell, Oxford, with permission.)

lessness, laboured breathing and fatigue. Other signs are weight loss, barrel chest, forced expiration with pursed lip breathing, prolonged expiration with I:E ratio at 1:3–1:4, and quiet breath sounds. Soft-tissue recession and other signs of laboured breathing are evident, fossae are prominent and the neck appears sculpted with the skin draped over the bones (Fig. 2.2), because of inspiratory effort and malnutrition with the associated decreased skin-fold thickness (Tobin, 1988). Patients may lean forwards on their elbows in order to force the diaphragm into a more efficient dome shape and stabilize the shoulder girdle for optimum accessory muscle action.

Gas delivery to areas of capillary destruction leads to a high $\dot{V}_A/\dot{Q}$ ratio, and airways obstruction leads to a low $\dot{V}_A/\dot{Q}$ ratio, but relative preservation of gas exchange is a feature of emphysema in the early stages, $\dot{V}_A/\dot{Q}$ match being maintained partly by capillary and airways damage compensating for each other, and partly by development of collateral ventilation (Morrell 1994).

The radiograph shows signs of hyperinflation (Fig 2.5), but CT scanning quantifies emphysematous changes more accurately (Morgan 1992), showing areas of low density, blood vessel attenuation and sometimes bullae. Airways obstruction causes expiratory flow limitation as shown by a reduced FEV_1. A low gas transfer distinguishes it from chronic bronchitis and is the most sensitive test for emphysema, a reduced TLCO becoming evident before X-ray or physical changes (Hodgkin 1993, p. 66).

3.2.3 Chronic bronchitis with emphysema

People with COPD can potentially demonstrate 89 symptoms (Kinsman *et al* 1983).

The blood gas picture is seen anywhere along a spectrum with the following extremes (Fig. 3.6):

- the 'pink puffer' (PP) patient maintains near-normal blood gases at the expense of breathlessness and weight loss,
- the 'blue bloater' (BB) patient abandons the fight for normal blood gases and feels less breathless, but pays for symptomatic relief with oedema, inadequate gas exchange and a mortality rate twice as

high as the PP patient (Clague and Calverley 1990). Some BB patients may tolerate a $PaCO_2$ of over 12 kPa (90 mmHg) for years (Hodgkin 1993, p. 436).

It was originally thought that repeated hypoventilation in BB patients desensitized their chemoreceptors to hypercapnia so that they became dependent on low oxygen tension as a stimulus to breathe. But more recent studies put the blame on respiratory muscle fatigue, the patient 'choosing' the wise option to hypoventilate (Bégin, 1991). PP patients sometimes show a tendency to rush at activities, and breathless management techniques are particularly effective (Chapter 6).

Half of all COPD patients aged over 50 years have cardiovascular disorders (Hodgkin 1993, p. 66) because of related pathology and the mutual association with smoking. Cardiac function plays a significant role in oxygen delivery in people with COPD. Despite preservation of blood gases and more efficient tissue oxygen extraction in the PP patient, oxygen delivery is impaired because of reduced cardiac output (Donahoe *et al* 1992). Low cardiac output prolongs pulmonary transit time, which further allows these patients to escape hypoxaemia. BB patients have more unsaturated arterial blood, but often have normal cardiac output and may be less hypoxic at tissue level. In other words, 'pink puffers' may be only superficially pink and 'blue bloaters' only superficially blue. These terms are hardly complimentary and are not appropriate bedside terminology, but are useful as graphic descriptions of individual responses to COPD.

Exacerbation of COPD occurs when the severity of signs and symptoms increases, especially breathlessness, airways obstruction and sputum production (Ball 1995). Causes are viral infection, sometimes bacterial infection, or non-microbial inflammation due to pollution or allergy, which may be moderated by steroids. Secretions may com-promise airway function (Wanner 1990), and physiotherapy is often required to help the patient clear secretions and reduce the work of breathing.

Medical management of COPD is discussed in Chapter 4, and physiotherapy management in Chapters 5 and 6.

3.2.4   Asthma

Asthma is more common, more serious and more treatable than is generally thought. Mortality increased by one-third during the 1980s (Lawrence 1995), and the disease kills on average five people a day in England and Wales (Finfer and Garrard 1993), many of them young. Asthma is now the only treatable life-threatening condition in the Western world with a rising death rate, with up to 86% of asthma deaths being preventable (GRASSIC 1994). People die because they, their relatives or doctors do not see asthma as a potentially fatal disease, or grasp the importance of prevention, or recognize deterioration.

Asthma is a chronic inflammatory condition of the airways, characterized by undue responsiveness to stimuli that are normally innocuous, a mechanism known as hyper-reactivity. It is distinguished by the variability and reversibility of its presentation, which makes evaluation of severity difficult. It shares with COPD the common pathology of small airways obstruction, but the differences are shown in Table 3.1. Patients suffer recurrent airway narrowing, which usually reverses spontaneously or with treatment.

Physical examination is a hit-and-miss affair because of the episodic nature of the condition and the fact that the symptoms of wheeze, breathlessness and cough are common respiratory complaints. Diagnosis is made from a history of recurrent acute attacks and confirmed by respiratory function tests. If the peak flow varies by 15%, either diurnally, after exercise, or after broncho-

Table 3.1 Distinguishing features of asthma and COPD

	Asthma	*Chronic bronchitis*	*Emphysema*
History	?Family history ?Allergy ?From childhood	Smoking Gradual history	
Provocation of symptoms	Weak stimulus, e.g. cold air	Strong stimulus, e.g. infection	
Variation of symptoms	Much	Little	
Cough at night	Wakes coughing	Wakes then coughs	None
Response to bronchodilators	Yes	Sometimes	Rarely
Response to steroids	Yes	Occasionally	Rarely

dilator treatment, this is considered diagnostic of asthma.

Causes and pathophysiology

A combination of genetic and environmental factors leads to the development of asthma. Predisposing factors include anxious parents, history of a stressful birth and a single gene which causes atopy. Atopy is predisposition to allergic disease and is the main risk factor for developing asthma. An atopic person may become asthmatic if exposed to the house-dust mite, other allergens or occupational pollutants. Asthma is more common in urban areas, implicating pollution (Cogswell 1994). Passive smoking or viral infection damage epithelium so it is more sensitive to allergens. Two phases of response occur (Fig. 3.7):

1. Sensitization stage (which only occurs in atopic people): exposure to allergens, especially in fetal or early life, stimulates production of excess immunoglobulin E (IgE) antibodies in the serum. IgE become fixed to mast cells, which then react to antigens and release bronchoconstrictor substances such as histamine.
2. Hyperreactive stage: continued exposure leads to chronic low-grade inflammation of the airways, causing bronchial hyper-reactivity. Once asthma has developed, removal from exposure to the allergen, if delayed, does not always prevent continuing asthma.

The mechanism for the persistence of asthma is thought to be localized because asthmatic recipients of transplanted lungs lose their asthma, while non-asthmatic patients who receive asthmatic lungs develop the disease (Corris and Dark 1993).

Once hyperreactivity is established, other factors which may or may not be related to the original cause can trigger an asthma attack, for example:

- exercise,
- allergenic foods, e.g. dairy products, eggs, wheat, nuts, additives, cola or other acidic drink,
- drugs, such as NSAIDs, beta-blockers, aspirin (Empey 1992),
- stress, through multiple CNS interactions (Busse 1995),
- chest infection, especially in infants,
- warm-blooded pets,
- pollen,
- car exhaust,
- premenstruation (Cross 1994),
- night time,
- hyperventilation (Groen 1979),
- frustrated expression of emotion (Groen 1979),
- weather, especially change in temperature (Rossi *et al* 1993),
- smoking.

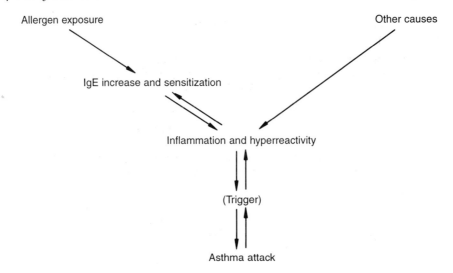

Figure 3.7 Development of asthma.

Some factors may be cause, effect or both. Anxiety, depression and social isolation are associated with asthma (Ramsay 1994), and gastro-oesophageal reflux (GOR) is common (Jack 1995) due to microaspiration of acid into the upper airway triggering bronchospasm, and/or reflux being caused by relaxation of the smooth muscle of the cardiac sphincter due to bronchodilators (Miles and Ayres 1993).

Allergic asthma, known as **extrinsic**, is common during early life in atopic people. **Intrinsic** asthma occurs with normal IgE levels, develops in adulthood, is more fulminant and less responsive to treatment.

Inflammation and hyperreactivity lead to airways obstruction by:

- mucosal oedema,
- bronchospasm,
- gelatinous mucus plugging.

The more severe the asthma attack, the greater the small airways obstruction (as shown by $\dot{V}_A/\dot{Q}$ mismatch), compared with large airways obstruction (as shown by spirometry). Small airways obstruction lasts longer than large airways obstruction, and it is suggested that more prolonged anti-inflammatory medication should be given than

would be indicated by spirometry alone (Ferrer *et al* 1993). Persistent inflammation leads to fibrosis of the airway walls and irreversibility.

Classification and clinical features

Mild chronic asthma manifests as an intermittent dry cough, often at night, or a morning wheeze once or twice a week. Peak flow varies by less than 25%. Even when asymptomatic, peripheral airways resistance can be fives times normal (Wagner 1992), and severe attacks are possible.

Severe chronic asthma means frequent exacerbations and symptoms that significantly affect quality of life. Peak flow varies by more than 25%. Daily anti-inflammatory drugs are required. The most severe form is unstable or brittle asthma, which shows greatly fluctuating peak flows, persistent symptoms despite multiple drug treatments, and unpredictable severe falls in lung function, often without a known precipitating factor (Garden and Ayres 1993).

Acute asthma reflects failure of preventive management or exposure to a noxious stimulus. The large airways are obstructed by bronchospasm and the small airways by oedema and mucus plugging. Asthma

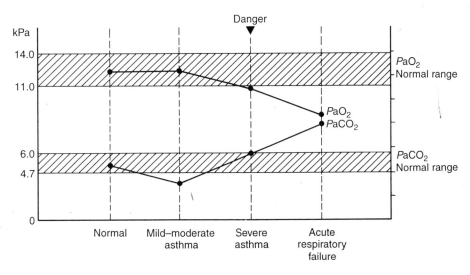

Figure 3.8 Progressive changes in blood gases during acute severe asthma. (From Smith, M. (1982) In case of emergency. *Nursing Mirror*, March 17, with permission.)

attacks are associated with breathlessness, rapid breathing and abdominal paradox. The work of breathing is increased by airflow resistance up to 15 times normal (Mador 1991) and hyperinflation to keep the narrow airways open (Wheatley 1990). Hyperinflation renders the diaphragm ineffectual and the inspiratory muscles are forced to work throughout inspiration and expiration. $\dot{V}_A/\dot{Q}$ mismatch reduces PaO_2, and rapid breathing reduces $PaCO_2$. If oximetry shows SaO_2 below 92%, respiratory failure is likely and blood gas monitoring is required (Carruthers and Harrison 1995).

The effort to breathe out against obstructed airways is reflected in prolonged expiration, as shown by decreased peak flow readings. Patients feel as if they are struggling to breathe through a narrow straw, and many are extremely frightened.

All one's strength, that one feels becoming weaker and weaker, is concentrated into one last effort to take one slight breath that will allow the respiration to continue.

Ruiz 1993

Severe acute asthma may present in one of two ways. Most commonly, the condition develops slowly, often after several weeks of wheezing. Alternately, the attack is sudden, especially if there has been poor drug control, and this so-called asphyxic or catastrophic attack can be fatal within minutes.

Deterioration can be deceptive, and paradoxically the patient may appear less distressed as the condition worsens. Medical help should be sought if the patient shows:

- respiratory rate > 25/min, then decreasing as the patient tires,
- ↑ $PaCO_2$ as the patient tires (Fig. 3.8),
- heart rate > 110, then bradycardia if the patient deteriorates,
- peak flow < 40% of the predicted value, or < 200 l/min if the predicted value is not known,
- ↓ response to bronchodilator, i.e. < 10% improvement in peak flow or FEV_1,
- difficulty in speaking,
- loss of wheeze, and silent chest on auscultation if the airflow is too slow to oscillate the airways, indicating worsening obstruction or failing ventilatory muscle

function, with decreased respiratory effort and exhaustion,
- pallor and sweating,
- pulsus paradoxus (the difference between the highest and lowest systolic blood pressure) < 10 mmHg,
- cyanosis, which represents a life-threatening attack (Carruthers and Harrison 1995),
- exhaustion, confusion, drowsiness, coma.

Very breathless patients cannot produce reliable peak flow readings, and for those too breathless to speak, the peak flow meter can exacerbate bronchospasm (Fanta 1992). Ventilatory failure during severe acute asthma is usually attributed to inspiratory muscle fatigue, but sudden deaths without obvious exacerbation of airflow obstruction have been associated with impaired respiratory drive related to depressed mood (Allen *et al* 1994).

Status asthmaticus is an imprecise term that is sometimes used interchangeably with severe acute asthma, but specifically describes an asthma attack prolonged over 24 hours, leading to dehydration and exhaustion. When the term is used accurately it does not mean the most dangerous form of acute asthma, which can lead to rapid death (Kallenbach *et al* 1993).

Exercise-induced asthma is present in 80% of asthma sufferers, and in some is the only manifestation. Hyperventilation during exercise, especially in cold weather, leads to evaporation, hyperosmolality and cooling of airway surface liquid, and then bronchospasm (Widdicombe 1992). Bronchospasm normally occurs 5–10 minutes after exertion, recovery is usually complete 30 minutes later, and a refractory period of about an hour follows in 50% of patients (Sterk 1993). Bronchospasm can also occur during exertion (Beck *et al* 1994). Warm-up and cool-down periods help to prevent the rapid airway rewarming which can cause oedema. Other preventive measures include β_2-stimulants or sodium cromoglycate taken 20 minutes before

exercise, and on cold days a scarf worn over the mouth to warm the inspired air.

Nocturnal asthma occurs in 80% of asthmatics (Douglas 1993), interferes with sexual intercourse and causes a marked early morning dip in peak flow (Fig. 3.9). Many people develop tolerance to nocturnal symptoms, and lack of awareness of the treacherous diurnal variation leads to underdiagnosis and avoidable deaths. Suggested trigger factors are either an exaggerated bronchial response to cold bedrooms, gastro-oesophageal reflux, reduced lung volume in the supine posture, allergens in bedding, the timing of drug administration or hormonal circadian rhythms.

Occupational asthma may take weeks or even years to develop. Symptoms usually worsen during the week and ease at weekends, but some patients may need several days of not working before improvement is noticed, which confuses the diagnosis.

Education and prevention

Self-management can prevent the majority of asthma deaths and allow most people with stable chronic disease to be largely free of symptoms rather than accept them as inevitable. Education based on booklets and peak flows improves knowledge but does not necessarily change behaviour, and personal instruction has been found the most effective approach (Make 1994). Substantial changes in behaviour have been shown, for example, by a brief three-hour education programme in the community for those recently discharged (Yoon *et al* 1993). Patients are more motivated when the emphasis is on management of symptoms rather than general knowledge (Osman *et al* 1994).

The advantage of education during hospitalization is that motivation is greatest during an acute episode. The disadvantages are that there is often little time, and information may not be easily absorbed during this anxious period. It is best to motivate patients

(a)

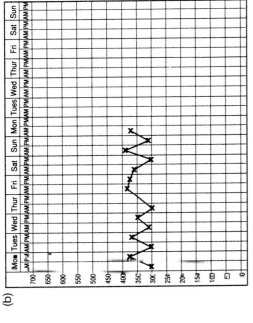

(b)

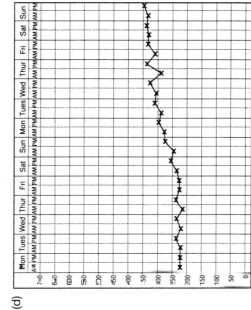

(c)

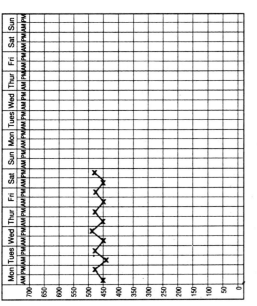

(d)

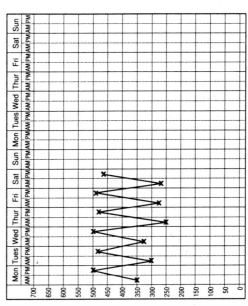

Figure 3.9 Serial peak flow readings: (a) normal diurnal variation, (b) increased diurnal variation indicative of chronic asthma, (c) early morning dip, representing nocturnal asthma and/or impending asthma attack, (d) steroid trial demonstrating significant reversibility. (From Hubbard, J. (1992) Use of the peak flow meter in asthma, *Resp. Dis. Pract.*, 9(4). Reproduced by kind permission of Hayward Medical Communications Ltd, 44 Earlham Street, London WC2H 9LA.)

in the acute phase, provide sufficient information for them to understand that prevention is the key, help them identify their own needs and offer some follow-up education. Collaborative self-management has shown the following outcomes (Make 1994):

- ↓ accident and emergency department visits and hospitalization,
- ↓ medication use,
- ↓ symptoms,
- ↑ compliance with treatment,
- ↑ quality of life.

Education should include the following:

1. Identification of precipitating factors using a diary (Fig. 3.10) to identify the individual pattern of asthma, then prevention when possible, e.g. intensive vacuum cleaning and special bedding to protect against house dust mite (Owen *et al* 1990), avoiding insecticides, keeping pets out of bedrooms, avoiding the not-uncommon scenario of an inhaler in one hand and a cigarette in the other.

2. For people with stable asthma, twice-daily peak flow readings are encouraged, using peak flow diaries available from drug manufacturers. Plans to short-circuit the referral system and self-admit to hospital should be prearranged if the peak flow is less than 40% of the patient's normal after medication. Comprehensive prehospital care can reduce asthma deaths to zero (Cochrane 1995).

3. For women with a family history of asthma, minimal intake of allergenic foods during pregnancy and while breast feeding, and similar care of the baby's diet in the first year of life.

4. Food exclusion diets in appropriate patients, which can reduce medication by over a half (Lewith 1995).

5. Understanding the action and administration of drugs, and the importance of taking preventive drugs, such as steroids, even when feeling well. At present fewer than half of asthmatics take their drugs as prescribed (Couriel 1994b).

6. Mastering relaxation (Freedberg *et al* 1987).

7. Stress reduction by techniques such as biofeedback (Peper 1992), meditation (Lehrer *et al* 1986), hypnotherapy (Morrison 1988a) or yoga (Singh *et al* 1990). Acupuncture can reduce the need for medication, and homeopathy is useful if the trigger is identified (Lewith 1995). Complementary therapies are reviewed by Lane and Lane (1991).

8. For those with nocturnal asthma, trying different sleeping positions, room temperatures, drug timings and a stress-free period before bed.

9. Avoidance of room humidifiers, which nurture the house dust mite and collect moulds.

10. Prevention of gastro-oesophageal reflux (p. 87).

11. Learning the warning signs of an exacerbation, e.g. reduced exercise tolerance, waking at night, prolonged wheeze after waking, declining or variable peak flows, reduced effectiveness of bronchodilator.

12. Individual written guidelines on how to respond to warning signs, and an understanding of when to increase drug dosage, take oral steroids, or seek medical assistance, e.g:

    (a) if the peak flow falls < 70% of the patient's normal, take regular bronchodilators and double inhaled steroids,

    (b) if the peak flow falls < 50%, start oral steroids and contact the doctor,

    (c) if the peak flow falls < 40%, seek urgent advice (Couriel 1994b).

ASTHMA DIARY
Times when I felt extra breathless or wheezy

Date	Time of day or night	What made me breathless or wheezy?	What did I do to help myself?	How much did it help?

Figure 3.10 Example of a diary for the self-management of asthma.

13. Advice for high-risk patients is to keep with them at all times their devices for self-administration of drugs, information bracelet (BTS 1990) and a note from their GP for ambulance personnel to administer unrestricted oxygen. Spare inhalers should be kept in the car and at work.
14. Joining an organization, such as the National Asthma Campaign, which provides diary cards and educational material (Appendix C).

Breathing techniques

Certain breathing manoeuvres can be used to aid relaxation and give patients some control. Patients can practice them regularly and put them into practice when an attack is anticipated. The emphasis is on gentle changes in breathing, not deep breathing which can exacerbate bronchospasm (Lim *et al* 1989). All patients should be encouraged to find their own forms of relaxation and stress management, e.g. the profound relaxation achieved with meditation has shown positive outcomes (Fried 1993, p. 234).

Girodo *et al* (1992) show how simple relaxed abdominal breathing can reduce the intensity of symptoms and increase physical activity. Innocenti (1974) describes how patients can gain control by learning to change back and forth between abdominal and upper chest breathing, and to alter, breath by breath, the rate and depth of breathing. Weissleder (1976) claims that asthmatic attacks can be aborted by teaching the 'complete breath technique', which consists of the following instructions, with the patient in supported sitting:

- listen to and feel the quality of your breathing, including any wheeze,
- inhale through your nose, slowly enough to eliminate the wheeze, while increasing the depth of your breathing tem-

porarily to compensate for the slow breath,
- adjust the rate as breathing becomes comfortable and there is less hunger for air, a hunger which will also be modified by feeling in control,
- observe and modify any muscle tension,
- gradually increase the depth of breathing in three different segments, progressing upwards from abdominal, lateral costal and upper chest expansion, then reduce the depth in reverse order,
- recheck muscle tension,
- progress to unsupported sitting and standing positions.

The physiotherapist can start by breathing alongside the patient, but the aim is for patients to recognize their ability to manage their own condition.

Exercise

Asthma and exercise have a difficult relationship. Exercise can directly trigger an acute episode, but numerous asthmatic athletes have won Olympic medals, and aerobic training, with bronchodilator prophylaxis, has shown the following outcomes:

- ↓bronchospasm, ↑peak flow, ↓wheeze (Dean *et al* 1988),
- ↓breathlessness (Cochrane and Clark 1990),
- ↑work capacity (Gong 1992),
- ↑confidence (Robinson *et al* 1992),
- ↓exercise-induced asthma by greater fitness, which reduces minute ventilation at high intensity work loads (Cochrane and Clark 1990).

Other physical measures

It has been claimed that the inspiratory muscles can be damaged during an acute attack and that this risk can be reduced by strengthening these muscles. Six months of inspiratory muscle training, using a pressure-threshold device for half-an-hour five days a week, showed evidence of reduced symptoms, medication use and hospitalization (Weiner *et al* 1992).

Some patients who are anxious or have poorly controlled asthma show muscle tension and poor posture. The physiotherapist can help the patient deal with anxiety, ask for a drug review and work on stretching and postural exercises. Patients who have developed a habitually hyperinflated chest as a carry-over from acute episodes benefit from advice to emphasize expiration (not to be encouraged during acute episodes, when hyperinflation is necessary to hold open the obstructed airways).

Coughing can relieve or exacerbate asthma (Young *et al* 1991) and the physiotherapist can advise on effective coughing or cough suppression (p. 139) as appropriate.

Outcome measures have traditionally comprised respiratory function tests, complication rates, hospitalization and death rates, but functional measures most usefully relate to physiotherapy outcomes. Quality of life questionnaires have been described by Rowe (1993) and Juniper (1993).

Drug management

Charts describing the step-by-step recognition and drug management of chronic and acute asthma are available (BTS 1993). Underuse, overuse and inappropriate use of drugs is common. Historically, treatment relied on the sticking plaster of bronchodilators for symptom relief, but it is now understood that medication should hinge on regular preventive medication in the form of mast cell stabilizers (p. 99) or steroids, with intermittent bronchodilators if symptoms recur.

Patients find bronchodilators attractive, but they do not prevent long-term inflammatory damage to the airways. The paradox is that they can be beneficial immediately but detrimental in the long run. Even in the acute state, over-reliance may delay seeking med-

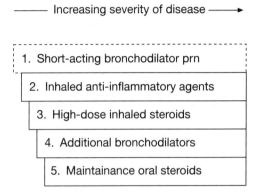

Increasing severity of disease ⟶

1. Short-acting bronchodilator prn
2. Inhaled anti-inflammatory agents
3. High-dose inhaled steroids
4. Additional bronchodilators
5. Maintainance oral steroids

Figure 3.11 Drug management of chronic asthma. If 'as required' inhaled bronchodilators (1) are needed more than once a day, inhaled anti-inflammatory drugs (2, 3) are given. If symptoms persist, a second bronchodilator (4) is given. A small percentage of people with severe chronic asthma need oral steroids (5).

ical assistance. In the chronic state, regular use, especially overuse, can smother symptoms so that a wheeze no longer acts as a warning to avoid the offending stimulus. Prolonged inflammation develops which can double hyperreactivity and increase morbidity and mortality (Cockcroft *et al* 1993). Surveys on asthma deaths invariably implicate underuse of steroids in the fatal attack (Neville *et al* 1991).

The frequency of the need for bronchodilators provides a useful marker for adjusting prophylactic treatment. A stepwise protocol is advocated for drug management (Fig. 3.11). Accurate monitoring is essential. After diagnosis, peak flow should be measured within 30 minutes of waking and in the evening, then drugs adjusted until either the normal predicted value or 'best peak flow' is achieved. If the initial value is less than 80% predicted, a two-week course of steroids, and sometimes bronchodilators, may be needed to find the 'best peak flow'.

People with acute asthma may need high concentrations of oxygen, high-dose nebulized bronchodilators in small frequent doses

(Bennett 1991) and oral or intravenous steroids (Neville *et al* 1991). Antibiotics are rarely indicated.

The characteristics of asthma make it susceptible to non-compliance with treatment. It is a chronic condition with long periods of remission, drug regimes may show no immediate benefit and inhalers are conspicuous and sometimes difficult to operate. Education that considers the patient's individual needs, health beliefs and lifestyle is likely to succeed, especially with adolescents.

Physical management of an asthma attack

Fear of an acute episode is reduced if the patient is given the following advice:

1. Sit upright, or lean slightly forwards resting the arms on a table, or sit astride a chair backwards with the arms resting on the chair's back.
2. Sit near fresh but not cold air.
3. Drink sips of warm liquid.
4. Breathe through the nose unless breathlessness makes this impossible.
5. If there is dizziness with tingling hands and feet, try to slow down the breathing.
6. Practise previously-learned techniques of relaxation, abdominal breathing and control over breathing. These should be begun at the first intimation of an acute episode.
7. Raise the resting respiratory lung volume by starting inspiration slightly early, which may help to open the narrowed airways (Innocenti 1974). The extra elastic work imposed by hyperinflation is offset by less airflow resistance so that total work is reduced (Wheatley 1990). However, many patients will have already achieved optimal hyperinflation spontaneously, and close observation of the patient's breathing pattern is required if this technique is chosen.

Relatives can be shown how to apply acupressure to the bronchospasm acupunc-ture points: CV.17 between the nipples, Co.4 on the dorsal thumb web, Li.3 on the dorsal space between first and second metatarsals, to be pressed or massaged alternately each side.

Vibrators over the chest wall can aid relaxation. Some find it helpful to cuddle a not-too-hot hot water bottle. Some benefit from rhythmic slow percussion to help promote relaxation. Other techniques to reduce the work of breathing are described in Chapter 5.

Mucus may or may not be a problem (Strunk 1993). Slow percussion has the benefit of both promoting relaxation and clearing secretions. If secretions are too thick to shift, warm humidification with normal saline may be indicated (Phillips and Millard 1994), but this can increase airflow resistance in children or those with severe airways obstruction, so close observation for desaturation or bronchospasm is required.

Patients who continue to tire will need mechanical assistance. Low-to-medium levels of CPAP will relieve the inspiratory muscles from their relentless work of holding open the obstructed airways (Shivaram *et al* 1987). If CPAP is not available, IPPB can be used to ease the work of breathing. If positive pressure aids are needed, the radiograph should be checked in case of pneumothorax. Mechanical ventilation for asthma is discussed in Chapter 11 and asthma in children in Chapter 12.

3.2.5   Bronchiectasis

Bronchiectasis is characterized by chronic irreversible dilatation and distortion of the bronchi. This originates from an inflammatory insult, e.g.:

- inhalation of unwanted material such as gastric contents or a peanut,
- severe respiratory infection, particularly if repeated.

The incidence of bronchiectasis is diminishing in countries where living standards are rising and children are vaccinated

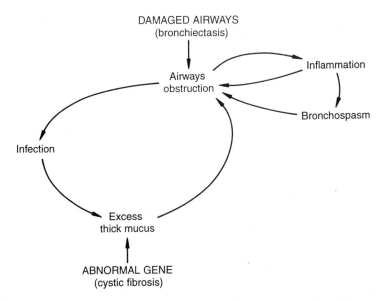

Figure 3.12 Vicious cycle that augments the processes of cystic fibrosis and bronchiectasis.

against diseases such as whooping cough and measles.

The **pathophysiology** involves destruction of the elastic and muscular components of the airway walls. This is most damaging if it occurs in early childhood before the respiratory tract is fully developed. The warm, moist environment within the lung combines with excess mucus to set up a vicious cycle of infection, destroyed cilia, disorganized airways, persistent inflammation and further obstruction (Fig. 3.12). Infection and inflammation release toxic chemicals which interfere with lung defences. Inflammation can cause bronchospasm, which augments the cycle. The process may be complicated by abscess formation. A third to a half of patients show progressive destruction (Munro 1992), leading to pulmonary hypertension and cor pulmonale.

Clinical features include coarse wheezes and crackles, due to secretions and collapsing airways on expiration (Piirilä *et al* 1991), finger clubbing, dyspnoea and fatigue. Coughing is less efficient than normal because of corrugated airways, but volumin-

ous quantities of purulent sputum are produced, sometimes with haemoptysis caused by mucosal ulceration. Radiological signs, if present, are usually localized, showing parallel tramlines representing thickened airway walls and cystic ring shadows representing dilated airways seen end-on. There may be patchy areas of overinflation, consolidation and atelectasis.

Medical treatment is based on the liberal prescription of antibiotics, which help control infection but not the persistent inflammation which may be progressively destroying the airways (Shum *et al* 1993). Other drugs are inhaled steroids, which reduce inflammation and the volume of sputum (Elborn *et al* 1992), and bronchodilators for patients with demonstrable hyperreactive airways. Surgical resection is occasionally indicated for localized and disabling disease.

Physiotherapy is by education in sputum clearance. Hydration must always be attended to, and an exercise programme may be sufficient for moderate disease, but other measures (Chapter 5) are needed for most patients. Much encouragement is needed to help patients set up a life-long programme that is both effective and suited to their lifestyle. Thereafter occasional checks are needed.

3.2.6   Cystic fibrosis (CF)

CF is a chronic progressive obstructive disorder affecting the exocrine glands. It is the commonest lethal inherited disease among white people. It is acquired as an autosomal recessive disorder, so that only people who have two faulty genes – one from each parent – develop the disease. Two carriers have a one-in-four chance of having an affected baby and a two-in-four chance that a baby will be a carrier. The pattern of CF management has been changed by identification of the rogue gene, prenatal diagnosis and transplantation. A child born with CF in the 1990s is expected to survive to middle age, but the disease is still eventually fatal, and treatment is aimed primarily at improving the quality of life. With skilled management, a high proportion of adults live fulfilled lives. The diagnosis is suspected if infants show failure to thrive or repeated chest infections. Suspicions are heightened if a blood test reveals increased levels of the antibody IRT (Harris 1991), and confirmation is by a test for abnormally salty sweat.

Pathophysiology

In most cells the abnormal gene is dormant, but in epithelial cells it is switched on. This impairs ion and water transport across epithelial surfaces of the body, causing dehydration of secretions and obstruction of various body lumens. In the gut there is malabsorption secondary to pancreatic insufficiency, and in the lungs sodium and chloride ions cannot escape from the epithelial cells into the airways in order to maintain hydration of mucus, which becomes thick and sticky.

The respiratory component determines the quality of life and is the usual cause of death. The lungs are structurally normal at birth,

then become caught up in a vicious cycle that is similar to that in bronchiectasis (Fig. 3.12), but set off by tenacious mucus which encourages bacterial adherence. CF is progressive, whereas the course of bronchiectasis varies.

Infection is commonly caused by bacteria, but viruses and fungi play undervalued roles. The patient's own inflammatory mediators directed against the colonizing organisms not only fail in their task, but actually cause tissue breakdown, a by-product of which is excess DNA within the cells, leading to even thicker secretions. The viscid mucus, instead of helping clear bacteria, impairs defence, and intractable infection becomes established in early life, leading to a smouldering course of bacterial colonization punctuated by exacerbations.

The range of bacteria is curiously restricted, but *Staphylococcus aureus* causes significant damage, and acquisition of *Pseudomonas/ Burkholderia cepacia* poses a particular threat because the organism is unresponsive to many antibiotics and its presence may herald rapid deterioration and premature death (Govan *et al* 1993). Preventive measures against *cepacia* include segregation and minimal social contact, at great personal cost for those who have previously socialized freely. Even sibling separation is tolerated by some families.

Aggravating factors are inflammation, especially in severe disease, and bronchospasm. Malnutrition contributes to impaired respiratory defence and is related to deteriorating lung function, leading to a spiral of decline in both. Pneumothorax occurs in up to 10% of children and 20% of adults, due to rupture of a subpleural bleb or bulla (Noppen *et al* 1994).

As more patients are surviving to adulthood, new clinical difficulties have arisen. Liver and gall bladder problems develop, pancreatic fibrosis can lead to diabetes and dehydration, and vasculitis can affect joints, skin and brain. Bronchial artery hypertrophy may lead to pulmonary haemorrhage. Respir-

atory and cardiac failure eventually super-
vene.

Clinical features

> *Coughing and spluttering like an old man does*
> *not endear one to the general public, and neither*
> *does the popular misconception that one is*
> *scattering infections round like confetti . . . My*
> *fingers are like spoons and I can't wear nail*
> *polish . . . It doesn't do too much for one's*
> *confidence to know that one has probably got*
> *halitosis – so I tend to talk to people sideways*
> *on . . .*
>
> Hall 1984

This fictionalized account of the experience of
CF underlines the antisocial nature of the
disease. Clinical features include incessant
coughing, delayed puberty, flatus, increasing
breathlessness and relentless weariness.
Breath sounds are clear in the early stages,
becoming wheezy as a bronchiolitis-like process develops in the small airways, then
exhibiting widespread crackles. Other signs
are similar to bronchiectasis, with the addition of small stature and sometimes hepato-
megaly and GOR. Growth is stunted because
of energy imbalance, energy supply being
reduced by malabsorption and often anor-
exia, and energy demand increased by excess
work of breathing. The fact that patients do
not often look ill means that they have to
cope with others not expecting them to suffer
fatigue and other invisible problems (Eigen
et al 1987).

The radiograph is normal at first, then
shows patchy opacities in the apical regions,
then signs of widespread bronchiectasis,
emphysema and, finally, cor pulmonale. If
chest pain occurs, it may be due to pleural
inflammation, strain from excessive coughing
or pneumothorax. Exacerbation is indicated
by weight loss or worsening respiratory signs
and symptoms.

Males are sterile. Women can have children at some medical risk to themselves, but
their child is unlikely by adolescence to have
a mother.

In later stages, FEV_1 declines, PaO_2 falls
and eventually $PaCO_2$ rises. The inexorable
deterioration is anticipated by patients, who
each respond in their individual way. They
often form strong attachments to each other,
which provide comradeship but can be
devastating when one of them dies.

Medical management

Prevention   Screening is possible at three
stages. Carrier screening helps when making
decisions about reproduction, and if two
carriers want to have a child, they can be
offered *in vitro* fertilization, genetic screening
and implantation of a healthy embryo. Prenatal diagnosis provides information on
which to base decisions about continuing a
pregnancy. Neonatal screening leads to early
diagnosis and more effective treatment.
Screening usually occurs only after the birth
of the first, unexpected, cystic child or if there
is a family history of CF.

Research into gene therapy is proceeding
at a dizzy pace and if successful could
provide a virtual cure for the disease by
halting it in its tracks. The accessibility of the
airway makes CF suitable for gene therapy,
which involves inhalation of a normal copy of
the gene to sufficient lung epithelial cells to
replace the defective gene. Treatment would
be required monthly because of the turnover
of these cells, and the damage that had
already occurred would not be reversible.

Education   When a baby with CF is born,
education for the parents should begin immediately:

- no smoking in the home,
- CF children are of normal intelligence and
    should go to normal schools,
- within their limitations they should take
    part in normal physical activities,
- they are not infectious,

- they should share with their healthy siblings the disciplines and standards of the family,
- the lifelong treatment routine is time consuming, and preplanning can ensure attention for siblings and prevent isolation for the family.

Self-help groups are valued by adolescents, young adults and parents.

Medication   At present the backbone of medical management is an unremitting onslaught against bacterial infection. Antibiotics are used aggressively, but complete eradication of infection is impossible. High doses are required to compensate for difficulty in reaching the lung through areas of poor perfusion or obstructed airways. Access is by peripheral or central venous line or subcutaneous venous reservoir (Davies *et al* 1991), often managed from home with back-up support. Nebulized antibiotics are preferred by some patients, but are time consuming, polluting and variable in effect (Mukhopadhyay *et al* 1994).

The drug DNase is a clone of the gene responsible for breaking down DNA, and when given as an aerosol can reduce secretion viscosity and improve pulmonary function by 10–15% (Hardy 1993). It is also helpful if there is intractable atelectasis (Shah *et al* 1994). Aerosolized alpha$_1$-antitrypsin helps replenish the patient's defences (Briars and Warner 1993). Aerosolized amiloride, a sodium channel blocker, helps restore normal hydration to secretions but requires up to four treatments a day and has been challenged as no better than inhaled saline (Middleton *et al* 1993). Anti-inflammatory therapy may reduce the inflammation associated with infection (Konstan *et al* 1990). Asthma is often present, and bronchodilators improve lung function if hyperreactivity can be demonstrated (Eggleston 1991). Mucolytic drugs are considered ineffective in CF (Fiel 1993).

Nutrition   Malnutrition is associated with poor survival (Heijerman 1993). Nutritional support is essential in childhood to prevent impaired growth, and a calorie intake up to 150% of normal is the goal. Enzyme supplements are usually required throughout life to make up for pancreatic insufficiency. Supplementary feeds may be used in advanced disease.

Surgery   Pneumothoraces are managed by chest tube drainage if minor, but recurrent pneumothoraces require thoracoscopic pleurodesis (Noppen *et al* 1994). More intrusive intervention precludes future lung transplants because of pleural adhesions.

Transplantation of heart, lung and/or liver can transform a chair-ridden patient into an active individual within weeks of the operation. Most of the pulmonary problems of CF can be eliminated because donor lungs do not have the genetic abnormality. But the obstacles are formidable, including the stress of waiting, life-long immunosuppressive drugs for the successful, and dashed hopes for the unsuccessful (Whitehead and Leval 1994). Selection criteria include life expectancy < 2 years, oxygen dependence, FEV_1 < 30% predicted, cor pulmonale and high motivation. The availability of transplantation has raised difficult moral issues. Gentle palliative management may now be supplanted by vigorous gastrostomy feeding, mechanical ventilation and other heroics to keep an increasingly desperate patient alive.

Patients must be free to make their own choices, especially in the later stages. Options include nocturnal oxygen therapy (Coates 1992), nasal ventilation (Regnis 1994) or palliation.

Physiotherapy

Once cystic fibrosis has been diagnosed, physiotherapy is started immediately, with the intention of minimizing the cycle of excess secretions and airway damage. Physiotherapy is the most gruelling and least tolerated aspect of treatment and shows adherence rates below 50% (Abbott *et al* 1994). Daily treatment regimes produce no immediate improvement in well-being, and sputum is the only reinforcement to encourage this repetitive task. Parents of CF children are compliant with treatment, but less than half of CF adults believe physiotherapy to be effective (Fong 1994), and some physiotherapists consider that it is not necessary for all patients (Samuels *et al* 1995). Treatment to clear secretions is best individualized according to patient preference, and should achieve maximum effectiveness with minimum burden on an already stressed family.

Physiotherapy should take place after any prescribed bronchodilator treatment to open the airways, and before nebulized antibiotics to encourage absorption through mucus-filled airways. Details of sputum clearance techniques are in Chapter 5, with aspects specific to CF outlined below.

Positive expiratory pressure, the active cycle of breathing techniques and autogenic drainage are popular because they allow independence.

If postural drainage is the chosen treatment, drainage time is about 15 minutes in younger children, more in older patients or if there are excessive secretions. Length of time depends on fatigue, patient preference, whether there are scant or copious secretions and the effectiveness of other measures. History and symptoms should be checked for GOR, because the head-down postural drainage position exacerbates symptoms and should be avoided (Button *et al* 1994). Percussion and vibrations can be included if they produce more sputum or the patient finds them effective. Some authorities consider them unnecessary (Sutton *et al* 1985), but the combination of all three techniques has shown positive outcomes (Reisman 1988).

Exercise has the advantage that most patients enjoy it and will actually do it

(Abbott *et al* 1994). It usually complements other techniques, but in less severe cases can be the primary treatment (Andréasson *et al* 1987). Patients with severe disease are less likely to benefit, partly because of fatigue and partly because little extra tidal volume can be superimposed on hyperinflated lungs. Swimming is especially beneficial, but patients should choose their favourite activity, which may be trampolining for children and weight-lifting or jogging for adults.

Exercise training has the added benefit of improving breathlessness, well-being, clinical status and lung function (Dodd 1991). For training, patients exercise to a pulse rate of 50–75% of that obtained during maximum exercise capacity, with the duration and frequency tailored to the individual but aiming at a minimum 30 minutes four times a week. Successful exercise training requires regular contact with a physiotherapist and commitment from patient and family.

Inspiratory muscle endurance is normally elevated because of the extra work required to breathe through obstructed airways, but it has been claimed that inspiratory muscle training improves exercise tolerance (Sawyer and Clanton 1993).

Interesting data have emerged suggesting that abdominal breathing with biofeedback can reduce airways obstruction (Delk *et al* 1993).

The optimal frequency for physiotherapy is not known (Eigen *et al* 1987), but it is usually performed twice daily, with variations depending on quantity of secretions and whether there is remission or exacerbation. Treatment is best continued until sputum is no longer expectorated or a rest is needed.

Both parents should be given advice and support until children are able to manage themselves, with a check on treatment techniques every three months. Early independence should be encouraged, with young children actively participating in their treatment, and 10-year-olds encouraged to stay with friends overnight and do their own treatment. Older children are advised against cough suppression, by which they sometimes conceal their illness from peers.

The 'best' treatment is not always the most effective in the teenage years, when it may not be followed. Management is best negotiated, with the physiotherapist 'complying' with the patient's wish rather than the other way round. People with CF are particularly worth listening to because they are medically streetwise and understand much about their treatment. When patients are hospitalized, motivation is enhanced by simple measures such as offering a choice of treatment times and techniques.

Outcome measures are based on quality-of-life measures such as exercise tolerance, questionnaires or well-being scales (Orenstein and Kaplan, 1991).

Precautions

Patients should not be prevented from coughing, but also not exhorted unnecessarily, because excessive coughing causes collapse of central airways with impairment of sputum clearance (Zapleta *et al* 1983), and may accelerate emphysematous changes. The active cycle of breathing provides a more controlled means of sputum clearance, although it still causes a degree of airway closure.

When using CPAP or nasal ventilation (Chapter 5), high pressures are not necessary for respite from fatigue and should be avoided because of the risk of pneumothorax.

If haematemesis develops from oesophageal varices associated with liver cirrhosis, all physiotherapy, except abdominal breathing, is contraindicated until bleeding is controlled.

Blood streaking of sputum is common in CF and should be disregarded, but frank haemoptysis should be reported and physiotherapy temporarily halted.

Measures to prevent cross-infection include separate treatment areas, scrupulous hand washing, single patient use of PEP and flutter devices and the covering of sputum pots.

Longer lifespans mean that osteoporosis is emerging as a problem in young adults (Bachrach *et al* 1994), sometimes represented by increased kyphosis. Loss of bone mineral is due to steroids, chronic respiratory acidosis and, for older patients, the limited diets that were advised in the past.

It is not known if short periods of oxygen desaturation are harmful, but those with an $FEV_1 < 50\%$ predicted are likely to desaturate during exercise. They need supervised exercise testing and should exercise at a level that avoids desaturating by more than 5% or an absolute level below 80% (Dodd 1991). In advanced disease, added oxygen allows longer periods of exercise and may limit pulmonary hypertension (Marcus 1992). Fluids and free access to the salt shaker are needed in hot weather because of the high salt concentration in sweat.

3.2.7   Primary ciliary dyskinesia

Primary ciliary dyskinesia is often misdiagnosed as CF. It is an inherited condition characterized by an uncoordinated and ineffectual ciliary beat, causing recurrent infection of ears, sinuses and lungs. It is suspected in children with a perpetually runny nose, glue ear and frequent chest infections. Regular physiotherapy delays the onset of bronchiectasis (Baum 1990).

3.2.8   Allergic bronchopulmonary aspergillosis

Aspergillosis is an infection manifesting mainly in the lung as allergic bronchopulmonary aspergillosis, which is an allergic reaction to the *Aspergillus* fungus. It occurs in 10% of people with CF, up to 20% of asthmatics and often in cavitating lung diseases, such as TB.

Patients present with malaise, weight loss, fever, haemoptysis and a cough productive of brown, rubbery mucus casts sometimes in the shape of the bronchial tree. The disorder may continue for years with episodes of pulmonary infiltration and wheezing, sometimes leading to fibrosis and cor pulmonale.

Treatment is by inhaled steroids (Seaton 1994), antifungal agents delivered bronchoscopically or percutaneously, or for those with adequate lung function, surgical resection (Jackson *et al* 1993).

3.3 RESTRICTIVE DISORDERS

3.3.1 Pneumonia

Pneumonia is acute inflammation of lung parenchyma, which fills alveoli with inflammatory products, creating consolidation. When alveoli are filled with something other than air, this is termed consolidation. The precipitating factor for pneumonia is a breach in lung defences by infective or chemical agents. The disease is a common cause of death because of its predilection for the elderly and immunosuppressed. Other risk factors are heart disease, acute stroke, poor nutrition, smoking and alcoholism.

Clinical features are fever, chills, breathlessness and often dehydration. If localized, the affected area shows decreased expansion, a dull percussion note, bronchial breath sounds, opacity on X-ray and sometimes a pleural rub. There may be a dry cough at first, which can become productive of purulent and sometimes rusty blood-stained sputum. The structure of the lung is preserved and complete resolution is possible, although sensitized nerve endings sometimes leave a dry, irritating cough.

Treatment is by oral or intravenous fluids, oxygen if indicated and antibiotics if there is bacterial infection. In the acute stage when consolidation is not yet resolved, physiotherapy is limited to positioning for $\dot{V}_A/\dot{Q}$ matching (p. 111) and sometimes CPAP if

hypoxaemia persists despite 40% oxygen (Brett and Sinclair 1993). There is overlap between different types of pneumonia, but the usual classifications are described below, with an explanation of modified physiotherapy when appropriate.

Bronchopneumonia

Bronchopneumonia is patchy and scattered, often favouring the lower lobes. It is common in the immobile and elderly. Early signs are dullness to percussion and barely-perceptible fine crackles which persist despite deep breathing. Physiotherapy is based on hydration and early mobility. Other measures may be needed to increase lung volume or improve gas exchange. When the disease is resolving, some patients need assistance or advice to clear secretions.

Lobar pneumonia

When pneumonia is confined to a lobe, localized pleuritic pain and bronchial breathing are added features. Physiotherapy is as above plus relief of pain, for example, by transcutaneous nerve stimulation.

Pneumocystis carinii pneumonia (PCP)

If a person's defence mechanisms are weakened by HIV or medication given after organ transplant, he or she is vulnerable to opportunist infection by organisms that are not normally pathogenic. PCP is a manifestation of this and is a common first AIDS-defining illness in people with HIV, especially in those who smoke.

Invading organisms damage the alveolar lining, and a foamy exudate interferes with gas exchange. Clinical features include a dry cough, breathlessness, hypoxaemia and the features of stiff lungs. Patients are wasted from diarrhoea, malabsorption, dysphagia and mouth ulcers. They may or may not be pyrexial, because immunocompromised people cannot always mount a fever in response to infection. Some patients may be reluctant to take a full inspiration in case it brings on coughing or pleuritic pain. Auscultation may be normal or show fine scattered crackles. The radiograph may be normal at first, if immune deficiency delays the appearance of an inflammatory response, but later signs are a perihilar haze, progressing to diffuse symmetrical shadowing and air bronchograms (Fig. 2.10). Reduced peak flows sometimes indicate a degree of bronchospasm. Sudden deterioration raises suspicions of a pneumothorax.

Drug treatment is most effective if started early. High-dose steroids, co-trimoxazole or pentamidine are given.

Physiotherapists are involved in the following ways:

1. Diagnostic procedures, such as bronchoscopy, can be avoided by using the more comfortable technique of inducing sputum from the lower respiratory tract for analysis. After starvation and mouth cleaning to reduce oral contamination, 20–30 ml of hypertonic (3–5%) saline is ultrasonically nebulized over 10–20 minutes. This irritates the airways to produce secretions, and the hypertonicity of the saline draws water into the airways (Miller *et al* 1991). The patient is asked to breathe through an open mouth during nebulization, to take occasional deep breaths and gargle with sterile water before coughing so that oral pathogens do not contaminate the specimen. Side-effects are bronchospasm, breathlessness, oxygen desaturation and nausea. TB is common in patients with HIV, and a well-ventilated room is needed to minimize cross-infection from coughing. Ideally, two sputum specimens are obtained because the second is thought to originate from deeper in the lung. The sputum should be clear, non-purulent and resemble saliva. A simpler diagnostic test is oxygen desaturation during exercise (Chouaid *et al* 1993).

2. Physiotherapists may be involved in administering nebulized drugs to the lung parenchyma. A nebulizer is needed that can deliver particle sizes of 2–5 μm and incorporates a filter to reduce environmental contamination. The room needs an extractor fan or venting system. It is best that patients lie down to ensure that the upper lobes are not excluded (Thomas *et al* 1990). The side-effects of coughing and bronchospasm can be reduced by prior bronchodilator inhalation (Harrison and Laube 1994).

3. Patients need support when in the grip of acute breathlessness because they are intensely frightened and often think that they are dying. Physical assistance is described on p. 154. Positioning depends on the patient's choice, but when breathlessness is severe, minimal handling is preferred. Reassurance can be given because although AIDS patients know that they have a fatal disease, death rarely occurs during episodes of acute breathlessness.

4. Help with mobilization may be needed because of weakness.

5. Immune function can be improved by relaxation and exercise which incorporates endurance and strengthening (Lang 1991).

6. Neuropathic pain can be relieved by massage, which is especially important in this group of people, to whom touch is still sometimes denied.

7. CPAP (p. 115) at pressures of 5–10 cmH$_2$O improves gas exchange in patients with severe PCP (Miller and Semple, 1991) and buys time for discussion with the patient about further treatment. If necessary, some patients may choose mechanical ventilation while antimicrobial drugs have time to work. Ventilated patients with PCP rarely have a secretion problem, and physiotherapy is based on

positioning for $\dot{V}_A/\dot{Q}$ matching, maintenance of lung volume and comfort.

Patients are prone to infections and extra care is needed with hand washing and sterilization of respiratory equipment. Patients are often undernourished, dehydrated and stressed. They need autonomy and attention to their many individual needs. In the later stages, they need particular attention to physical comfort.

People with AIDS may have other respiratory complications, such as lung abscesses and pleural effusion, and other problems such as diarrhoea, dry skin, oral herpes, Kaposi's sarcoma (p. 83) or a sore mouth, which may make eating difficult and oxygen therapy intolerable. Necrotic lung tissue may rupture and cause a pneumothorax, which is notoriously difficult to treat (Light 1993).

Body fluids known to contain the HIV are blood, semen, vaginal secretions and urine. The virus has not been found in normal sputum in enough quantities to pose a risk, but any sputum may contain blood and any patient may be HIV-positive. Precautions against transmission include covering cuts or abrasions with waterproof plasters, wearing gloves during contact with body fluids and wearing masks and protective eyewear during suction.

Nosocomial pneumonia

Pneumonia which develops in a patient hospitalized for over 48 hours is considered to be hospital-acquired or nosocomial pneumonia. It is the leading cause of hospital-related mortality (Heyland 1994) and involves a different spectrum of pathogens from community-acquired pneumonia. The disease may be caused by cross-infection between patients, usually carried by staff, or endogenous infection arising from other colonized sites in the patient, such as a tracheostomy or the gut. A major cause is misuse of broad spectrum antibiotics (Fiorentini 1992).

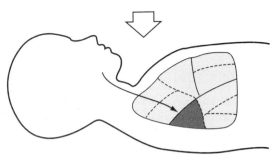

Figure 3.13 Area of aspiration pneumonia for a supine patient.

Legionella pneumonia

Pneumonia that occurs in local outbreaks, especially in relation to cooling systems, or develops after a trip abroad, raises suspicions of Legionnaire's disease, a community-acquired pneumonia with a mortality of 5–10%.

Aspiration pneumonia

People who have inhaled unfriendly substances, such as vomit or gastric acid, need immediate physiotherapy to clear their lungs. Aspiration (inhalation) sets up a vicious pneumonitis which corrodes the alveolar–capillary membrane and leaves a legacy of pulmonary oedema, haemorrhage, necrosis and the classic signs of pneumonia. Aspiration pneumonia should be suspected in anyone after a period of unexpected unconsciousness or in those with swallowing difficulties. The area most likely to be affected is the apical segment of the right lower lobe because this is dependent when the patient is supine (Fig. 3.13).

Signs of acute aspiration include coughing or choking, added sounds on auscultation, gurgly voice or loss of voice, tachycardia and sometimes change of colour. Chronic aspiration is caused by dysphagia or a poor gag reflex, and is suspected in patients with recurrent right lower lobe pneumonia, spiking temperatures, excess oral secretions, reluctance to eat or drink, weight loss or

GOR. Silent aspiration during sleep is common in elderly people (Kikuchi *et al* 1994).

3.3.2   Interstitial lung disease

The umbrella term 'interstitial lung disease' covers a bewildering array of conditions. Over 200 disorders, often related to immune disturbances and/or exposure to toxic agents, are associated with generalized inflammatory changes, to which the lungs are particularly susceptible. Inflammation leads to alveolitis, which may resolve or progress to fibrosis, leading to thickened alveolar septa and small, stiff lungs. Stiff lungs lead to increased elastic recoil (usually) and fewer functioning alveoli (always). Smoking augments the lung injury. Examples are described below.

- **Fibrosing alveolitis** is the commonest interstitial lung disease and kills half of its sufferers within five years of diagnosis (Bois 1992). It may have no obvious cause or may be the end result of other disorders, including those described below (which may or may not be classified separately). There is widespread fibrosis of the alveolar walls and eventually severe impairment.
- **Asbestosis** is lung fibrosis which can occur 20 years after asbestosis exposure.
- **Pneumoconiosis** is lung fibrosis caused by inhaling mineral dust such as coal.
- **Bird fancier's** or **farmer's lung** are allergies which produce fever and malaise some hours after exposure. Lung fibrosis may develop if the patient and offending antigen do not remove themselves from each other.
- **Systemic lupus erythematosis** (SLE) is a connective tissue disorder characterized by exacerbations and remissions, including joint pain. The lung may become involved by developing pleurisy, pleural effusion and fibrosis.
- **Scleroderma** is a connective tissue disorder which is confined to the skin at first, but often progresses to internal organs including the lung.
- **Rheumatoid disease** is a systemic disease of connective tissue, manifesting usually as inflamed joints and sometimes including 'rheumatoid lung', i.e. pleural effusion, nodules, predisposition to infection and fibrosis.
- **Sarcoidosis** is a multisystem disorder of unknown cause, often presenting in young people with widespread variation in severity including sometimes lung fibrosis.

Clinical features

The lungs have a large reserve capacity and the following symptoms only emerge after considerable injury has occurred:

1. Shallow breathing to ease the elastic load, and rapid breathing to sustain ventilation.
2. Dry unproductive cough.
3. Fine end-inspiratory crackles on auscultation, due to sudden opening of peripheral airways.
4. X-ray signs of irregular 'ground glass' lung fields at first, then a reticular or honeycomb appearance as alveoli are pulled apart to form cystic spaces (Fig. 2.9). In advanced cases the shrinking lung pulls up the diaphragm to an exaggerated dome shape.
5. PaO_2 is reduced due to $\dot{V}_A/\dot{Q}$ mismatch, and $PaCO_2$ is reduced due to rapid shallow breathing. Hypercapnia is rare even in severe disease.
6. Respiratory function tests show impaired gas transfer and reduced lung volumes, both static (VC and TLC) and dynamic (FEV_1).
7. Dyspnoea may become progressively incapacitating.

Treatment

Early diagnosis is possible with CT scanning. Patients may not respond to medication, but symptoms are sometimes alleviated by immunosuppressive drugs or steroids. Oxygen may be helpful, and portable oxygen can improve exercise tolerance. Single lung transplant offers hope for people with severe irreversible disease.

Physiotherapy is aimed at reducing the work of breathing (Chapters 5 and 6) and maintaining functional activities within the limits of dyspnoea, desaturation and fatigue. Help with positioning is appreciated in the late stages. In the unlikely event of a patient being mechanically ventilated, bag-squeezing should be used minimally because the non-compliant lungs are at risk of pneumothorax.

3.3.3 Pleurisy

Pleurisy is inflammation of the pleural membranes, sometimes associated with lobar pneumonia. The parietal pleura is highly sensitive, and pleurisy causes a wicked localized pain, leading to rapid shallow breathing and pleural friction rub. The pain can sometimes be eased by heat or transcutaneous nerve stimulation.

Dry pleurisy may or may not develop into a pleural effusion. This brings relief from symptoms as the raw pleural membranes are separated by fluid.

3.3.4 Pleural effusion

The pleural space normally contains 7–14 ml of fluid (Bartter 1994). Pleural effusion is excess fluid in the pleural cavity, caused by disturbed osmotic or hydrostatic pressure in the plasma, or changes in membrane permeability. Twenty-five per cent of pleural effusions are due to malignancy (Bartter 1994); other causes include heart, renal or liver failure, abdominal or cardiac surgery, pneumonia or TB.

Clinical features include a stony dull percussion note, decreased breath sounds over the affected area, and increased vocal resonance over the upper level of the fluid. A fluid line on X-ray is usually confirmatory, often tracking up the pleura laterally or seeping into the fissure. CT scanning distinguishes pleural effusion from pleural thickening. A large effusion displaces the mediastinum and causes breathlessness.

General treatment is directed at the cause, plus symptomatic relief of breathlessness by needle aspiration (thoracocentesis), performed slowly to avoid 're-expansion pulmonary oedema' (Kam *et al* 1993). Surgery may be needed for a thickened restrictive pleura.

Malignant invasion of the pleura is less responsive to treatment, but can be palliated by repeated aspiration, although most effusions re-accumulate within one to three days. Other options include chest tube drainage with local instillation of drugs, the more comfortable pleuroperitoneal shunt, or pleurodesis (Reid and Rudd 1993).

Physiotherapy is limited. Deep breathing exercises cannot expand lungs under pressure from fluid (Dechman *et al* 1993), but mobilization of the patient helps to prevent atelectasis, and positioning can be used to optimize gas exchange. People with moderate unilateral effusion benefit from side-lying with the fluid uppermost, because both ventilation and perfusion are greater in the lower lung, thereby optimizing $\dot{V}_A/\dot{Q}$ matching. Large effusions show improved PaO_2 with the effusion downwards to minimize compression of the unaffected lung (Chang *et al* 1989).

Transudates are clear, low-protein, straw-coloured pleural fluids associated with heart failure and fluid imbalance. **Exudates** are cloudy, high-protein fluids associated with malignancy and infection. **Haemothorax** is blood in the pleura and is managed by treating the cause, plus tube drainage if necessary.

Empyema is pus in the pleural cavity following nearby infection. It is often a complication of pneumonia, bronchiectasis, abscess or chest surgery. The patient may be asymptomatic or toxic, depending on the offending organism and volume of pus. Early intervention for acute empyema reduces the risk of chronicity and protracted treatment. Local and systemic antibiotics are indicated. Pus can be drained and the lung re-expanded by continuous drainage into an underwater seal system (p. 192) or, for easier mobility, into a drainage bag. The pus may be thick and require aspiration with strong suction or lavage. Other options are open drainage with rib resection, or for an established empyema with a thickened pleura, a full thoracotomy with decortication (Kaplan 1994). Patients needing surgery are often malnourished and debilitated.

3.3.5   Pneumothorax

When the pneumothorax happened I was totally conscious of the puncturing of the thorax, the unbearable pain, the cold sweat, being afraid that the final moment would come quicker than the help that you could give me.

Ruiz 1993

The relationship between the lungs and chest wall is normally maintained by negative pressure which sucks together the two layers of pleura. If either layer is ruptured, air rushes into the pleural space, causing a pneumothorax. The lung shrivels towards the hilum in proportion to the amount of air rushing in, not necessarily symmetrically. Air continues to escape into the pleura until pressure is equalized or the collapsing lung seals the offending hole.

Clinical features are diminished breath sounds, characteristic X-ray signs (Fig. 2.7), rapid breathing by a reflex arc with afferents carried in the vagi, and pain in 75% of patients (Light 1993).

Types of pneumothorax

Spontaneous pneumothorax   The apex of the upright lung is subject to greater mechan-ical stress than the base because the weight of the lung pulls down on it. A spontaneous pneumothorax often occurs in this region, especially in tall, thin young men who are thought to grow faster than their pleura is able to keep up with. Although 'spontan-eous', many patients are smokers and have blebs on X-ray (Light 1993).

Secondary pneumothorax   A pneumo-thorax may occur secondary to puncture from a fractured rib, inaccurate insertion of a cannula, high-volume positive pressure vent-ilation, or rupture of an emphysematous bulla.

Tension pneumothorax   A pleural tear sometimes functions as a valve so that air enters the pleural space but cannot escape, causing a pneumothorax under tension. Increasing pressure displaces the media-stinum and impairs venous return, causing respiratory distress and circulatory collapse. Recognition and management are discussed on p. 263.

Treatment

To drain or not to drain? This depends on the size of the pneumothorax and medical opin-ion. Usually, a small symptomless pneumo-thorax can be left to heal itself, a moderate first pneumothorax is managed by needle aspiration, and a pneumothorax over 20% or causing breathlessness requires tube drainage over several days.

Chest tube drainage (p. 192) may require suction to help oppose the pleural surfaces and seal the leak more rapidly, but sudden lung re-inflation is avoided to prevent re-expansion pulmonary oedema. Once the air leak has ceased, i.e. when there is no more bubbling in the drainage bottle, the drain is clamped for 24 hours and then removed, provided there is no recurrence, as indicated by X-ray. High levels of inspired oxygen will speed resolution by increasing the absorption of pleural air fourfold (Light 1993). Recurrence is less likely if sclerosing agents are instilled through the chest drain. Surgical intervention (p. 185) is necessary if these measures fail or if the condition is bilateral.

Physiotherapy is based on mobilization and regular position change. Lying on the side of the pneumothorax may help seal the leak and facilitate lung expansion (Zidulka *et al* 1982), but this is uncomfortable if there is a chest drain, and might cause desaturation with a large pneumothorax because of $\dot{V}_A/\dot{Q}$ mismatch (p. 111).

Mobilization should be particularly rigorous if the cause is, for example, a stab wound (Senekal 1994), but not too enthusiastic immediately after surgery in case the pleura becomes unstuck.

Precautions include avoidance of positive pressure techniques (CPAP, intermittent positive pressure breathing or bag-squeezing) if there is no chest drain.

3.3.6 Neuromuscular and skeletal disorders

Impairment of respiratory drive, muscle power or rib cage mechanics restricts expansion and reduces vital capacity. These conditions may also impair secretion clearance because of a weak cough and reduced mechanical movement of the lung (Mier *et al* 1990).

Pathophysiology and clinical features

Skeletal disorders such as kyphoscoliosis upset the configuration of the diaphragm and force it to work from an inefficient position against the load of a stiff chest wall.

Ankylosing spondylitis is a systemic disease which affects breathing because of a rigid thoracic cage and kyphotic spine. Chest wall compliance is impaired, but lung compliance and diaphragmatic movement are preserved, although occasionally fibrosis and bullous disease damage the lung. The chest

X-ray shows apparent hyperinflation because the chest wall becomes fixed in an inspiratory position.

If a patient has generalized muscle weakness, this usually involves the respiratory muscles. Respiratory muscle weakness may go undetected if limb weakness reduces mobility, and ventilatory failure may arrive unexpectedly (Tobin 1988). The most important step in assessment of inspiratory muscle weakness is to think of it as a possibility.

Bilateral paralysis or severe weakness of the diaphragm show the following signs:

• orthopnoea unexplained by heart disease,
• accessory muscle activity unexplained by lung disease,
• paradoxical inward abdominal motion during inspiration, especially in supine when the impaired diaphragm is unable to counteract the weight of the abdominal contents,
• postural fall in VC of about 50% in supine compared with upright (Tobin and Yang 1990),
• symptoms of nocturnal hypoventilation, such as disturbed sleep, morning headache and daytime somnolence,
• less-specific symptoms, such as breathlessness or recurrent chest infections.

Bilateral diaphragmatic paralysis is like removing a portion of the chest wall. When upright, patients exhale by contracting the abdominal muscles, which push up the diaphragm, then relaxing them to allow passive inspiration. Breathing difficulties worsen during sleep.

Unilateral diaphragmatic paralysis shows nocturnal hypoxaemia due to $\dot{V}_A/\dot{Q}$ mismatch in supine, unilateral abdominal paradox on sniffing, and one raised hemidiaphragm on X-ray, this last sign being more obvious than with bilateral paralysis.

Severe cases of neuromuscular and skeletal disorders may lead to type II respiratory failure which is characteristically associated with hypercapnia (p. 88). Cor pulmonale may develop.

Physiotherapy

Treatment for excess work of breathing or sputum retention may be needed (Chapter 5), but specific measures are described below.

Upright positioning to facilitate breathing is advised for patients with muscle weakness, and manual support will assist coughing (p. 139). Regular position change and incentive spirometry help to prevent atelectasis.

Swallowing dysfunction is suspected if there is excess salivation, lack of elevation of the larynx on swallowing and deterioration after meals. Risk of aspiration is reduced by avoiding neck extension, maintaining head and chest elevation, and periodic turning from side to side. Dysphagia may lead to weight loss, which further limits mobility, and dehydration, which further limits secretion clearance. Swallowing problems often develop insidiously, but dysphagia usually parallels or shortly follows the development of speech problems. A speech therapist can provide an accurate assessment.

Hypertonic abdominal muscles may occur with some neurological conditions, which inhibits full inspiration and further reduces lung volume. Postures which encourage inhibitory control over spasticity will modify this.

Severe muscle weakness leads to hypercapnia, initially during sleep (Green and Moxham 1993). Nasal ventilation may be appropriate in certain circumstances. Some patients with progressive diseases may accept mechanical assistance if respiratory deterioration is due to a temporary relapse, but if deterioration is progressive, weaning may be impossible. For non-progressive neuromuscular disease, ageing may reduce lung function to the point where mechanical assistance can make life more comfortable.

If respiratory failure is due to bulbar weakness, the airway needs protection and some patients will accept intubation or tracheostomy with a cuffed tube, which will partially prevent aspiration and allow for mechanical ventilation. Impaired communication, due to the disease or mechanical ventilation, can be the most devastating aspect for the patient and family, and a reliable communications system is essential.

3.4   OTHER DISORDERS

3.4.1   Cancer

Lung cancer has shown the greatest rise in mortality for any tumour in the UK this century (Spiro 1993). It is the most common cancer for men worldwide, and is showing an alarming increase in women. Tumour cells usually invade the central airways at bronchial bifurcations, which are the areas most vulnerable to bombardment by inhaled carcinogenic agents.

Clinical features are breathlessness, haemoptysis, clubbing, cough, unresolving pneumonia, weight loss and pain. Recurrent pneumonia in a smoker is a suspicious sign. A large tumour of a main bronchus may produce no radiological change until the lung collapses, but stridor or monophonic wheeze may be heard. Hoarseness indicates involvement of the recurrent laryngeal nerve, which may impair speech and cough.

General treatment is aimed at inflicting the greatest damage to the cancer with the least damage to the patient, but the disease is usually disseminated at presentation and five-year survival is under 10% (Michie 1994). Surgery, radiotherapy and chemotherapy meet with limited success, especially for small cell lung cancer. Other tumours (squamous cell, large cell and adenocarcinoma) may be operable if localized.

Malignant airways obstruction can be palliated and sometimes a lung can be temporarily reexpanded by cryotherapy, laser resection, localized radiotherapy, stenting to splint open the airway or a combination of these (Rudd 1994). Stenting may cause an irritating cough, which can be eased by nebulized bronchodilators.

A spreading tumour may obstruct the superior vena cava, causing oedema, headache, difficulty breathing, sometimes stridor and faintness on bending down. Drugs, radiotherapy and raising the head of the bed may temporarily relieve the symptoms.

Kaposi's sarcoma (KS) is a vascular tumour which affects the skin and connective tissue, and occurs in immunocompromised people. Pulmonary KS affects the parenchyma, lymph nodes or pleura, and manifests as hypoxaemia, pleural effusion, nodular signs on X-ray, breathlessness and sometimes respiratory failure. Up to a quarter of people with AIDS develop KS (Miller *et al* 1992), representing late-stage disease and a poor prognosis.

Mesothelioma arises in the mesothelial cells of the peritoneum, pericardium or pleura. It is caused by asbestos exposure and is always fatal. In the pleura it is associated with malignant pleural effusion and chest pain.

Physiotherapists may be involved at any stage of cancer from sputum induction (Khajotia 1991) through surgery to care of patients in the terminal stages. Weakness and fatigue are common accompaniments to the disease and its various treatments.

3.4.2 Abscess

Lung abscess is a focal collection of pus within the lung parenchyma, caused either by inhalation of septic material or airway blockage. It leads to cavitation and necrosis. Patients may have a swinging pyrexia, and the X-ray often shows a ring shadow and fluid line (Fig. 2.12). Medical treatment is by antibiotics. Physiotherapy is effective if the abscess is open, postural drainage being safe so long as the correct antibiotic is given and positioning is accurate and thorough to avoid dissemination of infection.

3.4.3 Sleep apnoea

Sleep apnoea occurs when breathing stops for periods of more than 10 seconds during sleep. Nocturnal oxygen saturation may drop to 75%, which stimulates the cortex, and the subsequent arousal is accompanied by spectacular snoring. A typical night includes 300–400 such events (Davies and Stradling 1993). The patient's quality of life is affected by morning headaches due to CO_2 retention, daytime sleepiness, poor concentration and a disgruntled spouse. The condition may lead to respiratory failure, cor pulmonale, and pulmonary and systemic hypertension (Okabe 1995). It often goes unrecognized, and physiotherapists may be the first to suspect the condition. Sleep apnoea is less common in women, possibly because progesterone is a respiratory stimulant. Ten per cent of patients with sleep apnoea have COPD, usually those with the blue bloater pattern (Chaouat 1995). The condition is exacerbated by smoking (Wetter 1994) and high alcohol intake (Jalleh 1993).

Obstructive sleep apnoea (OSA) is due to nocturnal upper airway obstruction despite respiratory effort, and worsens as the night progresses (Charbonneau 1994). It is the commonest form of the condition and is usually associated with obesity, which virtually chokes patients in their own fat when muscle tone wanes at night.

Restrictive sleep apnoea occurs in people whose breathing is already impaired by disorders such as scoliosis, ankylosing spondylitis or diaphragmatic paralysis. For those who have little respiratory reserve, the normal inhibition of accessory muscle action during sleep leads to apnoea.

Central sleep apnoea is caused by abnormal central nervous system control of breathing,

described on p. 43, which are often apparent before clinical signs.

Treatment of LVF is by dealing with the cause where possible, plus oxygen, venodilator drugs to reduce filling pressures and diuretics. The role of the physiotherapist is limited to giving symptomatic relief by positioning the patient upright, with support of the feet to prevent the inexorable slide down the bed. The supine posture, that anathema for physiotherapists, is particularly unhelpful for patients with an enlarged heart because of compression of the left mid- and lower lung zones (Wiener *et al* 1990). If mechanical ventilation is necessary, patients rarely require physiotherapy other than positioning and attention to limbs.

Right ventricular failure is caused by LVF, valvular disease of the left heart or chronic hypoxic conditions, such as COPD, which lead to pulmonary hypertension and impaired emptying of the right ventricle. The term **congestive heart failure** means right and left heart failure with congestion in the pulmonary and systemic circulations.

Pulmonary embolus (PE) is a blood clot in the pulmonary vasculature. Secondary blood supply from the bronchial circulation usually keeps lung tissue viable, but this blood exudes into alveoli, causing haemoptysis and an inflammatory reaction which manifests as a sharp, localized pleuritic pain, pleural rub, breathlessness and pallor. Massive embolism causes circulatory collapse. PE is difficult to diagnose clinically, but is suspected in anyone who complains of chest pain and breathlessness, especially if there is hypoxaemia, haemoptysis, pleural rub or evidence of deep vein thrombosis (p. 172). X-ray signs are non-specific, but occasionally a wedge-shaped lesion can be identified. A $\dot{V}/\dot{Q}$ scan shows a perfusion defect (Fig. 2.14). Immediate management is by giving oxygen and placing the patient supine, thus boosting venous return to the left heart which is deprived of pulmonary artery flow (Gray 1992). Treatment is by heparin infusion or, in

severe cases, embolectomy. It is unlikely that any physiotherapy treatment could dislodge the clot and, if so, the clot would move safely with the blood flow into a smaller vessel, but liaison with medical staff is advisable before active intervention because of the unstable nature of the condition.

Renal disease

Kidney disease and its treatment affect most body systems, the respiratory system being influenced by any of the following:

- fluid overload, leading to pulmonary oedema and sometimes pleural effusion,
- breathlessness associated with metabolic acidosis or pulmonary oedema,
- muscle wasting due to steroids and uraemia,
- opportunistic chest infection due to steroids and other drugs following transplantation,
- sleep apnoea associated with end stage renal disease (Kimmel *et al* 1989).

Patients in renal failure are supported by one of the following:

1. Haemofiltration, which removes toxins and excess fluid slowly and requires moderate anticoagulation.
2. Renal dialysis or haemodialysis, which is faster and can cause rapid BP changes, pulmonary and systemic inflammatory changes, wheezing, hypoxaemia due to capillary blockage, and bleeding due to anticoagulation.
3. Peritoneal dialysis, in which alkaline solution is run into the peritoneum, left there until waste products have passed into it through the semi-permeable peritoneum, then drained out. This procedure causes minimal haemodynamic disturbance, but restricts basal ventilation and is now less used. Physiotherapy should coincide with the end of the emptying cycle to ensure free diaphragmatic movement.

Precautions when working with patients on renal support are to treat lines for vascular access with respect, to be watchful of fluid volume changes or hypertension and to be aware of the risk of bleeding if patients are anticoagulated.

Liver disease

The connection between liver disorders and respiratory care include the following:

* tracheal suction is performed with caution if there is a danger of clotting disorders associated with liver dysfunction or, for nasopharyngeal suction, oesophageal varices associated with portal hypertension,
* impaired manufacture of albumin may disturb fluid balance,
* portal hypertension and reduced albumin cause ascites, which splints the diaphragm and leads to a restrictive lung defect,
* encephalopathy reduces the patient's ability to co-operate,
* cerebral oedema causes hyperventilation, which sometimes requires mechanical ventilation (Cowley 1993),
* asterixis is associated with liver disease,
* bilirubin in the plasma of jaundiced patients limits the accuracy of oximetry,
* some patients with grossly enlarged livers are immobile and may not even be able to roll.

Patients admitted for liver transplant are often severely debilitated. A 'Mercedes-Benz' incision incorporates a double subcostal incision and laparotomy, and close teamwork is required for effective pain relief. Postoperative complications include right basal atelectasis, pleural effusion, liver rejection and the long-term effects of immunosuppressive drugs.

Liver transplantation reverses most lung function abnormalities. It is indicated for end-stage cirrhosis, acute fulminant hepatitis or other form of liver failure. Rehabilitation is surprisingly rapid once the toxin-producing liver has been removed. Indeed, some patients may be so poisoned by their own liver that the offending organ is removed even if no donor is immediately available.

When caring for people who have alcoholic liver disease or liver damage from intended paracetamol overdose, physiotherapists need to put aside judgements about 'self-inflicted' conditions.

Sickle cell disease

Sickle cell disease deforms red cells into a sickle shape. Acute vascular occlusion leads to a sickle cell crisis, causing pulmonary vaso-occlusion and excruciating ischaemic pain. Other complaints are cough, breathlessness, chest infection or infarction and atelectasis. Physiotherapy may be indicated for these problems, or if the patient needs assistance with mobilization because of anaemia and fatigue. Epidural analgesia or other potent pain relief is advisable (Yaster *et al* 1994).

Gastro-oesophageal reflux

GOR is the involuntary passage of gastric contents into the oesophagus due to a neuronally-mediated reflex (Ing *et al* 1992). It often occurs at night, especially in people with chronic aspiration or asthma, children with spastic cerebral palsy, people with poor oral health or at the extremes of age. If allowed to enter the airways, the gastric contents cause acid damage to the mucosa. GOR is suspected if there is chronic cough or recurrent chest infection.

Symptoms include heartburn, nocturnal cough, discomfort on swallowing, morning hoarseness and regurgitation with a bitter taste in the mouth, especially after large meals, recumbency or stooping. There may be recurrent pulmonary infiltrates on X-ray. Confirmation of the diagnosis is by endoscopy, barium swallow or pH monitoring (Miles and Ayres 1993). Management is by raising the head of the bed at night, avoidance of late evening meals, large meals, stooping, bending, smoking, alcohol or caffeine, weight reduction if appropriate, drug review and avoidance of aminophylline, which relaxes the cardiac sphincter.

3.4.7 Chest infection

Infection from viruses, bacteria or fungi can occur anywhere from the upper respiratory tract to the lung parenchyma. These are known non-specifically as chest infections. The term encompasses anything from acute bronchitis, a common and usually self-limiting viral infection of the upper bronchial tree, to life-threatening pneumonia. Features include fever, malaise and cough.

Chest infections are a common cause of exacerbation of lung disease, causing excess secretions and impaired mucociliary clearance (Wilson 1988). Those people most at risk are the young, the old, the immunocompromised and those with chronic lung disease. Antibiotics may help bacterial and some fungal infections, but are ineffective against viral infections. Physiotherapy is required if patients are unable to clear their secretions.

3.4.8 Respiratory failure

The main function of the respiratory system is to secure gas exchange, and **respiratory failure** is the inability to maintain blood gases within certain limits. Type I (hypoxaemic) respiratory failure is failure of oxygenation, represented by a $PaO_2 < 8$ kPa (60 mmHg). It is due to failure of the gas exchanging function of the respiratory system and can be acute, e.g. pneumonia, or chronic, e.g. COPD.

Type II (hypoxaemic and hypercapnic) respiratory failure is failure of ventilation, represented by a $PaCO_2 > 6.7$ kPa (50 mmHg) as well as $PaO_2 < 60$ mmHg. It is caused by failure of the respiratory pump and can be acute, e.g. severe acute asthma, or chronic, e.g. advanced COPD. Type II failure is also known as ventilatory failure, and is the outward clinical manifestation of muscle weakness or fatigue. If acute, it is accompanied by a fall in pH because there has been no time for renal compensation.

The process of respiration includes components other than gas exchange in the lung, but the term 'respiratory failure' is reserved for disorders that result in a disturbance of arterial blood gases only. Respiratory insufficiency is when adequate gas exchange is maintained but at great cost to the breathing mechanism (Pilbeam 1992, p. 76).

RECOMMENDED READING

BTS (1993) Guidelines for management of asthma: a summary. *Br. Med. J.*, **306**, 776–82.

Cochrane, G.M. (1995) Acute severe asthma. *Thorax*, **50**, 1–2.

Gross, N.J. (1990) Chronic obstructive pulmonary disease: current concepts and therapeutic approaches. *Chest*, **97**, 19S–23S.

Henderson, A. (1994) Chronic respiratory failure. *Practitioner*, **238**, 345–50.

Hunninghake, G.W. (1995) Approaches to the treatment of pulmonary fibrosis. *Am. J. Respir. Crit. Care Med.*, **151**, 915–18.

MacFarlane, J. (1995) Acute pneumonia in the hospital patient. *Hosp. Update*, 19–23.

McClure, J. (1993) The role of physiotherapy in HIV and AIDS. *Physiotherapy*, **79**, 388–93.

Michie, J. (1994) An introduction to lung cancer. *Physiotherapy*, **80**, 844–7.

Parker, A.E. and Young, C.S. (1991) The physiotherapy management of cystic fibrosis in children. *Physiotherapy*, **77**, 584–6.

Woodhead, M.A. (1992) Management of pneumonia. *Respir. Med.*, **86**, 459–69.

4. *General management*

4.1 INTRODUCTION

Although rehabilitation for people with respiratory disability has been slow to respond to the changing needs and expectations of patients, respiratory medicine itself has been transformed in the past 20 years, both by technical advances and by an understanding that for these to be effective, patients must become central players in their own care. This chapter looks at current knowledge in respiratory medicine.

4.2 OXYGEN THERAPY

Throughout the past 200 years, oxygen has been much used and sometimes abused. Oxygen is an odourless colourless drug that has side-effects and specific risks, but with rational prescription, precision of administration and objective monitoring, it is a potent therapy for the respiratory patient.

Oxygen must be medically prescribed, with the flow rate and method of delivery specified, but all team members need to be involved because it is notoriously mismanaged. Studies have shown 21% inappropriate prescription, 86% inadequate monitoring and 56% inaccurate administration (Leach and Bateman 1993). In one postoperative survey, the mask stayed in place on only one out of 20 patients (Baxter *et al* 1993).

4.2.1 Indications

Supplementary oxygen should normally be prescribed only for hypoxaemia, i.e. resting PaO_2 below 8 kPa (60 mmHg) or SaO_2 below 90%. Supplemental oxygen is also needed for potential hypoxaemia, such as before and after suction, and when bronchodilator drugs or mucolytics are administered for the first time in case of adverse effects.

Postoperatively, oxygen prescription depends on the patient and type of surgery. Postoperative hypoxaemia may be only transient, but for people with lung disease or those who have had heart or lung surgery, oxygen may be required for longer than expected, especially at night (p. 171).

For long term oxygen therapy, nocturnal monitoring is needed for accurate prescription because daytime oxygen saturation bears little relation to nocturnal saturation (Mohsenin 1994).

Contrary to tradition, oxygen is not indicated for uncomplicated myocardial infarction without hypoxaemia (Leach and Bateman 1993), nor should it be used as a tonic for breathlessness (Stewart and Howard 1992). Breathlessness and hypoxaemia often coexist but have different mechanisms, and oxygen for resting breathlessness is considered an expensive placebo (Leach and Bateman 1994). The following exceptions may apply:

• supplementary oxygen may reduce breathlessness during exercise in a proportion of patients, independent of resting PaO_2 (Leach and Bateman 1994), but oxygen is unhelpful before or after exercise (Williamson 1993),
• terminally ill patients who are breathless may find some relief with oxygen therapy.

Many patients are both hypoxaemic and breathless, but oxygen should be prescribed for the hypoxaemia, not the breathlessness. A subjective feeling of wanting air is not an indication for oxygen, and prescription 'as required' makes no physiological sense. People do not feel a physical need for oxygen as they do for food because chemoreceptor signals are not consciously appreciated (Holland 1991). Education is more beneficial than the psychological crutch of an expensive drug.

Oxygen should be administered continuously unless hypoxaemia has been demonstrated only in specific situations such as sleep, eating or exercise (AARC 1992a).

4.2.2   Limitations

Oxygen therapy is not just aimed at making the patient pink. It does not improve ventilation, nor does pushing oxygen into the throat guarantee its arrival at the mitochondria. Tissue hypoxia is often assumed when there is a low PaO_2, but this can be misleading if oxygen delivery is hindered, for example by polycythaemia, impaired cardiac output, anaemia or hypoperfusion.

If hypoxaemia is due to physiological shunt, benefit from oxygen therapy is limited because the shunted blood does not 'see' the oxygen. A shunt above 50% renders oxygen therapy virtually useless.

4.2.3   Complications

1. High concentrations of inspired oxygen may impair the respiratory drive in people with acute hypercapnic COPD (p. 93).
2. Oxygen toxicity is an inflammatory response of lung tissue following exposure to 100% oxygen for between 40 hours and seven days (Heulitt 1995). All organs can be harmed by excess oxygen, but the lung is exposed to the highest PO_2. Oxygen toxicity impairs the actions of cilia, macrophages and surfactant, and the patient experiences substernal pain, cough and dyspnoea. Vital capacity drops, and a syndrome of stiff lungs and progressive hypoxaemia develop. The risk of oxygen toxicity is increased by high-volume ventilation and malnutrition, but pre-existing lung disease affords some protection (Durbin 1993). If oxygen toxicity is suspected, monitoring by PaO_2 is advisable because the shape of the dissociation curve means that measurements of SaO_2 at high levels of oxygenation are relatively insensitive.
3. Blindness may be caused if neonates are given high concentrations of oxygen (Chapter 12).
4. For mechanically ventilated patients who are receiving low tidal volumes and low cycling pressures, 'absorption atelectasis' can occur if more than 70% oxygen is given (Pilbeam 1992, p. 239). Absorption

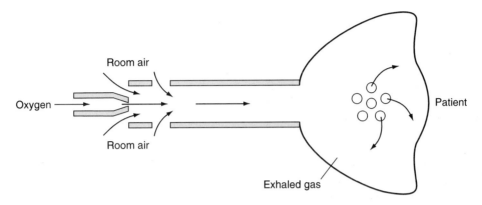

Figure 4.1 High flow fixed performance 'venturi' mask.

of oxygen from the alveoli exceeds re-plenishment of alveolar gas during inspiration, and the lungs are no longer held open by a cushion of inert nitrogen.

5. Discomfort can be caused by drying of mucous membranes, eye irritation or a sense of being smothered. The sight of a patient attempting to 'oxygenate' his or her forehead is a familiar sign of this problem.

6. Oxygen is not addictive, but dependency occurs when patients rely on their oxygen unnecessarily.

7. Oxygen creates a fire hazard by supporting combustion.

Smoking is banned.

4.2.4 Delivery devices

The nasal specs caused so many problems; they kept falling out or were too tight. They were one of the most uncomfortable appliances, yet better than the mask which seemed to suffocate you.
Ludwig 1984

Low flow (variable performance) masks

These masks, also known as simple masks, deliver only a portion of the patient's inspired gas. They provide a flow rate that is less than the patient's inspiratory flow and allow room air to be sucked in through the edges of the mask to dilute the oxygen. The fractional inspired oxygen concentration (F_1O_2) varies with the patient's own flow: the more rapid the ventilation, the lower the F_1O_2. This provides inaccurate (uncontrolled) oxygen, but flow rates of 6–8 l/min provide approximately 40–50% oxygen (Gribbin 1993). The flow rate should be maintained above 6 l/min to avoid rebreathing CO_2. These masks are suitable when accurate concentrations are not necessary, e.g. after routine surgery.

High flow (fixed performance) masks

These masks, also known as venturi masks, flood the patient with a prescribed gas mixture at flow rates greater than the individual's demand, even for breathless patients with high inspiratory flows. This minimizes rebreathing of expired air from the mask, even if it is loosely fitted, and delivers a relatively accurate F_1O_2, as specified on the mask. Oxygen rushes from a nozzle and entrains an exact proportion of room air so that a fixed concentration is delivered. This concentration depends on the size of the entrainment ports and oxygen flow through the nozzle (Fig. 4.1).

Venturi masks can deliver up to 60% oxygen, but are more accurate at lower percentages (Fulmer 1984). Large capacity masks are often used because they act as reservoirs to prevent a fall in F_1O_2 for breathless patients. Humidification is not required for venturi masks (p. 131). These masks are used for:

- patients needing an accurate F_1O_2, e.g. hypercapnic COPD patients who are dependent on their hypoxic drive and need controlled oxygen therapy (see p. 93),
- breathless patients.

High-and low-flow masks relate to high and low accuracy, not to high and low-F_1O_2.

Nasal cannulae

Cannulae are low-flow systems which deliver oxygen directly into the nostrils. The accuracy of nasal cannulae is variable (Bazuaye *et al* 1992), and the patient's flow rate and breathing pattern affect the inspired oxygen, but the following are approximate figures (Branson 1993):

- 1 l/min provides 24% oxygen,
- 2 l/min provides 28% oxygen,
- 3 l/min provides 32% oxygen,
- 4 l/min provides 36% oxygen.

Flows above 6 l/min add little to the F_1O_2 and may cause drying and irritation. Mouth breathers are partly accommodated by entrainment of oxygen into the reservoir of the nasopharynx during expiration, but F_1O_2 is higher with the mouth closed (Dunlevy and Tyl 1992). Nasal cannulae are cheap, comparatively comfortable and prevent rebreathing of expired air. Drying of mucus membranes is reduced by giving patients a supply of lanolin (not Vaseline which is oil-based and reacts with oxygen). The flow rate can be marked on the flow meter with tape to remind patients and others of the correct setting.

Indications for nasal cannulae are:

- long-term oxygen therapy so that talking, coughing and eating are unhindered,

- confused patients,
- patients who find masks uncomfortable,
- in combination with a mask, for patients who need a high, if inaccurate, concentration of oxygen, e.g. in severe acute asthma,
- hypoxaemic patients using an incentive spirometer, inspiratory muscle trainer, ultrasonic nebulizer and for certain patients using a jet nebulizer (p. 104).

Nasal catheters

These devices are inserted deep into one nostril. They have several holes near the tip so that the force of the oxygen flow is diffused and does not harm the mucous lining. Some have a sponge which holds the device in place, but this invites infection if it is not changed every eight hours. They are impractical in infants because they occlude most of the nasal airway, and are usually not tolerated by older children, but are less likely to be dislodged than cannulae.

Transtracheal oxygen catheters

These devices are introduced surgically directly into the trachea, percutaneously or through a tunnelled route, for long-term oxygen therapy. They are suited to patients who are sufficiently motivated to follow a regimented protocol of self-care. Advantages are:

- less dead space and reduced flow rates by up to 50%, which reduces oxygen consumption by over a half and extends portable oxygen use (Haas and Haas 1990, p. 130),
- high flow rates without irritating nasal mucosa, which is useful for patients with severe hypoxaemia,
- reduced hospitalization, improved exercise tolerance and quality of life (Hoffman 1994),
- high patient compliance due to its unobtrusive presence.

Disadvantages are:

- the need for surgical placement, risking infection, subcutaneous emphysema, haemoptysis, displacement and dermatitis,
- mucus ball formation, although this is reduced by regular irrigation with saline.

Reservoir masks

For high levels of oxygen, a system incorporating a one-litre reservoir bag can be used. During exhalation the bag fills with oxygen and during inhalation this oxygen enriches the inspired gas (Branson 1993). A non-rebreathing system has a valve between mask and bag to prevent expired CO_2 entering the bag, delivering 55–90% oxygen at 6–15 l/min. A partial-rebreather has no valve and about one-third of the expired CO_2 enters the bag, allowing delivery of 35–60% oxygen at 6–15 l/min (Bolgiano 1990). Reservoir masks cannot be humidified. The flow rate must be sufficient to keep the bag inflated during inspiration.

Tents

Humidified oxygen is still occasionally delivered to children over one year old via tents, which are isolating, uncomfortably wet and deliver fluctuating levels of oxygen. Oxygen escapes each time the edges are untucked, but if undisturbed, levels of 50% oxygen can be achieved, although CO_2 retention then becomes a problem.

Head boxes

Tents have been largely superseded by head boxes, which are clear plastic boxes placed over the heads of babies to control the delivery of humidified oxygen. They are more acceptable to infants, but care should be taken to direct the gas flow away from the baby's face and to ensure that the edges of the box do not rub the skin. Alternatives are oxygen chairs, which incorporate a plastic canopy or hood to enable oxygen to be delivered to an upright baby.

4.2.5 Acute oxygen therapy

People with a hypercapnic exacerbation of COPD should be given controlled oxygen in order to preserve their respiratory drive, especially if a normal pH indicates compensated acid-base status. Sustained hypercapnia has left them dependent on a low PaO_2 as a ventilatory stimulus, and uncontrolled oxygen may deliver a too high F_IO_2, causing hypoventilation, drowsiness and severe respiratory acidosis which can be lethal. Patients without hypercapnia are not at risk (Fulmer 1984).

Simple low-flow masks are inadequate for these patients. Nasal cannulae are sometimes used, but hypoventilating patients will entrain little room air and can receive dangerously high F_IO_2 levels (Davies and Hopkin 1989), so if cannulae are necessary for patient comfort, close monitoring is required. Controlled oxygen is best delivered by a high-flow venturi mask.

Hypercapnic COPD patients show a wide variation in their response to oxygen. Those with a $PaO_2 < 6$ kPa (45 mmHg) and elevated $PaCO_2$ require monitoring to show whether 24%, 28% or 35% oxygen is indicated. Patients start with 24% or 28% oxygen by venturi mask, then blood gases are taken after 30 minutes. If the $PaCO_2$ rises no more than slightly and stabilizes, the F_IO_2 can be increased. If the $PaCO_2$ rises excessively, the F_IO_2 must be reduced. If this leaves the patient unacceptably hypoxaemic, ventilatory support is required by mechanical or chemical means (Fig. 4.2).

Small amounts of oxygen can relieve hypoxaemia in these patients because reactions take place on the steep part of the oxygen dissociation curve. In practice, the

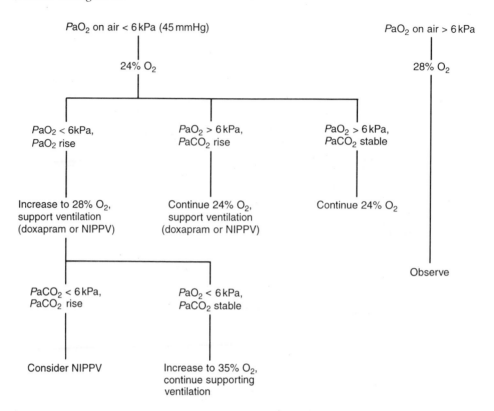

Figure 4.2 Flow chart of controlled oxygen therapy for exacerbations of COPD, showing how PaO_2 and $PaCO_2$ relate to the need for supplementary oxygen and ventilatory support. Arterial blood gases are taken 30 minutes after each therapy change, and treatment adjusted accordingly. A more detailed flow chart can be found in Gribbin (1993).
Doxapram: respiratory stimulant drug.
NIPPV: nasal intermittent positive pressure ventilation.

danger of giving too much oxygen is usually overestimated, with patients often deprived of much-needed oxygen. Hypoxaemia kills more people than hypercapnia.

Intermittent oxygen therapy given in the acute phase of COPD, especially for hypercapnic patients (Fig. 4.3), is like pulling a drowning man out of the water and then pushing him under again. CO_2 is stored in the body in larger quantities than oxygen, so if the inspired oxygen is allowed to fall, CO_2 crowds out oxygen and causes a sharp drop in PaO_2 (Collins 1976).

Patients with acute problems other than exacerbation of COPD, e.g. those with pneumonia or acute asthma, need generous levels of 60% or more oxygen.

Patients on acute oxygen therapy should not have their mask removed except for expectoration or other brief reason, especially hypercapnic COPD patients and people after heart surgery when the body is adjusting to its new haemodynamic status. During recovery, oximetry can be used to monitor withdrawal of oxygen therapy (King and Simon 1987).

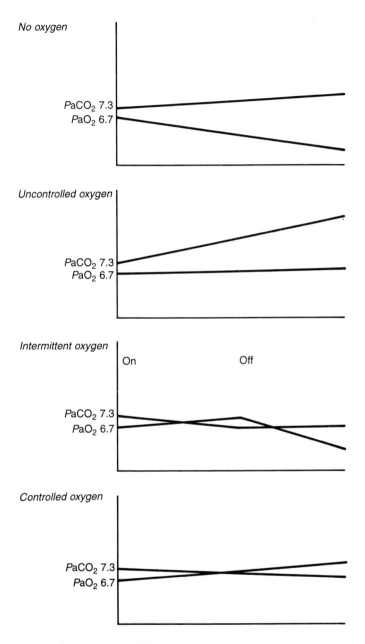

Figure 4.3 Effects of different forms of oxygen administration on blood gases (in kPa) in COPD patients in acute hypercapnic respiratory failure: (a) continued deterioration, (b) blunting of respiratory drive leads to further $PaCO_2$ retention, (c) gradual hypercapnia and rapid hypoxaemia, (d) normalization of blood gases.

4.2.6   Long-term oxygen therapy (LTOT)

A proportion of well-motivated people with severe COPD benefit from carefully managed home oxygen therapy. Outcomes (Leach and Bateman 1994) include ↓ mortality, ↑ sleep and quality of life, ↓ exacerbations and ↓ hospital admissions, which is significant considering that one month's LTOT costs less than one day in hospital (Fulmer *et al* 1984). Improvement stems mainly from reduced nocturnal desaturation, thus relieving pulmonary hypertension and improving haemodynamics (Fletcher 1994). People with chronic hypoxaemia due to other diseases may also benefit (Petty and O'Donohue 1994).

LTOT is prescribed after comprehensive drug review and extended monitoring to assess oxygen saturation during sleep, rest and exercise. The following criteria apply (Donner and Howard 1992):

- chronic stable hypoxaemia with $PaO_2 <$ 7.3 kPa (55 mmHg) breathing air, on two samples taken at least three weeks apart,
- with $PaO_2 <$ 8.7 kPa (65 mmHg), haematocrit above 55%,
- severe nocturnal or exercise hypoxaemia despite daytime normoxaemia,
- $FEV_1 < 1.5$ l,
- mental impairment, e.g. short-term memory loss,
- severe exercise limitation.

Patients usually under-use their oxygen therapy (Make 1994) due to lack of education. Patients should understand that oxygen should be used for as long as they can manage. The minimum effective prescription is for nocturnal oxygen, but over 12 hours daily is preferable and near-continuous oxygen is ideal (Hodgkin 1993, p. 215). The flow rate is set to achieve a PaO_2 of at least 8.7 kPa (65 mmHg) without a rise in $PaCO_2$ by more than 1.3 kPa (10 mmHg), and will generally be between 1.5–2.5 l/min. This can be increased by 1 l/min during sleep or exercise

if appropriate. Monitoring is advisable at first with 24-hour domiciliary oximetry, and ongoing home care support is mandatory. Administration is by:

- oxygen cylinders, which are cumbersome, require repeat prescriptions and regulator changes, are dangerous if not secured carefully and rapidly run out of oxygen,
- oxygen concentrator, which is cheaper if life expectancy is more than three months (Leach and Bateman 1994) but is noisy, cannot be modified for portable use and needs regular maintenance,
- liquid oxygen, which is expensive and not available on the NHS in the UK, but is versatile, easily portable and preferred by patients who are mobile or employed.

Portable cylinders are problematical because at low flow rates improved exercise capacity may be cancelled out by the work of carrying the cylinder, and high flows empty the cylinder in 20–30 minutes (Leach and Batemen 1994). Exercise performance may not be improved even if desaturation is reduced (Keilty 1994). Portable oxygen should be recommended only if a double-blind comparison of a six-minute walk (breathing cylinder air or oxygen), demonstrates a 50% gain in exercise tolerance or breathlessness using a visual analogue scale (Leach and Bateman 1994). The flow rate should be sufficient to prevent desaturation and is usually about 4 l/min. Portable cylinders are best wheeled on a shopping trolley or custom-built walker. Transtracheal catheters and other oxygen-conserving devices are available to increase efficiency (Hoffman 1994).

Domiciliary oxygen means that the disease is visible and can no longer be denied. Veteran patients on long-term oxygen therapy are often willing to talk to new patients and their carers who may feel dismayed at the prospect of a life spent tethered by the nose to bulky equipment.

4.2.7 Hyperbaric oxygen therapy

Hyperbaric oxygen therapy involves a patient being pressurized to greater than atmospheric pressure in a chamber. High pressure oxygen does not improve tissue oxygenation under normal circumstances, but several conditions are responsive to hyperbaric oxygen therapy, including the following:

1. Carbon monoxide poisoning, which hinders the oxygen-carrying capacity of haemoglobin. Hyperbaric oxygen helps to compensate by increasing the transport of dissolved oxygen.
2. Gas gangrene, whose anaerobic organisms are unhappy in the high PO_2 environment created by hyperbaric oxygen.
3. Crush injuries, ischaemia and burns (James *et al* 1993).

4.2.8 Helium/oxygen therapy

A helium/oxygen mixture called Heliox replaces the nitrogen in air with helium, creating a mixture that has one-third the density of air. This can more easily bypass an obstruction and is used in acute asthma (Kass 1995) or to relieve stridor or upper airway narrowing caused by a tumour or burns.

4.3 NUTRITION

Breathing and eating are basic life processes that are intimately related in their physiology, emotive associations and mechanics. Both obesity and malnutrition impair lung function (Chen *et al* 1993), but nutrition is still a neglected area of respiratory medicine despite its importance being well documented. Malnutrition often reaches 'marasmic proportions' in COPD (Donner and Howard 1992). Forty-seven percent of stable patients have shown nutritional abnormalities (Sahebjami 1993) and malnutrition exceeds 50% in hospitalized patients (Fitting 1992), especially in those at the emphysematous end of the COPD spectrum.

Physiotherapists need to work closely with the health care team, otherwise they will be working uphill with an unnecessarily compromised patient. The following facts will support their argument:

- malnourished people are unable to improve muscle function and exercise tolerance without weight gain (Fitting 1992),
- well-nourished patients with stable COPD show no evidence of chronic fatigue (Similowski 1991).

4.3.1 Causes of poor nutrition

1. Eating becomes a chore rather than a pleasure for breathless people because the combined actions of eating and breathing are in competition.
2. A normal-sized meal can interfere with diaphragmatic mechanics, especially when accompanied by air-swallowing associated with breathlessness.
3. Appetite is reduced by smoking, sputum, depression or medication.
4. Exercise limitation discourages the preparation of healthy food.
5. Desaturation during meals can be caused by the breath-holding required for swallowing and the increased metabolic activity associated with digestion and assimilation.
6. Increased work of breathing raises calorie requirements.
7. Oxygen therapy or mouth breathing can dry the mouth and make eating difficult.
8. Hypoxaemia itself impairs nutrition (Donahoe *et al* 1992).
9. Hospitalized patients have added obstacles, such as unappetizing food, missed meals due to tests or procedures, the effect of illness on appetite and the low priority given to nutritional support. Allison (1995) has shown that 40% of general patients are malnourished on admission and become more so during their stay.

4.3.2   Effects of poor nutrition

Nutritional depletion aggravates the emphysematous process (Sahebjami 1993) weakens inspiratory muscles, increases the oxygen cost of breathing (Donahoe *et al* 1992), increases the risk of infection (Fitting 1992), decreases exercise capacity (Schols *et al* 1991), causes depression and apathy (Allison 1995), damages lung tissue (Sridhar 1995), impairs ciliary motility, impairs respiratory drive, depletes surfactant (Ryan *et al* 1993) and reinforces this whole unhappy process by blunting hunger.

4.3.3   Management

Nutrition therapy should be a routine preventive measure for all people with COPD and not left until debilitated patients have cannibalized the protein from their own respiratory muscles. Education includes the following suggestions:

- eat multiple small meals, preferably six times a day,
- clean your teeth or use a mouth wash before meals if inhaled drugs or sputum have left a bad taste,
- if breakfast is difficult, try liquidizing it,
- eat fruit and vegetables every day to improve intake of vitamin C, which helps prevent infection, reduces inflammation and mops up oxidants in tobacco smoke (Sridhar 1995),
- take liquids separately from meals,
- avoid hard or dry food, or add sauces such as gravy or custard,
- avoid gas-forming foods,
- make use of high-energy drinks, such as homemade milk shakes and fresh fruit juice,
- meals should be leisurely, enjoyable and taken sitting up with elbows on the table to stabilize accessory muscles.

Patients can be advised to experiment with reducing or abstaining from:

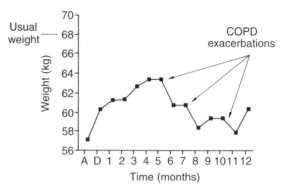

Figure 4.4 Weight of a patient with severe COPD, showing beneficial effect of nutritional support and detrimental effect of exacerbations. A = admission, D = discharge. (Source: Donahoe, M. and Rogers, R.M. (1990) Nutritional assessment and support in COPD. *Clin. Chest Med.*, **11**, 487–504, with permission.)

- dairy foods, which many patients claim increases the viscosity of their mucus, a claim which now has some objective validity (Enderby 1995),
- caffeine, which has a potentiating role in peptic ulceration, to which people with COPD are susceptible (Hodgkin and Petty 1987),
- additives, spicy food and alcohol (Hodgkin 1993).

Alcohol increases pulmonary hypertension and hypercapnia in COPD (Jalleh *et al* 1993), causes snoring in normal people, sleep apnoea in snorers (Chan 1990), and impairs ciliary action and immune function in everyone else (Hodgkin 1993, p. 113).

Supplementary feeds provide concentrated nutrition orally or nasogastrically, and are useful for patients with exacerbation of disease. Patients with advanced disease may need supplementary feeding even in the chronic state (Fig. 4.4). Nasogastric feeds are best given at night to encourage daytime eating. Slow continuous infusions help to prevent excess metabolic activity which can increase energy expenditure by 24% and cause desaturation (Ryan *et al* 1993). High-fat, low-carbohydrate formulae should be used for respiratory patients because the normal high-carbohydrate feeds can increase CO_2 production, oxygen consumption and breathlessness for up to 1½ hours (Kuo *et al* 1993). Oximetry during and after meals will identify patients who need supplementary oxygen while eating, although this may not be acceptable if nasal cannulae diminish the sense of smell and reduce enjoyment.

Physiotherapists may be the first to identify the need for nutritional guidance and give basic advice, but a dietitian is required for accurate assessment and treatment. Respiratory patients can show a complicated pattern of weight loss, fluid retention, obesity and masked malnourishment. Body water can be altered by oxygen therapy (Donahoe *et al* 1992), and body weight is not an inadequate measuring tool.

4.4 DRUG THERAPY

Medication is normally prescribed by doctors and administered by nurses, but physiotherapists are involved in requesting and sometimes administering respiratory drugs. Patients with respiratory diseases tend to be subjected to blind polypharmacy, so physiotherapists should become informed of the indications, side-effects and delivery systems of different drugs (see Table 4.1).

4.4.1 Drugs to prevent inflammation

The mechanism of allergic asthma can be influenced by mast cell stabilizers, which hinder the release of inflammatory mediators and decrease bronchial hyperreactivity. They protect against allergic and exercise-induced asthma, but do not reverse an established attack. They can only be inhaled, should be used prophylactically and regularly, and are particularly effective in exercise-induced and childhood asthma, for which they should be the first-line medication. They take two to six weeks to reduce inflammation and up to three months to alter bronchial reactivity (Fawcett 1995).

4.4.2 Drugs to treat inflammation

Corticosteroids are hormone-based agents which are used as prevention in respiratory medicine, suppressing the inflammatory reactions that set off bronchospasm, oedema and mucus hypersecretion. They are not thought to alter the ultimate course of the disease (Phelan 1994).

Steroids are commonly used as prophylaxis for asthma, with increased dosage during infection or allergen exposure. They help about 20% of people with COPD (Clarke 1991), sometimes even those who do not respond to bronchodilators. People with bronchiectasis and restrictive diseases such as fibrosing alveolitis may also benefit from steroids. For accurate prescription, a home trial with serial peak flow measurements (Fig. 3.9) is necessary because of spontaneous fluctuations in airway calibre (Wiggins 1991). Side-effects are listed in Table 4.1, with further points discussed below:

1. Systemic side-effects are reduced by using the inhaled route. Local side-effects can be minimized by using a spacer, inhaling slowly, and afterwards rinsing the mouth, gargling or cleaning the teeth. Toothbrushes should be renewed frequently. If using a mask, the face should be wiped afterwards.
2. In children, inhaled steroids are sometimes thought to retard growth, but it is contested that poorly controlled asthma has a greater effect on growth (Barry 1994). Fluticasone, which is twice as potent as other steroids, does not appear to affect growth (Russell 1994).
3. In children, high doses cause adrenal suppression (Ninan *et al* 1993).
4. The risk of bone demineralization is lessened by vitamin D supplements.
5. Severe asthma may require intravenous or oral steroids, which bring significant side-

Table 4.1 Medication for airways obstruction

Drug	Delivery	Side-effects
Mast cell stabilizers		
Sodium cromoglycate (Intal) Nedocromil sodium (Tilade)	Inhaler/nebulizer	Throat irritation
Corticosteroids		
Beclomethasone (Becotide, Beclovent) Budesonide (Pulmicort) Fluticasone (Flixotide)	Inhaler/nebulizer	Hoarse voice Oropharyngeal candidiasis
Prednisone Prednisolone	Oral	Osteoporosis Fluid retention ↑ infection risk
Hydrocortisone	Intravenous/oral	Obesity Muscle atrophy Bruising in the elderly Hyperglycaemia Cataract Delayed healing Retarded growth
Bronchodilators		
β_2-agonists Salbutamol (Ventolin) Terbutaline (Bricanyl) Salmeterol (Serevent)	Inhaler/nebulizer Slow release capsule Intravenous	Tremor Tachycardia
Anticholinergics Ipratropium (Atrovent)	Inhaler/nebulizer	Dry mouth
Xanthines Theophylline Aminophylline	Intravenous Oral Slow release capsule	Headache Gastric ulcer Insomnia Nausea and vomiting Arrhythmias Nasty taste

effects with long-term use. Increased breathlessness due to steroid-induced muscle atrophy may be mistakenly ascribed to deterioration of the disease and lead to increased steroid dosage (Gallagher 1994).

Concern about side-effects tempts prescribers to nibble ineffectively at the problem with low-dose therapy. Both undertreatment and side-effects can be minimized by high dosage and early weaning (acute disease), or alternate day dosing (chronic disease), and by taking the drug first thing in the morning. Patients as well as doctors may become 'steroid phobic'.

4.4.3 Drugs to treat bronchospasm

Response to bronchodilators is usual in asthma, occasional in chronic bronchitis and rare in emphysema. All patients on broncho-dilators should have a peak flow chart until the response is confirmed, and patients under review need a drug trial (Spence 1991) with peak flow and symptom monitoring. This will identify reversible bronchospasm, defined as improvement in peak flow or FEV_1 by at least 15% or by 150 ml (Dekker *et al* 1992). Measurements are taken 10 minutes after salbutamol and 20 minutes after ipratropium bromide (Rimington *et al* 1994). A drug trial also pinpoints which drug, combination of drugs, dosage and route of administration are indicated.

Both sympathetic (adrenergic) and para-sympathetic (cholinergic) receptors have been identified in bronchial smooth muscle.

Sympathomimetics are versatile drugs which mimic the action of the sympathetic nervous system, stimulating β_2-receptors in the bronchial smooth muscle and dilating the airways, especially the smaller airways. β_2-stimulants are also known as β_2-adrenergics or β_2-agonists. Examples are:

- salbutamol: onset of action seven minutes, peak effect 20 minutes, duration of action four to eight hours,
- salmeterol: onset 15 minutes, peak one hour, duration 12 hours.

The long-acting β_2-stimulants, such as sal-meterol, can be prescribed regularly, have a greater effect on quality of life (Juniper 1995), and are particularly useful in controlling nocturnal asthma and protecting against the effects of brittle asthma. The short-acting drugs, such as salbutamol, should be taken symptomatically rather than regularly, apart from prophylactic use before exercise-induced bronchospasm.

β_2-stimulants are prescribed freely and sometimes mindlessly. Unnecessary use can worsen the course of COPD (Postma 1991)

and increase the risk of death from asthma (Barrett 1995). The side-effect of trembling hands and tachycardia can impair function in severely breathless people.

Anticholinergic (antimuscarinic) drugs, such as ipratropium, cause bronchodilation by blocking the effect of acetylcholine on autonomic nerve endings. They primarily affect the larger airways and have a slow onset of 30–45 minutes. They tend to be used for older people, those with COPD or those who do not respond to β_2-stimulants. However, individuals show different response patterns and may respond better to β_2-stimulants, anticholinergics or both together.

Theophylline and its derivatives, such as aminophylline, are part of the xanthine group of drugs which have an interesting variety of effects. They bronchodilate, reduce inflammation, moderately boost inspiratory muscle action and the immune system, improve gas exchange and lung function (Mulloy 1993), promote mucociliary clearance and reduce pulmonary hypertension (Banner 1994). It now seems likely that bronchodila-tion is less responsible for the anti-asthma properties of these drugs than the effects on the inflammatory or immune responses.

The theophyllines are too insoluble to be given by inhalation, and precise dosage is required because of side-effects. Slow-release preparations are used to control nocturnal asthma and continuous intravenous therapy can be used for people with brittle asthma. Clearance rates are increased in smokers and children, and decreased in elderly people and those with viral infection or heart failure.

If both β_2-stimulants and anticholinergics are prescribed, the anticholinergic is taken first to open up the large airways and pro-vide better access for the β_2-stimulants (Mathewson 1993). If both bronchodilator and preventive drug are prescribed, the bronchodilator should be taken first to ensure maximum penetration of the preventive drug. However, complicated instructions can demotivate patients, and it is more important that the drugs are taken than that the exact sequence be adhered to.

4.4.4   Drugs to treat breathlessness

Breathlessness in chronic lung disease becomes significant to the patient when roughly half the ventilatory capacity of the lungs is already lost. Little of this function is recoverable, which often leads to an attitude of therapeutic defeatism. This is not totally justified.

Sometimes the cause of breathlessness can be treated, for example by diuretics, broncho-dilators or steroids. Drugs that act directly on breathlessness are limited. Anticholinergics can reduce a degree of breathlessness in some patients (Spence and Hay 1993). Morphine reduces respiratory drive, lessens anxiety and may reduce breathlessness; the risk of respiratory depression is reduced by a slow-release preparation and titration to the individual's need (Light 1989). Buspirone is an anxiolytic without sedative effect and can reduce breathlessness and increase exercise tolerance (Argyropoulou 1993).

4.4.5   Drugs to treat infection

An antibiotic is indicated if a patient's condition is caused by bacterial infection and if the organism responsible is sensitive to the antibiotic prescribed. Prophylactic antibiotics do not reduce exacerbations of COPD (Clarke 1991) and should be used only for people with chronic sepsis, such as cystic fibrosis or bronchiectasis. Sputum specimens may be requested for identification of the organism, but are often of limited value because of contamination with upper respiratory tract flora.

Antibiotics are administered orally, intra-venously or by special nebulizers which can cope with viscous solutions and have an exhalation filter. Access to the affected site may be hampered by obstructed airways and damaged vasculature. Side-effects include skin reactions and the emergence of resistant organisms because of interference with the friendly flora of the respiratory tract.

4.4.6   Drugs to help sputum clearance

First-line expectorants are systemic hydration, inhaling warm moist air or drinking a steamy cup of tea. If drugs are needed, they should be aimed at improving mucus transport or thinning secretions, not at irritating the airways so that more sputum is produced.

Mucus transport is enhanced by vitamin C (Silver and Foster 1990), a mucolytic-expectorant called iodinated glycerol (Petty 1990), and to a lesser extent by the β_2-stimulants, especially salmeterol (Rusznak 1991). Amiloride is a weak stimulator of mucociliary clearance (DiBenedetto 1990). The volume of sputum expectorated can be reduced by inhaled oxitropium (Tamaoki 1994), inhaled indomethacin (Tamaoki 1992) or inhaled steroids (Elborn *et al* 1992).

Acetylcysteine is a mucolytic that tends to be viewed as a form of iatrogenic smoking because of its irritant effect on the airways. It has a nasty smell and taste and needs to be accompanied by a bronchodilator because it can cause bronchospasm (Judson 1994). However, it can reduce the viscosity of non-infected secretions (Empey 1993b) and reduce exacerbations in people with COPD, possibly by increasing antioxidant protection (Hansen 1994). When nebulized, air should be used as the driving gas because the drug is inacti-vated by oxygen.

4.4.7   Drugs to inhibit coughing

To suppress a non-productive and irritating cough, medication is available if physical means (p. 138) are to no avail. Codeine or the opiates can be given in end-stage interstitial lung disease or cancer, for example, but may have unacceptable side-effects. The pheno-thiazines are non-opioid central acting anti-tussives, which also show antihistamine properties (Charpin and Weibel 1990). Nebu-lized local anaesthetics, such as lignocaine, block sensory nerve traffic and provide tem-porary relief at night (Trochtenberg 1994), but patients cannot eat or drink until the drug wears off. A cough caused by asthma or ACE-inhibitors can be reduced by nedocromil sodium (Hargreaves 1995), and a post infec-tion cough by ipratropium (Holmes *et al* 1992).

'Cough mixtures' may unhelpfully contain both expectorant and suppressant, but are strong placebos and the sugar content is thought to soothe irritated airways tran-siently.

4.4.8 Drugs to improve ventilation

Respiratory stimulants should be used with caution so as not to override the protective function of fatigue. They do not reverse the underlying cause of ventilatory failure.

Doxapram stimulates ventilation but at the cost of central nervous system stimulation, increased work of breathing and extra breath-lessness. An infusion is sometimes tolerated by drowsy patients with post-anaesthesia hypoventilation, or to prevent mechanical ventilation (Hirschberg 1994). It is sometimes used with acute oxygen therapy for patients who cannot reach satisfactory oxygen satura-tions without excessive hypercapnia, although Gribbin (1993) advises against this.

Almitrine is a chemoreceptor agonist which increases ventilation, reduces hyper-capnia and can increase PaO_2 by 0.7–1.3 kPa (5–10 mm/Hg) (Winkelmann 1994), but the side-effects of breathlessness and neuropathy make it unacceptable at present. Diaphrag-matic contractility is improved by drugs such as theophylline and tricyclic antidepressants, but often with unacceptable side-effects.

4.4.9 Drugs to relieve oedema

Diuretic agents, such as frusemide, promote kidney excretion of salt and water, relieving oedema associated with, for example, cor pulmonale. Potassium-conserving diuretics are preferred in order to reduce the risk of arrhythmias. Over-enthusiastic use of diur-etics can lead to volume depletion, loss of calcium and potassium, arrhythmias (Hell-man 1994) and reduced fluid intake in patients who have stress incontenence (a common complaint in elderly patients with a chronic cough). It may also be worth tolerat-ing a little oedema to give the heart a good head of steam.

4.4.10 Drugs to reduce pulmonary hypertension

General vasodilators have unacceptable side-effects such as systemic hypotension, reduced cardiac output and oxygen desatura-tion. Apart from oxygen, the only satisfactory drug to selectively reduce pulmonary hyper-tension and ease the work of the right heart is nitric oxide (Moinard 1994). This is inhaled for 10 minutes, but needs frequent repetition which limits its use at present.

4.4.11 Delivery devices

Are respiratory drugs best ingested or inhaled? Inhaled therapy delivers an aerosol-ized drug directly to the respiratory tract. The advantages are:

- rapid onset of action,
- local delivery in large doses to maximize effects and minimize toxic side-effects,
- delivery of drugs that might not be active by other routes (Manthous 1994).

Disadvantages are:

- exclusion of obstructed airways from the drug, which can cause patchy distribu-tion in people with COPD or acute severe asthma (Lipworth 1995),

- reduced effectiveness in breathless people whose rapid airflow favours deposition in the upper airways only,
- loss of much of the drug to the atmosphere, stomach and pharynx, although high doses compensate for this and nebulizers such as the Ventstream can be used which deliver high dosages (Lipworth 1995).

Large particles ($> 12 \mu m$ in diameter) are lost in the mouth and pharynx. Small particles ($< 2 \mu m$) are deposited in the alveoli and are used for antibiotic and pentamidine delivery. Particles from 2–$12 \mu m$ target the bronchi and bronchioles and nebulizers producing this size are used for bronchodilators and steroids (Manthous 1994). The tasks of patient education and assessment for delivery systems may fall to the physiotherapist.

Inhalers

Pressurized inhalers deliver an aerosol by creating a suspension of active drug in a propellant.

The metered dose inhaler (MDI) is portable and cheap, but many patients find it difficult to co-ordinate inhalation with manual triggering of the device. Keeley (1994) claims that poor inhaler technique is the main cause of failed drug treatment. The principles of good technique are the following:

1. Shake the inhaler, hold it upright and remove the cap.
2. Sit upright; exhale fully.
3. Seal the lips around the mouthpiece, breathe in through the mouth, pressing the top of the cannister just after initiating the breath; inhale slowly and deeply.
4. Hold the breath for five seconds before exhaling.
5. If more than one dose is prescribed, 30 seconds should be allowed between puffs because each puff cools the cannister and reduces its efficiency. In cold temperatures, the cannister should be prewarmed in the pocket.

Other inhalers such as the autohaler (Fig. 4.5) co-ordinate drug release with inhalation. Details of technique are available from the manufacturers.

Dry powder inhalers release powdered drug on inspiration and require minimal co-ordination and no breath-holding. The disadvantages are that some children and people with bronchospasm cannot generate the required flow to release the drug, and the powder is sensitive to moisture unless stored in foil blisters. Individual disadvantages are that the Rotahaler and Diskhaler are fiddly to operate, and the Turbohaler has no carrier powder or propellant to indicate to the patient that the dose has been delivered.

Spacers are chambers between the patient and inhaler which show the following advantages:

- propellants and large particles drop out in the chamber, thus reducing local side-effects of steroids (Everard et al 1992),
- aerosol momentum is slowed so that less is lost by impaction on the back of the throat,
- less co-ordination is required between drug release and inhalation because the drug remains suspended in the spacer until the patient breaths in, although maximum dosage is gained with early inhalation (O'Callaghan 1993),
- high doses can be delivered during an acute episode.

Spacers should always be used for children using steroids (Barry 1994), and aerosols can be delivered to infants by a soft face mask attached to a spacer (Everard et al 1992). The large pear-shaped spacers, such as the Nebuhaler or Volumatic, are cumbersome, but they simulate the aerosol cloud from an inhaler and are the most efficient type. Bronchodilation can be further enhanced by using a PEP device (p. 136) at 10–15 cmH$_2$O connected to the spacer (Frischknecht 1991).

Problems for patients with inhalers are:

- difficulty in understanding instructions,

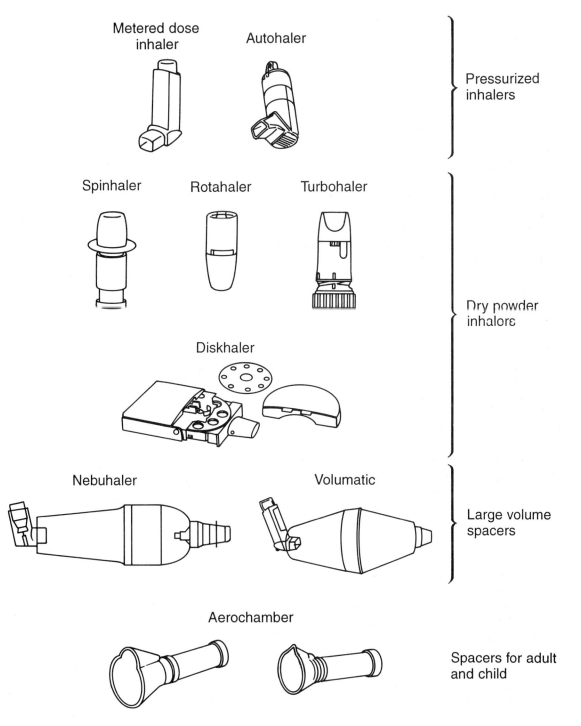

Figure 4.5 Inhaler devices.

- the need for co-ordination and/or manual dexterity,
- confusion about when to use which inhaler, e.g. mistaken use of steroids on a symptom-related basis.

Nebulizers

A jet nebulizer transforms a drug in solution into a mist of droplets that can be inhaled. Oxygen or air is forced at high velocity through a narrow tube, sucking the dissolved drug into the gas stream and impacting it on a baffle to create droplets.

Method

1. If the patient does not need oxygen, use an air compressor because the higher the relative humidity of the driving gas, the more stable the particle size (Hodgkin 1993, p. 209).
2. Select a mouthpiece if possible, because nose breathing filters the drug and reduces lung deposition by one-quarter (Salmon *et al* 1990), and aerosol escaping from a mask can cause eye irritation. If the patient prefers a mask or is too breathless to use a mouthpiece, ask the patient to mouth-breathe through the mask.
3. Have the patient sitting upright in a chair or in side lying, to maximize basal deposition. Some nebulizers do not function sideways.
4. Fill to 4 ml, diluting with normal saline if necessary, and set the flow rate to 6–8 l/min (Hodgkin 1993, p. 209), unless a compressor is used, which has a preset flow rate.
5. Advise the patient:
   (a) to intersperse tidal breathing with deep breathing and breath-holds at end-inspiration to improve deposition (Hess 1994),
   (b) when using a mouthpiece, not to obstruct the excess air inlet, which

can create excess pressures in the system,
   (c) after use, to wash and rinse the inside to prevent encrustation by salt from the saline, then dry with a tissue or air from the compressor to minimize infection risk.

Drugs can be mixed in the nebulizer except for ipratropium bromide with budesonide. Tapping the device when the liquid is beginning to fizz increases the delivered dose by 38% (Everard *et al* 1994); this is unnecessary with the high doses used for bronchodilation and simply extends treatment time, but is useful for drugs such as antibiotics. Adding a PEP device appears to improve the effectiveness of nebulizer delivery (Gradwell 1994).

For home nebulizer therapy, laboratory measurements are not adequate (Hosker 1995) and a three-week home trial is needed for patients who remain symptomatic despite regular inhaler use. A typical trial would comprise nebulized saline, nebulized salbutamol and then nebulized salbutamol/ipratropium mixture six-hourly, each for one week. Symptoms and twice daily peak flows are monitored, and a positive nebulizer trial is defined as a 15% increase in peak flow during a week on active treatment compared with the week on saline (Goldman *et al* 1992). The first dose is best administered in hospital in case of side-effects such as cardiac arrhythmias. Trials can also be done with steroids or other delivery methods, such as an MDI with spacer. If patients use nebulizers at home, they must be given adequate assessment, advice and back up servicing.

Disadvantages and precautions

1. There is a wide variation in aerosol output and treatment time between different nebulizers (Loffert 1994).
2. Nebulization cools the inspired gas, creating a risk of bronchospasm.
3. Angina or hypoxaemia may occur with nebulized salbutamol (Simpson 1993).

4. 'Horrifying tales' of bacterial contamination and inadequate servicing have been reported when used at home (Lane 1991).
5. Patient compliance may be hindered by a lengthy time to complete nebulization.
6. Patients may rely on repeated use when airways are acutely obstructed and nebulization is ineffective, possibly leading to increased asthma deaths (Lane 1991).
7. The inspired gas must be accurate. Acutely hypoxaemic asthmatic patients require high F_IO_2 levels, and acute hypercapnic COPD patients may require air, sometimes with oxygen via a nasal cannula.

Indications

The following may be suited to nebulizers:

1. People who are too breathless to use an inhaler, such as during an asthma attack, so long as overreliance does not occur when medical assistance is indicated.
2. Antibiotics and antifungal drug delivery.
3. Delivery of high drug doses if these cannot be delivered by inhaler, e.g. for some people with severe COPD, a quarter of whom benefit from high-dose bronchodilation (Hosker 1995).

Inhaler or nebulizer?

Patients often love nebulizers. They look impressive, do not need respiratory gymnastics for co-ordination, and produce more rapid results because 10–50 times the drug dose is prescribed compared with inhalers. The reason for this excessive difference in dosage is unclear (Lewis 1985), but there is no reason why large quantities cannot be delivered by inhalers with spacers. According to Hess (1994), nebulizers are less convenient, less efficient and twice as expensive as inhalers.

Children may fare better with inhalers because nebulized bronchodilators can paradoxically increase wheezing (Yuksel 1994).

The device needs to adapt to a child's lack of co-ordination, low inspiratory flow rate, short inspiratory time and reduced ability to breath-hold. The following are suitable:

- metered dose inhaler – 10 years upwards,
- dry powder inhaler (which needs a high inspiratory flow rate) – 5 years upwards,
- inhaler with spacer – 3 years upwards,
- inhaler with spacer and mask – 0–2 years (Cogswell 1994).

Children may need to tilt up the large spacers during inhalation to open the valve. Masks may be frightening for babies, and it helps if the cheek is stroked gently with the mask first, or if it is used when the baby is asleep, or if the parent holds the mask. A useful stand-by in case other equipment does not work is a disposable coffee cup with the inhaler inserted through a hole in the bottom, but care should be taken that the drug does not blow into the child's eyes.

4.5 BRONCHOSCOPY AND BIOPSY

Access to the bronchial tree for diagnostic or therapeutic purposes is gained with a fibreoptic bronchoscope, which is passed through the nose and into the airway under local, nebulized or general anaesthesia. Diagnostically, biopsies or washings can be taken to locate malignant lesions or identify parenchymal lung disease. Therapeutically, foreign bodies can be removed and tumours or stenoses treated.

Bronchoscopy is rarely justified as a substitute for physiotherapy in clearing secretions (Brooks-Brunn 1995) because it only reaches the larger airways, cannot cope with tenacious secretions, does not reverse the underlying process and is complicated by hypoxaemia, discomfort, bronchospasm, infection, haemorrhage, pneumothorax, subcutaneous emphysema or arrhythmias. However, bronchoscopy may be appropriate if there is intractable sputum retention with no air bronchogram on X-ray, i.e. with blocked central airways. To re-expand atelectatic areas, it is best combined with selective insufflation of air (Susini *et al* 1992) or followed by physiotherapy.

Bronchoalveolar lavage involves washing up to 200 ml of warmed saline through the bronchoscope when it is wedged into a bronchus, then aspirating this along with fluid and cells from the lower respiratory tract for diagnostic or research purposes. Hypoxaemia and other side-effects are greater with lavage than for bronchoscopy alone.

RECOMMENDED READING

Barrett, T.E. (1995) Inhaled β-adrenergic receptor agonists in asthma: more harm than good? *Am. J. Respir. Crit. Care Med.*, **151**, 574–7.

Cahalin, L.P. and Sadowsky, H.S. (1995) Pulmonary medications. *Phys. Ther*, **75**, 397–414.

Crompton, G. (1995) Drug delivery: matching devices to patients. *Practitioner*, **239**, 206–8.

Goldman, J.M., Teale, C. and Muers, M.F. (1992) Simplifying the assessment of patients with chronic airflow limitation for home nebulizer therapy. *Respir. Med.*, **86**, 33–8.

Hobbs, J. (1995) On patients and inhalers. *Respir. Dis. Practice*, **12**(1), 8–12.

Leach, R.M. and Bateman, N.T. (1993) Acute oxygen therapy. *Br. J. Hosp. Med.*, **49**, 637–44.

Leach, R.M. and Bateman, N.T. (1994) Domiciliary oxygen therapy. *Br. J. Hosp. Med.*, **51**, 47–54.

Lin, Y.-Z. (1995) Metered dose inhaler and nebuliser in acute asthma. *Arch. Dis. Child*, **72**, 214–18.

Paton, J. (1994) The safety of inhaled steroids in childhood asthma. *Practitioner*, **238**, 322–4.

Rees, J. and Price, J. (1995) Treatment of chronic asthma. *Br. Med. J.*, **310**, 1459–63.

Sridhar, M.K. (1995) Nutrition and lung health. *Br. Med. J.*, **310**, 75–6.

Thompson, J. (1994) Misuse of metered-dose inhalers in hospitalized patients. *Chest*, **105**, 715–17.

5. *Physiotherapy management*

5.1 INTRODUCTION

What is respiratory physiotherapy? And does it work? Chest physiotherapy is not the tip, tap and cough that commonly passes as its definition. It includes problem identification and management by education, pain relief, accurately controlled activity, use of mechanical aids and listening to patients in distress. It is ineffective to intervene with a process as personal as breathing without attention to the person as a whole.

It is also ineffective to improve a patient's condition without maintaining that improvement. Rather than ticking off a patient's name in a notebook, on-going management is needed in the form of liaison with nursing staff or relatives and, for hospital-based patients, maintenance of positioning and brief follow-up checks during the day.

Another step towards effectiveness is to avoid routine. It is comfortable to work to a recipe, but it demeans the profession. There is a sorry lack of objective data on how and if

respiratory physiotherapy works, but this chapter will relate techniques to the available evidence.

5.2 METHODS TO INCREASE LUNG VOLUME

Loss of lung volume takes a variety of forms.

1. Atelectasis is collapse of anything from a few alveoli to the whole lung. Physiotherapy is indicated to treat or prevent atelectasis if it is caused by or anticipated as a result of immobility, poor positioning, shallow breathing or postoperative pain.

2. Consolidation causes loss of functioning lung volume. It is not directly responsive to physiotherapy, but may, depending on the cause, be prevented from worsening by, for example, hydration, positioning or mobilization.

3. Pleural effusion, pneumothorax and abdominal distension are outside the

lung but intrude on lung volume. Physiotherapy does not influence the cause, but the patient's condition may be improved by positioning.

4. Restrictive disorders of the lung or chest wall reduce lung volume, but are less responsive to the measures discussed in this chapter.

By improving lung volume, there is reduced airways resistance and increased surface area for gas exchange. Assessment and outcome evaluation are by breath sounds, percussion note, X-ray and sometimes SaO_2, although this relates to other variables.

When increasing lung volume, the distribution of the extra air should be directed to poorly-ventilated lung regions. In postoperative patients, for example, this is usually the lower zones.

5.2.1 Controlled mobilization

The most fruitful technique for increasing lung volume is exercise (Dean 1994). This combines the upright posture, which encourages basal distribution of air, with natural deep breathing. It is the first line treatment for patients who are able to get out of bed.

To ensure accuracy, the level of activity is controlled so that the depth of breathing increases only slightly (to prevent tension), then the patient is asked to lean against a wall to get his or her breath back, while being discouraged from talking. Relaxed standing minimizes postural activity of the abdominal muscles, allowing the diaphragm to move freely. The controlled 'slight breathlessness' is therefore used therapeutically, not wasted as shallow apical breathing.

Patients who are not able to walk can use controlled activity by simply transferring from bed to chair, then get their breath back by relaxing against the back of the chair. Even when patients have simply turned into side-lying in bed, they can be encouraged to relax in an appropriate position while they get

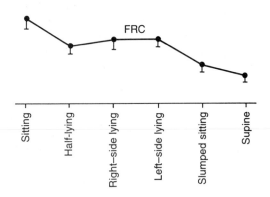

Figure 5.1 Functional residual capacity as a percentage of the sitting value (sitting = sitting upright with legs dependent):
* 90% in left-side lying, inclined towards prone,
* 88% in right-side lying, inclined towards prone,
* 86% in half-lying (propped up at 45°),
* 76% in slumped sitting (not propped up),
* 71% in supine.

(Source: Jenkins, S.C., Soutar, S.A. and Moxham, J. (1988) The effects of posture on lung volumes in normal subjects and in patients pre- and post-coronary artery surgery. *Physiotherapy*, **74**, 492–6, with permission.)

their breath back. At the opposite end of the spectrum, some patients will need to climb stairs before achieving the right level of breathlessness.

Once patients understand these principles and can identify the feeling of 'slight breathlessness', they can practice on their own, using walking and their normal functional activities as a medium for improving lung volume. Regular graded exercise can be encouraged and monitored by the physiotherapist.

5.2.2 Positioning

Changing a patient's posture may not seem a dramatic technique, but this simple action often prevents recourse to more time-consuming or tiring techniques. Positioning should be an integral part of all respiratory care, especially when prophylaxis is the aim. It is used in its own right or in conjunction with other techniques, and no physiotherapy treatment should be carried out without consideration of the position in which it is performed.

Lung volume is related to displacement of the diaphragm and abdominal contents, and most volumes are responsive to positioning. FRC increases sequentially from supine to standing (Fig. 5.1).

The following principles apply:

1. Patients who are confined to bed should spend a proportion of their time on their side, lying well forwards so that their diaphragm is free from abdominal pressure (Fig. 5.2). Compared to supine, this position not only increases lung volume, but also improves gas exchange and reduces the work of breathing (Dean 1993). It can also be used for sleeping.

2. Half-lying in bed rapidly becomes the slumped position for most patients as they slide down the bed. This should be avoided unless necessary for a specific medical reason or to reduce pain. Manoeuvres to increase volume, such as deep breathing, are ineffective in half-lying because of competition from the abdominal contents.

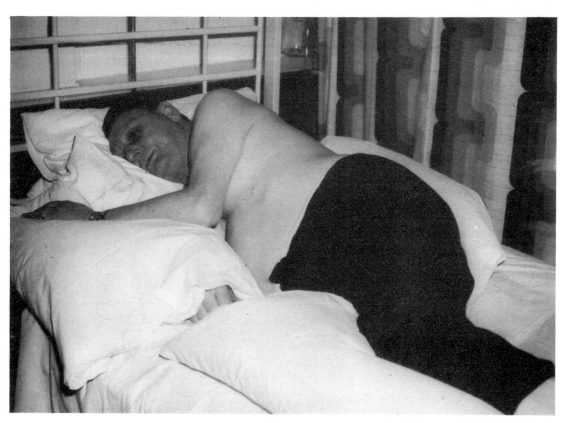

Figure 5.2 Side-lying position, with the patient comfortable, supported and rolled forwards to relieve the diaphragm from abdominal pressure. The pillow under the head is off the shoulder.

3. The supine position is least helpful for lung volume, especially in elderly people and those with respiratory disease.
4. When sitting a patient out after treatment, a foot stool is inadvisable unless the patient has ankle oedema, a recent vein graft or requests it.

The $\dot{V}_A/\dot{Q}$ ratio is also responsive to positioning. Ventilation and perfusion are usually well matched because the better ventilated lower areas of lung are also better perfused (p. 9). People with one-sided pneumonia, thoracotomy or other unilateral disorder show an accentuation of the normal downward ventilation gradient if they lie on their side with the affected lung uppermost. Perfusion is, as always, greater in dependent areas, and $\dot{V}_A/\dot{Q}$ match is therefore enhanced in this position, often resulting in a dramatic improvement in gas exchange (Fishman 1981).

The rule of thumb that the affected lung should be uppermost is relevant for other situations as well as for optimizing gas exchange. For example, it promotes comfort following thoracotomy or chest drain insertion, and facilitates postural drainage when indicated. Atelectatic areas are best positioned uppermost to encourage expansion. Exceptions to the 'bad lung up' rule are:

*   recent pneumonectomy (p. 185),
*   large pleural effusion (p. 79),
*   bronchopleural fistula in case any unsavoury substances drain into the unaffected lung,
*   occasionally, if there is a large tumour in a main stem bronchus, positioning the patient with this side uppermost obstructs the bronchus, causing breathlessness and desaturation.

Other functions are affected by positioning, for example:

*   lung compliance increases and work of breathing decreases progressively from supine to standing, because the dia-

phragm has to work less hard against the load of the viscera.
*   airflow resistance is lower in side-lying compared to supine (Barnas *et al* 1993).

After treatment, the physiotherapist should explain to nursing staff why the patient has been left in a specific position, and that this should be maintained until the patient wants to move or it is time to turn. Night staff should be included in educational programmes, and an oximeter can be used to demonstrate the effectiveness of positioning. Accurate positioning and regular position change should be incorporated into a patient's management plan 24 hours a day.

5.2.3 Breathing exercises

Breathing exercises to increase lung volume should be performed in cycles of three or four breaths so that (1) maximum effort is put into each breath, (2) dizziness from overbreathing is avoided and (3) shoulder tension is discouraged.

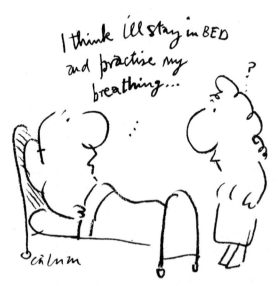

Once inflated, alveoli stay open for about an hour, so that patients should be asked to perform at least 10 deep breaths every waking hour (Bartlett *et al* 1973). This is a tall order for those whose minds are distracted by the events and uncertainties of hospital life, so patients are best advised to remember their exercises by linking them to the arrival of food and drink trolleys or routines such as hourly fluids.

Deep breathing   Low-volume areas of lung are relatively non-compliant, so optimum conditions are needed to ensure that deep breaths do not just fill easily inflated regions but reach poorly ventilated regions, which are often the lower lobes. The following will facilitate this:

- accurate positioning, usually side-lying inclined towards prone,
- comfort and relaxation,
- relief of pain, nausea, dry mouth, fatigue, anxiety,
- avoidance of distractions or conversation,
- minimal breathlessness, e.g. patients must have time to get their breath back after turning.

Patients are then asked to breathe in deeply, comfortably and slowly through the nose, and sigh out through the mouth. A demonstration is often the best way of explaining an action that is normally automatic. Some patients respond better when asked to take a long breath rather than a deep breath. Breathing through the nose warms and humidifies the air but doubles resistance to airflow, so some patients prefer to mouth-breathe.

People usually breathe deeper when they breathe slower. This reduces airway turbulence and encourages distribution to dependent regions (Reid and Loveridge 1983). Breathless people require a special approach and should not be asked to breathe slowly (p. 156).

The physiotherapist's hands can be placed over the basal area for monitoring purposes and for patient reassurance, but not with any assumption that this magically redistributes ventilation to the underlying lung. 'Local-ized' breathing exercises do not make physiological sense because humans are unable to deform individual portions of the chest wall selectively (Martin *et al* 1976), but patients can still be found obediently performing strap exercises, unilateral breathing (which usually involves subtle side flexion) and basal costal breathing. Even if localized breathing was physically possible, the way in which the two layers of pleura slide on each other means that the lung would respond generally rather than locally to an increase in volume. Distribution of ventilation is related only to position, gas flow, lung volume and pathology (Menkes and Britt 1980).

Between each cycle of breaths, it takes a few moments for the patient to resume a relaxed rhythm and be ready for the next cycle. The breathing rate and pattern should be checked, and the patient may need praise or a change in instruction before proceeding. Patients should not be engaged in conversation while regaining their rhythm.

Deep breathing increases lung compliance, reduces $\dot{V}_A/\dot{Q}$ mismatch, decreases dead space, replenishes surfactant (Melendez 1992) and can prevent desaturation (Ruggier *et al* 1994). The term 'thoracic expansion exercises' is synonymous with deep breathing, but inhalation must be assured as well as thoracic expansion, and if this terminology is used with patients it needs to be explained.

End-inspiratory hold

Air can be tempted into poorly ventilated regions by interspersing every few deep breaths with breath-holds for three seconds at full inspiration, which may boost collateral ventilation and distribute air more evenly between lung segments. Observation will identify whether this is effective and comfortable or, conversely, if it disturbs the breathing pattern. Accurate instruction and close observation are needed to prevent shoulder girdle tension. This technique is unsuitable for breathless people who should not be asked to hold their breath.

Single percussion

When a patient is breath-holding at full inspiration, a single manual percussion manoeuvre with one hand sends an oscillating wave through the lung that in some patients further encourages alveoli to open.

Sniff

Even after a full inspiration, it is often possible to squeeze in a wee bit more air and further augment collateral ventilation by means of one sniff at end-inspiration. Sceptical patients can be won over by a reminder that however packed a rush-hour underground train seems to be, an extra person can always be crammed in. A sniff also promotes a diaphragmatic pattern of muscle recruitment.

Abdominal breathing

Augmented abdominal movement during inspiration leads to slower, deeper breathing, less turbulence, reduced dead space and shoulder girdle relaxation. In the past, the term 'diaphragmatic breathing' was used to describe this pattern, but greater abdominal excursion does not imply greater diaphragmatic contribution to breathing (Gosselink 1995). The term 'breathing control' is synonymous with abdominal breathing.

It is useful to think of encouraging rather than teaching this form of breathing so that it becomes a natural outcome after certain instructions rather than an effort. The patient is asked to relax comfortably, starting in a symmetrical position, such as sitting. The manoeuvre is first explained and demonstrated unhurriedly, avoiding words like 'push', 'pull', 'try' and 'harder'. If relaxed abdominal breathing has not started naturally, then the patient is taken through the following instructions:

- rest the dominant hand on your abdomen, with elbows supported and, keeping your shoulders relaxed, allow the hand to rise gently, while visualizing air filling the abdomen like a balloon (the area to be expanded is sometimes best identified by first sniffing, which protrudes the abdomen),
- sigh the air out,
- gradually increase the depth of breathing while maintaining relaxation,
- check that the shoulders remain relaxed and heavy,
- progress to side-lying and relaxed standing if appropriate.

Variations include:

- putting the other hand on the non-moving upper chest to compare it with movement of the abdomen,
- imagining a piece of elastic round the waist stretching during inhalation,
- incorporating incentive spirometry in order to give feedback to the patient on the larger volume inhaled (Peper 1992).
- for non-surgical patients, positions can be taken up in which it is almost impossible not to breathe abdominally, for example, in standing placing the hands on the back of the hips with elbows pushed backwards or, for the energetic, taking to the floor on all fours.

Abdominal breathing increases lung volume but it is not thought to alter the distribution of ventilation (Martin *et al* 1976), but the slow deep breathing that it incorporates favours airflow to dependent regions (Fixley 1978).

Neurophysiological facilitation

Non-alert patients breathe shallowly and monotonously and tend to develop patchy atelectasis, which is best prevented by positioning. Neurophysiological facilitation is more short term, but is useful for spontaneously-breathing patients who are unable to turn, e.g. following acute head injury. This technique uses tactile and proprioceptive stimulation to increase reflexly the rate and depth of breathing (Bethune 1991). Examples are:

1. **Perioral pressure**, which is firm pressure applied just above the patient's lip and facilitates a deeper than average breath. The pressure is maintained for as long as the patient is required to deep breathe, but often the effect is continued for some minutes afterwards.
2. **Intercostal stretch**, which is pressure applied bilaterally downwards to the upper border of a rib in order to stretch the intercostal muscle and increase gradually the depth of breathing.

Rib springing

A more crude technique is rib springing, which is chest compression followed by overpressure and quick release at end-expiration. This may cause a deeper subsequent inspiration, but heavy pressure can cause airway closure.

5.2.4 Mechanical aids

If previous measures are ineffective, a variety of mechanical aids are available to increase lung volume. Physiotherapists are ideally suited to match people to machines because of their patient-handling skills and understanding of physiology.

Incentive spirometry

The flow and volume achieved by a sustained deep breath can be facilitated by an incentive spirometer, which gives visual feedback on performance. Inspiration should be slow and controlled. This is encouraged in the Coach by holding a marker steady between two arrows (indicating flow), and sustaining an end-inspiratory hold while a disc descends (indicating volume). In the Triflo two out of three plastic balls should be raised and the breath sustained while holding them up. The third ball is a control and should not be raised because this causes tension. It is still possible to cheat by taking short sharp breaths, especially with the Triflo. A suggested protocol is the following:

1. A demonstration is given using a separate device.
2. Patients should be relaxed and positioned as for deep breathing, in either side-lying or sitting upright in a chair.
3. After sealing the lips around the mouthpiece, the patient inhales slowly and deeply. Throughout the procedure the patient watches the incentive spirometer, but the physiotherapist watches the patient in order to monitor the breathing pattern.
4. After exhalation, shoulder girdle relaxation is rechecked.

Those on oxygen should have the mask kept close to their nose when using the device, or nasal cannulae can be used. People with tracheostomies can be accommodated with a connecting tube. Once the technique is faultless, patients are asked to practise 10 times an hour.

The same effect can theoretically be obtained without the device, but the incentive of using a device often results in greater inhaled volume and more controlled flow. However, individuals vary, and observation of chest expansion shows whether a sustained maximal inspiration is best with or without an incentive spirometer. An advantage is that its presence on the bedside locker acts as a memory aid. A disadvantage is that it is unsuitable for breathless patients.

Continuous positive airway pressure (CPAP)

For spontaneously breathing patients who cannot muster the breath for incentive spirometry, assistance to lung inflation and improved gas exchange can be given by pneumatically splinting open the airways with continuous positive pressure. A CPAP device delivers a constant flow of gas during both inspiration and expiration which exceeds the flow rate of patients even when they are breathless. It is like patients putting their head out of the window of a car moving at speed.

The system   The components needed to generate and withstand the high flows and pressures of a CPAP system are illustrated in Fig. 5.3. A flow generator connects to the oxygen supply, entrains air through a filter to give 30–100% oxygen, and generates a gas flow of up to 120 l/min. For generators not equipped with variable oxygen, a fixed flow of 30% oxygen is produced.

   The patient breathes through a face mask, nasal mask, mouthpiece (for intermittent use) or T-piece (for intubated patients). Positive pressure is maintained by a threshold resistor, known as a CPAP or PEEP valve, which is independent of flow. Preset valves provide constant pressures from 2.5–20 cmH$_2$O. A spare valve at 5 cmH$_2$O above the threshold pressure acts as a pop-off safety valve in case the system becomes obstructed. An oxygen analyser monitors the F_1O_2, and an oximeter monitors the patient's response. A humidifier is not necessary if a nasal mask is used, treatment is brief and the patient is well hydrated. More often, a humidifier is required, which has to be highly efficient to cope with the high flows generated, or else two humidifiers can be incorporated into the system (Harrison *et al* 1993).

Method   Suggested guidelines are the following:

1. Patients using a full face mask should be in a high dependency area or kept under constant observation because of the danger of vomiting and difficulty in expectoration.
2. A valve is chosen that provides a pressure low enough to be comfortable, but high enough to maintain adequate gas exchange, usually starting at 5–12.5 cmH$_2$O.
3. The system is set up, allowing patients to assist with putting on the mask if possible in order to reduce anxiety. Simultaneously the on/off dial is turned on.
4. The flow and oxygen are turned up. The flow should be sufficient to maintain an open CPAP valve, even during a deep breath. This can be checked by ensuring that there is a continuous gas outflow from the valve throughout the respiratory cycle, and ensuring that the mask has a firm but comfortable seal. Fine tuning trims the flow to just above the patient's peak inspiratory flow, without causing distress, so that there is just a small outflow at the valve on inspiration.
5. The outflow should be rechecked after the patient has settled, because relaxation changes the breathing pattern. The oximeter should be rechecked after changing the flow, and F_1O_2 adjusted if appropriate.
6. Regular checks should be made of the mask seal and comfort, the valve, oximeter and the fluid level and temperature of the humidifier.

   The high flow means that it is usually immaterial if air escapes through the mouth when using a nasal mask. However, if excessive air escapes, the mouth can be closed by a chin strap or soft collar. Some patients prefer periodic CPAP, in which the device is applied, say, every hour for 30 breaths.

Effects   When the above steps are followed and comfort assured, CPAP can increase FRC (Fig. 5.4), improve gas exchange, prevent atelectasis and avoid the need for intubation and mechanical ventilation (Keilty and Bott 1992). A sustained pressure of > 15 cmH$_2$O is required to re-expand atelectatic lungs (Andersen *et al* 1980).

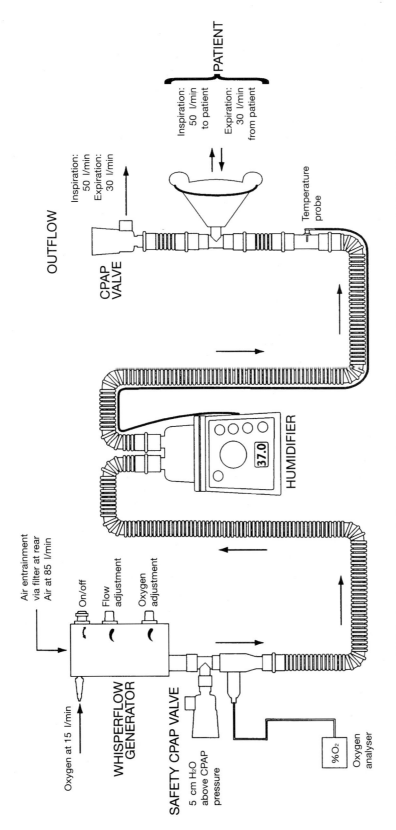

Figure 5.3 CPAP circuit set up to deliver approximately 33% oxygen. (Diagram courtesy of Medicaid Ltd.)

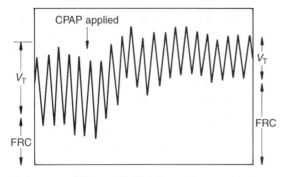

Figure 5.4 Effect of CPAP on lung volumes. V_T = tidal volume, FRC = functional residual capacity.

Complications A mouthpiece creates few problems, but is limited in effectiveness and can only be used intermittently. A full face mask is associated with the most complications. A nasal mask aims for maximum effectiveness with minimum complications and allows the patient to talk and cough. Complications with nasal or full face masks are the following:

1. Discomfort is common, and uncomfortable patients restrict their depth of breathing. Individual adjustment of the mask is needed to prevent discomfort, claustrophobia or gas blowing into the eyes. The bridge of the nose should be protected before rather than after a pressure sore has developed, especially in patients who are hypotensive, hypovolaemic or have thin skin due to ageing or long-term steroid therapy. If the mask seal is inadequate, it often helps to put the dentures in. Nasal masks feel less suffocating than a full face mask.

2. For patients unable to remove the mask rapidly by themselves, there is danger of aspiration of gastric contents. A nasogastric tube and head elevation reduce the risk, but patients should be oriented and not suffering from nausea or vomiting. A nasogastric tube may interfere with the mask seal, but this can be managed by adjusting the mask, compensating with higher flows or pressures, or by using a Medicaid customized bridge (see CPAP, Appendix C).

3. Some patients find exhalation difficult, especially if there is loss of lung or chest wall elasticity, and this might force them to use more active expiration. If this cannot be remedied by adjusting the dials, CPAP should be discontinued.

4. CO_2 retention can occur if a hypercapnic patient breathes with a small tidal volume due to a high pressure valve, especially with a small mask.

5. Because of the tight mask seal, a high F_1O_2 is readily achieved. This can obscure a deteriorating condition because it is easy to keep nudging up the inspired oxygen to maintain oxygen saturation. If a progressively increasing percentage of oxygen is found to be necessary, the patient is in danger because removal of the mask may precipitate desaturation. If the patient is not already in an intensive care unit, transfer is advisable.

6. At pressures $> 20–25\,\mathrm{cmH_2O}$, gas can be forced into the stomach, causing discomfort and restricted breathing. The risk is reduced with a nasogastric tube.

7. Eating and drinking are contraindicated because high flow may cause aspiration, but patients using a nasal mask can drink carefully through a straw.

8. With a full face mask, coughing without removing the mask can create high pressures. This can damage the ears and, in people with emphysema or late-stage CF, risk creating a pneumothorax.

9. Cardiac output response varies. Pressures of $5–10\,\mathrm{cmH_2O}$ have no effect in most people, but for those with severe heart failure, cardiac output can be increased by reducing afterload (DeHoyos 1995).

Precautions CPAP should not normally be used in the presence of:

- an undrained pneumothorax,
- subcutaneous emphysema,
- bullae,
- bronchopleural fistula,
- recent oesophageal or bronchial surgery,
- large tumour in the proximal airways, because inspired air under pressure may be able to enter but not exit past the obstruction,
- facial trauma.

Intermittent positive pressure breathing (IPPB)

The slings and arrows of fashion have not been kind to IPPB, attitudes swinging from hero-worship to ostracism. This modality has been scrutinized mercilessly in the literature and found wanting, usually because it has been used in the wrong way for the wrong patients. IPPB is simply assisted breathing with a pressure ventilator such as the Bird (Fig.5.5) or Bennett. Inspiration is triggered by the patient and expiration is passive.

Indications   Patients with volume loss who are drowsy, weak or fatigued may benefit from IPPB. Patients who are unwilling, restless or in pain do not. Pain is not a contra-indication in itself, but if atelectasis is caused by pain, it is best to deal with the pain because muscle splinting will prevent the patient accepting positive pressure. Sputum retention may or may not be an indication, depending on the cause, e.g. it may help certain people with neurological problems. Excess work of breathing can also be eased by IPPB (p. 125).

Method   The nebulizer is filled with saline and tested by activating the machine with the manual control. The inspiratory sensitivity determines how much negative pressure the patient must generate in order to receive a breath, and is set low enough for the patient to trigger into inspiration with ease ('Is it easy to breathe in?'). The flow rate is set as low as is comfortable to ensure minimal turbulence and optimum distribution of ventilation, but breathless patients need a high flow rate for comfort ('Is that enough air?'). The inspiratory pressure should be set according to patient comfort ('Is that blowing too hard?'). As a rough guide, using the Bird Mark 7, sensitivity and flow rate can be set at about 7, pressure at about 10, and each adjusted until synchronized with the patient's breathing pattern and comfort. Patients with restrictive disorders need a higher pressure.

If the aim is to increase volume to the lung bases, the patient is positioned comfortably in side-lying with the most affected lung uppermost. After turning into this position, the patient is allowed to get his or her breath back, then asked to hold the mouthpiece firmly with the lips. Measures that decrease lung volume, such as the head-down tilt or vibrations, should be avoided during IPPB. Patients are told that they will feel air blowing into their lungs and reassured that the procedure can be stopped by request at any time.

A small breath is taken and the machine allowed to do the rest, without the patient prematurely stopping inspiration by blowing into the mouthpiece. When the patient has settled, the pressure can be gradually increased. The physiotherapist's job is to:

- adjust the pressure and occasionally adjust the flow rate to compensate because flow governs the speed with which the preset pressure is reached,
- reassure and advise the patient to allow the air to fill the lungs and not to actively breathe out,
- observe the abdomen for unwanted active expiration,
- observe the face for discomfort,
- observe rib cage excursion to ensure that expansion is improving.

While the physiotherapist watches the patient, the patient may like to watch the

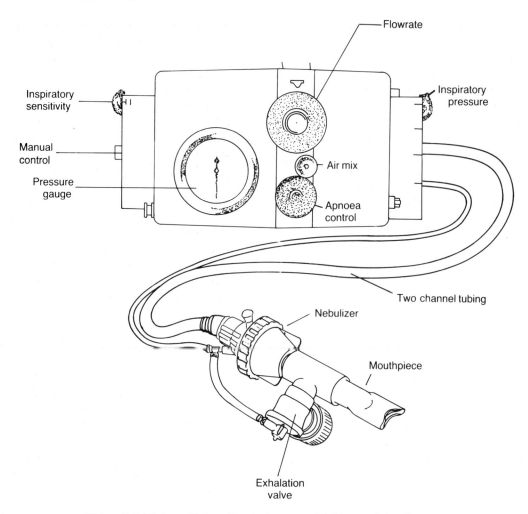

Figure 5.5 Bird ventilator. **Inspiratory sensitivity** regulates the ease with which the machine triggers into inspiration. The **flowrate** controls the rate at which gas is delivered to the patient, and acts as the on/off switch. **Inspiratory pressure** is the pressure that must be reached in the lungs before the machine cycles from inspiration to expiration, as recorded on the pressure gauge. This function can be overridden by the **manual control**. The **apnoea control** cycles the machine automatically and must be off during physiotherapy.

pressure gauge. Active expiration causes it to exceed the preset pressure, while an inadequate seal at the mouth means that the system is unable to reach that pressure. Prolonged expiration indicates the need to check for leaks at the mouth, reduce the pressure or increase the flow rate.

With the Bird, the air-mix switch is pulled out to entrain air, delivering 40% oxygen to the patient. For patients who require higher levels of oxygen, approximately 100% oxygen is delivered by pushing the air-mix switch in, or more fine adjustments can be achieved with an oxygen blender attachment. The flow rate will need to be increased with these modifications.

Some patients may need assistance in co-ordination at first with the manual control. A mouth flange can be used to improve the mouth seal, and a mask is necessary for semiconscious people. A mask is frightening for some patients, who need explanations, reassurance and the freedom to say no.

If the Bennett is used instead of the Bird, the flow and sensitivity adjust automatically, and the air-mix switch is pushed in instead of out for 40% oxygen.

The physiotherapist needs to be present throughout in order to make the fine adjustments needed for accurate treatment. IPPB is best used intensively for short periods of time, after which other techniques, such as positioning or, if necessary, CPAP can be used to maintain the lung volume achieved.

Effects and complications If the patient is relaxed, comfortable and well positioned, and the controls skilfully adjusted, IPPB should increase lung volume, although this only lasts for about an hour (AARC 1993a). Compared with CPAP, positive pressure is intermittent and typically reaches higher pressures, so that it tends to increase tidal volume, whereas CPAP tends to increase FRC. In practical terms, IPPB is best for opening up collapsed lung, and CPAP is best for maintaining increased lung volume.

IPPB also improves ventilation and gas exchange, and if the patient does not attempt to assist the machine, reduces the work of breathing (Bott *et al* 1992). However, IPPB has certain disadvantages compared with other mechanical aids:

1. Inappropriately used, the extra volume is distributed preferentially to areas already well ventilated, because of the passive nature of inspiration and absence of normal diaphragmatic activity (Celli *et al* 1984), hence the importance of positioning the atelectatic area upper-most. IPPB is less effective than spontaneous deep breaths (Bynum *et al* 1976), which is why patient selection must be accurate to avoid including those who are able to deep breathe effectively.

2. The breath is not sustained at end-inspiration.

3. As the machine is pressure-cycled, less volume is delivered to areas of poor compliance.

4. The forceful nature of inspiration increases the impaction of aerosol in the throat, so that IPPB is not the ideal medium for drug delivery.

5. It is possible that hypercapnic COPD patients may lose their hypoxic respiratory drive because of the 40% oxygen delivered by most IPPB machines, but this is not a risk if an adequate tidal volume is delivered (Starke *et al* 1979). If necessary, air can be given as the driving gas instead of oxygen, with monitoring of SaO_2.

7. As with CPAP, gastric distension may occur, which can be reduced in side-lying.

A side-effect that can sometimes be used to advantage is that techniques such as IPPB, incentive spirometry and even deep breathing can make patients slightly breathless. These patients can be positioned for optimum distribution of ventilation, then allowed to get their breath back undisturbed. This uses the same principle as controlled mobilization.

Precautions These are similar to those for CPAP. IPPB tends to be less comfortable postoperatively than CPAP because it causes more chest movement.

Table 5.1 compares the different mechanical aids.

Table 5.1 Comparison of mechanical aids to increase lung volume

Incentive spirometry
Full patient participation
End-inspiratory hold
Physiologically sound distribution of ventilation
Minimal supervision
Minimal infection risk
Quiet
Cheap

CPAP
Face or nasal mask
Used continuously or periodically
Can accommodate breathless patient
Can accommodate tired patient
Can accommodate uncooperative patient
Used for raising FRC rather than tidal volume
Patient can talk and cough (nasal mask)
Positive pressure is continuous

IPPB
Mouthpiece or face mask
Used periodically
Can accommodate breathless patient
Can accommodate tired patient
Can accommodate semiconscious patient
Used for raising tidal volume rather than FRC
Positive pressure on inspiration only

Table 5.2 Measures to optimize the balance between energy supply and demand

Measures to $\uparrow$ energy supply	*Measures to $\downarrow$ energy demand*
Nutrition management	$\uparrow$ Sleep, $\downarrow$ stress
Oxygen therapy	Positioning/breathing re-education
Fluid and electrolyte management	Mechanical assistance
O_2 delivery to inspiratory muscles (e.g. haemoglobin, cardiac output)	Exercise training Inspiratory muscle training

5.3 METHODS TO DECREASE THE WORK OF BREATHING

Work of breathing (defined on p. 5) is increased with breathlessness. Chapter 6 describes the management of chronic breathlessness in detail. This section provides an overview and emphasizes acute breathlessness, although there is much overlap.

Patients are often caught in the pincer of decreased ventilatory capacity and increased ventilatory requirements. The basic principle of reducing the work of breathing is, therefore, to optimize the balance between energy supply and demand, as summarized in Table 5.2.

Measures to increase energy supply are discussed in Chapter 4.

5.3.1 Sleep

There's no peace, no let up with this thing, you can't even escape when you go to bed, it's with you 24 hours a day.

patient quoted by Williams 1993

The only treatment for fatigue is rest. This can be achieved in various ways, but most satisfactorily by sleep. One of the cruel ironies of breathlessness is that it often interferes with sleep. Fragmentation of sleep impairs respiratory performance, blunts response to hypercapnia and hypoxaemia and reduces inspiratory muscle endurance (Neilly 1992). Sleep deprivation in respiratory patients is due to breathlessness and coughing, and is aggravated in hospitalized patients by noise and anxiety. Physiotherapists should avoid waking patients unnecessarily, ensure that their treatment does not cause fatigue and contribute to the teamwork required to allow adequate sleep.

5.3.2 Stress reduction

Relaxation is achieved indirectly by positioning, sensitive handling and reducing unnecessary muscle tension. Some of the relaxation and stress reduction strategies described in Chapter 6 can be used for people who are acutely breathless.

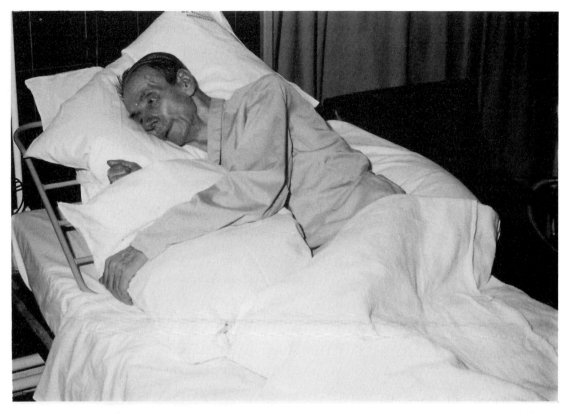

Figure 5.6 High-side lying. The head-rest is relatively low to prevent the patient slipping down the bed and to avoid kinking the spine.

5.3.3 Positioning

Many breathless people automatically assume a posture that eases their breathing, but others need advice to find the position that best facilitates their inspiratory muscles. Patients with a flat diaphragm may benefit from positions which use pressure from the abdominal contents to dome the diaphragm so that it can work with greater efficiency. Upper limbs are best supported but without tense shoulders. Suggested positions should fix the shoulder girdle and facilitate accessory muscle action, e.g.:

1. High-side-lying (Fig. 5.6).
2. Sitting upright in a chair with supported arms.
3. Sitting leaning forwards from the waist, with arms resting on pillows on a table, to dome the flattened diaphragm.
4. For some patients, lying flat may give relief by improving the efficiency of the diaphragm. Occasionally patients even like a slight head-down tilt.
5. Standing relaxed, leaning forwards with arms resting on a support such as a window sill.
6. Standing relaxed, leaning backwards against a wall with the legs slightly apart, chest forwards and relaxed, arms dangling.
7. Standing relaxed sideways with the shoulder girdle fixed against a wall and leg supported by the wall.

Individuals should experiment with different positions. Some find the forward leaning positions claustrophobic, others unpredictably desaturate in different positions. Oximetry can be used as biofeedback.

If breathlessness is due to pulmonary oedema, the upright supported sitting position is preferred because hydrostatic pressure is more relevant then diaphragmatic mechanics.

Some severely distressed people are relieved by being held closely and rocked. The combination of support and rhythmic movement soothes and relaxes them.

5.3.4 Breathing re-education

If patients do not spontaneously adopt an efficient breathing pattern, they may benefit from instruction in abdominal breathing (p. 114), but without progress to side-lying because the aim is not to increase lung volume. Other forms of breathing re-education are described on p. 156, but for some patients in the grip of acute breathlessness, this is like a person with normal lungs attempting to alter his or her breathing pattern while running upstairs.

5.3.5 Mechanical aids

> *From our very first night she made a quite startling difference to my life. Just one night converted me to the joys and thrills of home ventilation.*
>
> Brooks 1990

Non-invasive mechanical support can provide inspiratory muscle rest for people who are burdened with excessive work of breathing in both the acute and chronic state. Ventilation is delivered by positive pressure via mask or mouthpiece, or by negative pressure using the natural airway. Compared with mechanical ventilation via intubation or tracheostomy, patients find non-invasive ventilation comfortable, easier for speech and swallowing, safer and more convenient (Bach 1994).

Effects

For acute patients, mechanical assistance unloads the inspiratory muscles, reduces breathlessness and, in COPD, can reduce mortality (Bott *et al* 1993). For chronic patients, mechanical rest over a period of months allows fatigued muscles to recover and improves their endurance, although the underlying disorder is unchanged. Continuing improvement suggests that there is a gradual resetting of the respiratory centre so that ventilation improves. Patients often fall asleep as soon as the procedure begins, indicating relief of sleep deprivation.

Indications

Patients who may benefit from mechanical support include those with the following:

- severe chronic obstructive or restrictive respiratory disorder, e.g. advanced hypercapnic COPD, kyphoscoliosis, neuromuscular disorder,
- exacerbation of COPD or CF, especially with a rising $PaCO_2$,
- acute asthma, to reduce the effort of maintaining active hyperinflation by imposing passive hyperinflation,
- in tandem with acute oxygen therapy when $PaO_2 > 7$ kPa (52 mmHg) cannot be maintained without $PaCO_2$ rising above 10 kPa (75 mmHg) (Donner and Howard 1992),
- those weaning from mechanical ventilation or awaiting transplantation,
- those requiring mechanical ventilation but refusing intubation.

For people with chronic disease, nocturnal ventilation is used when possible because this compensates for the loss of accessory muscle activity during sleep and is less disruptive to everyday life. These patients may well be up and about in the daytime, but live in a precarious balance that leaves them unable to respond to an increase in energy demand.

Compared to intubation or tracheostomy, non-invasive mechanical ventilation does not protect the airway and provides no direct access to the trachea for suction.

For the first time in months I felt reasonably clear-headed, my thinking felt keener, I no longer fell asleep in mid-sentence, my headaches disappeared . . . Over the following months, as my strength slowly returned, my posture and balance noticeably improved.

Brooks 1990

IPPB

Work of breathing can be reduced by IPPB so long as the patient is relaxed and does not attempt to assist the machine. The upright supported sitting position is often preferred, and the flow rate should be turned up to fit in with the breathing rate of a breathless patient. The instructions on p. 119 are followed, but the pressure dial is not turned up gradually because the aim is not to increase lung volume. IPPB is indicated only for people with acute disease because supervision is needed.

CPAP

In hyperinflation conditions, CPAP takes over the work of sustained inspiratory muscle activity during inspiration. On expiration, CPAP keeps the airways open and allows greater gas emptying (Greenwald 1993). To reduce breathlessness, pressures of 4–5 cmH$_2$O may be adequate (O'Donnell 1994). In acute asthma, the pressure should be carefully titrated to the individual's response to ensure that hyperinflation is maintained but not increased.

CPAP has been advocated for patients with exacerbation of COPD (Mezzanotte 1994), but if poorly tolerated can cause desaturation (Elliott *et al* 1994), so is best attempted only if

mechanical ventilation is threatened and if IPPB or NIPPV (see below) are not available.

Nasal intermittent positive pressure ventilation (NIPPV)

Acute or chronic inspiratory muscle fatigue can be relieved by NIPPV, which delivers a predetermined volume or pressure by nasal mask either automatically or in response to patient effort. Full face masks can also be used but are less comfortable and may retain CO$_2$.

Effects   Patients with acute respiratory failure can be spared intubation and mechanical ventilation, one study showing happily alert patients having their blood gases corrected in five hours (Lapidus *et al* 1993). High concentrations of oxygen can be entrained even with hypercapnic COPD patients because of the safety backup of a pre-set breathing cycle irrespective of respiratory drive.

For patients with chronic disorders, this form of inspiratory muscle rest can provide relief from symptoms of hypoventilation, such as insomnia, morning headaches, dyspnoea, poor concentration and low exercise tolerance. Sustained normalization of blood gases enhances respiratory muscle performance and can reverse pulmonary hypertension (Fernandez 1991). NIPPV can increase vital capacity (Pehrsson 1994) and prolong life (Muir 1993). Patients are encouraged to use the ventilator regularly, sometimes just at night, until symptoms and blood gases are optimal. Improvements have been found with periods of rest from eight hours a week to 4–10 hours a day (Axen 1991). Complications include discomfort and leaks from the mask, any of which may disturb sleep. Gastric distension can occur with volume-control machines, but becomes less of a problem with time.

For patients needing long-term respiratory support, NIPPV facilitates discharge home and can show cost savings of 200% a year (Bach 1994). With rehabilitation and education, many patients can provide much of their own care, so long as a comprehensive maintenance service is available.

Technique As with IPPB and CPAP, the variables on a nasal ventilator are adjusted according to comfort and SaO_2. If patients do not want a chin strap or collar, mask leaks can be compensated for by large minute volumes (Elliott *et al* 1992). Success rates are high if patients are acclimatized and carefully educated.

Machinery A volume- or pressure-controlled machine can be used (p. 220). The advantages of pressure control are the comfort of a limited peak pressure and compensation for leaks. The advantage of volume control is that ventilation can be maintained in patients who have restrictive disorders. However, individual patients have their own preferences.

It is best that patients trigger the inspiratory cycle to prevent inspiratory muscle atrophy. Machines should have a sensitive trigger, short response time, variable flow rate, be capable of delivering large tidal volumes and be quiet and portable. Oxygen can be entrained, and some have a PEEP option. Patients with CF or bronchiectasis need a humidifier or heat-moisture exchanger.

Mouthpieces are used for those needing pressures above 25 cmH$_2$O because high pressures make nasal masks uncomfortable and allow unacceptable leaks. Some ventilator-dependent patients prefer mouthpieces in the daytime while using a mask at night. Some prefer them throughout the 24 hours, using a lipseal device.

CPAP is especially useful for people with hyperinflated chests or type I respiratory failure. NIPPV or IPPB are especially useful for people who are exhausted, hypercapnic or have type II respiratory failure.

Bilevel positive airways pressure (BiPAP)

The BiPAP machine delivers continuous pressure with independent control of inspiratory and expiratory pressures. With bilevel positive pressures, a lower pressure on expiration is often more comfortable than the unrelenting pressure of CPAP.

The machine delivers not just BiPAP itself, but can be adjusted to deliver CPAP or NIPPV. It can be set to provide the following:

- a spontaneous mode, which superimposes inspiratory and expiratory pressures on the patient's own breathing, i.e. BiPAP,
- a spontaneous/timed mode, which delivers breaths if the patient does not breathe after a set time interval,
- a timed mode, which is fully controlled ventilation.

Inspiratory positive airway pressure, set with the IPAP button, is usually started at about 8 cmH$_2$O and increased in increments of about 2 cmH$_2$O until there is minimum active inspiration and optimum gas exchange. Expiratory positive airway pressure, set with the EPAP button, is usually started at about 3 cmH$_2$O and increased in increments of about 2 cmH$_2$O for optimum comfort. With IPAP and EPAP set at the same pressures, CPAP is delivered. Adjuncts include a heat-moisture exchanger, entrained oxygen, PEEP and a stand-by button if the patient needs to talk or cough.

The effects of BiPAP include improved sleep, reduced breathlessness and increased exercise capacity (Renston 1994). The machine is flow-triggered, pressure-controlled and flow-cycled (p. 220). It adjusts spontaneously for leaks, which do not have to be eliminated by ruthless tightening of the mask. Some machines are unable to generate sufficiently high pressures to cope with poorly compliant chests.

Oscillators

Oral high frequency oscillation delivers high-flow bursts of gas, either through a mouthpiece or externally by generating an oscillating pressure at the chest wall (Hardinge 1995). It is expensive but comfortable and reduces the work of breathing by overriding spontaneous ventilation. It may encourage clearance of secretions.

Negative pressure ventilation

> *The kind of life lived by a patient under conditions of vigorous response to a challenge is infinitely preferable to a crunching, desperate winding down.*
>
> Cousins 1981

Negative pressure ventilators enclose part of the patient's body, apply negative pressure externally and suck air into the lungs through the patient's natural airway. They are suitable for patients who find positive pressure machines uncomfortable and restrictive of communication, or for those who cannot move their hands to their face. Advantages are that there is no mask, no gastric distension, and distribution of ventilation mimics normal breathing. Disadvantages are awkwardness of the machinery, and the risk of obstructive sleep apnoea in some patients because of upper airway collapse on inspiration (Hill 1994).

The tank ventilator encloses all of the patient except the head in an airtight iron lung. Disadvantages are size, noise, inaccessibility of the patient and some patients' fear of suffocation. Jackets and the rigid cuirass, which apply negative pressure over the chest and abdomen, are less efficient but more convenient (Bach 1994).

Patients in tanks may require physiotherapy because of immobility and ineffective cough. If the machinery is new to the patient, education and reassurance are necessary. Veteran patients usually know more than the physiotherapist about what they need and how they like to be handled. If secretions are a problem, they may find vibrations and percussion helpful, in prone with the lid shut and alternate side-lying with the lid open. A rotating tank can be used for turning. Otherwise the lid is opened and the patient turned manually with, if necessary, a positive pressure device applied temporarily at the mouth. Coughing is assisted manually through the portholes. Treatment in prone requires a person to sit by the patient's head to watch his or her colour. If the patient vomits, pressure must be equalized immediately by opening a porthole because of the danger of aspiration.

Motivated patients can be taught to master the art of glossopharyngeal breathing (Bach 1994). They gulp stepwise boluses of air into the lungs and can create a respectable tidal volume with six to nine mouthfuls of 60–100 ml. This allows those with no measurable vital capacity a few hours of ventilator-free time to enhance independence and provide a safety margin in case of ventilator failure.

Other ventilators

The rocking bed uses gravity to replace the function of an inert diaphragm by cyclically displacing the abdominal contents. It is most effective and comfortable when rocking is achieved entirely in the head-up position (Hill 1994). For immobile patients skin breakdown is reduced because of the variation in pressure.

The pneumobelt is used in sitting and standing only. For expiration, it inflates a bladder over the abdomen to push up the diaphragm. For passive inspiration, it allows diaphragmatic descent.

Some patients benefit from a combination, e.g. rocking bed at night and NIPPV by day.

Long-term tracheostomy

Long-term invasive ventilation may be appropriate for some patients with neurological conditions or, occasionally, COPD patients who have been unable to wean from mechanical ventilation (Muir *et al* 1994). A cuffed tracheostomy tube is necessary if airtight ventilation is required, for example if there is a risk of aspiration, but uncuffed or deflated cuffs can be used for the following:

- to allow spontaneous breathing at will or in case of ventilator failure,
- to permit speech, if there is a speaking valve attachment,
- for full ventilation provided the ventilator is volume cycled and can deliver three times the volume of air that would be required using a cuffed tube.

Tracheostomies can be managed at home if the patient or carer is educated to deflate and inflate the cuff, change and clean the tracheostomy tube and suction aseptically. If there is difficulty in replacing the tube, assistance must be available because the stoma can close within hours.

5.4   METHODS TO CLEAR SECRETIONS

5.4.1   Sputum in perspective

Question 1

Does sputum matter? Does it matter in the short term, e.g. can it obstruct breathing? Does it matter in the medium term, e.g. does it correlate with lung function or quality of life? Does it matter in the long term, i.e. is it implicated in the natural history of disease?

If secretions in the superficial airways are seen and heard to obstruct breathing, they need to be cleared. But the evidence that sputum clearance improves lung function is underwhelming, there being little correlation between secretions and airflow obstruction (Baldwin 1994; Bateman *et al* 1979; Peto *et al* 1983). For the long term, there is scant research, but in COPD there is little relation between secretions and mortality (Wiles and Hnizdo 1991).

However, for septic conditions the following must be considered:

- mucociliary clearance is impaired by some diseases,
- uncleared secretions are prone to infection,
- chronic infection damages airways.

Therefore, on balance, sputum does matter for patients with an acute secretion problem. It appears not to matter greatly for people with COPD, who indeed rarely complain of this and are usually quite capable of clearing their own chests unless weak or fatigued (although they need advice if symptoms are troublesome). For people with chronic sepsis, such as CF or bronchiectasis, a recent literature review suggests that secretion clearance slows deterioration in pulmonary function over time (Williams *et al* 1995). Despite the scepticism with which we must view the literature, at present we must assume that sputum does matter for these patients, especially as few researchers would care to investigate the effects of depriving, say, a sample of children with CF of their physiotherapy for a lifetime.

Question 2

How do we evaluate our techniques? The literature is a minefield when trying to measure sputum clearance. Studies *in vitro*, or in people with normal lungs, bear little relation to clinical practice. Studies that do not correct for cough alone are suspect because most physiotherapy techniques to clear secretions include coughing. Studies that do not follow-up secretion clearance for several hours after treatment only evaluate the immediate effects (Mortensen *et al* 1991). Studies that measure sputum volume or sputum weight are of limited value because they do not compensate for saliva or swallowed secretions (Hasani *et al* 1994; Mortensen *et al* 1991). Mucus transport is best measured by labelling inhaled radioactive aerosol and monitoring clearance by gamma camera (Mortensen *et al* 1991).

Question 3

Does physiotherapy make a difference? The effectiveness of mucus clearance in the large airways can be measured by the FEV_1, but the procedure itself alters bronchial status quo by shearing secretions off the airway wall. A less crude test is specific airways conductance, which measures airways obstruction without a forced expiration. For this we have one aged study to rely on, which suggests that conventional chest physiotherapy reduces airflow obstruction in the short term (Cochrane *et al* 1977). Tests of small airways function would be the most accurate.

Effectiveness also depends on accurate identification of the patient's problem. Is it quantity or quality of secretions? Is the patient weak, in pain or dehydrated? Is clearance impaired by hypoxia, infection, damaged airways, cigarette smoke, anaesthetic agents or a mixture of these?

The following section assumes that patients need physiotherapy if they have sputum retention or excess secretions which they cannot clear without advice or assistance.

5.4.2 Hydration, humidification and nebulization

The mucociliary escalator provides a frontier against the onslaught of 10 billion particles inhaled every day, but this depends on the maintenance of a layer of watery fluid that supports the cilia. Dehydration is a pulmonary insult which immobilzes cilia more than death (Clarke 1989), as well as causing mucosal drying, inflammation and ulceration.

The bronchial tree is normally fully saturated with water vapour from just below the carina onwards, but to prevent or treat dehydration, the following can be administered:

- systemic hydration by oral or intravenous fluids,
- humidification by inhalation of a vapour,
- nebulization by inhalation of an aerosol,
- heat–moisture exchange using a filter.

Classification

Hydration Dehydration leads to thick secretions and can impair oxygen delivery. Systemic fluid intake is not only the cheapest and safest expectorant, but is more effective than inhaled moisture, which is largely baffled out in the upper airways. Systemic hydration should always be the priority.

Some respiratory patients suffer dehydration by restricting their own fluid intake. They may be anxious after developing stress incontinence due to chronic cough. They may have frequency due to diuretics. Hospitalized patients may not be near the toilet. Many patients find it beneficial to drink six to eight glasses of water a day (Haas and Axen 1991, p. 224), so long as this is comfortable and correlates with medical management. If patients then find that expectoration is easier, this can be incorporated into their lifestyle, a jug of water being readily available as a reminder.

Hot weather, fever and exacerbation of disease increase requirements, and hospitalized patients are affected by the change in environment and routine.

Liquid diets and blenderized meals are not recommended for rehydration because they have a significant osmotic load and do not provide free water.

Some conditions may be complicated by acid-base or electrolyte disturbance, kidney dysfunction, pulmonary oedema or diuretic therapy, and liaison with medical staff is then advisable.

Humidification A steam inhalation delivers steam from near-boiling water to the patient via a mouth piece. Some patients find it beneficial, but the container is easily knocked over and is unsafe unless the patient is protected by a plastic sheet and is under supervision.

A **hot water humidifier** produces a vapour by passing gas over heated sterile liquid. The gas can also be bubbled through the liquid, but this increases resistance. Some equipment incorporates a heater in the tube to the patient in order to prevent condensation.

When used with non-intubated patients, the convoluted passages of the nose and mouth condense the vapour into large drops which cannot easily reach the lungs. The main use of hot water humidifiers, therefore, is to provide humidification for patients with endotracheal or tracheostomy tubes, or to aid expectoration for patients with a dry mouth.

To ensure safety, the humidifier should:

- be kept below the patient to prevent condensed water tipping into the airway,
- be kept heated continuously in order to maintain an unfriendly environment for bacteria,
- incorporate an over-heating safety device.

A **cold water humidifier** bubbles cold gas through cold water. This is unable to achieve relative humidity greater than 50% at body temperature (Darin 1982), is insufficient even to prevent insensible water loss (Hodgkin 1993, p. 207) and was condemned as 'dangerously inadequate' over two decades ago (Graff and Benson 1969). Its only indication is for the few patients on dry oxygen who feel that it makes their mouth more comfortable. Otherwise it simply increases airflow resistance and grows bacteria, although the patient is rarely infected because of the inefficiency of the device. Cold water humidifiers are still used, marketed in craftily-designed devices that mimic a nebulizer, due to the untiring enthusiasm of the sales representatives.

Nebulization Nebulizers to moisten airways use the same mechanism as those used for drug delivery, but are larger and used continuously. Sterile liquid is converted into an aerosol, whose droplets are small enough to navigate the nose and mouth and thus reach the airways.

The **jet nebulizer** commonly uses a cold liquid because heat is not necessary for this mechanism, but heated nebulizers are available which combine the advantages of vapour and aerosol. A venturi device allows different percentages of oxygen to be delivered.

The **ultrasonic nebulizer** transmits vibrations through a liquid to produce a 2–10-fold greater output than a jet nebulizer (Phillips and Millard 1994). Advantages are its efficiency and silence, while disadvantages are expense and, for patients with excess work of breathing, increased airflow resistance due to the dense aerosol. Oxygen can be added with a nasal cannula. Other staff should be advised that a physiotherapist should be available when it is used in certain patients in case they cannot clear the increased volume of secretions.

Heat–moisture exchange A filter can be fitted over a tracheal tube to act as an artificial nose. This is known as a heat–moisture exchanger (HME), a condenser humidifier or a Swedish nose. It functions by recycling exhaled heat and moisture. It is inadequate for patients needing more active humidification, but convenient for many mobile patients and, for limited periods, for mechanically ventilated patients. Hygroscopic HMEs increase moisture output more than conventional HMEs by conserving moisture in the expired air chemically (Branson *et al* 1993).

Tents and head boxes are discussed on p. 93.

Effects

The superficial gel layer of the mucus blanket acts as a protective barrier between the body and the atmosphere, but is not totally waterproof and can absorb some inhaled moisture (Conway 1992b).

Complications

1. Ubiquitous hospital bacteria enjoy nothing more than stagnant humidifier water, especially if it is lukewarm, so heated humidifiers should not be allowed to cool and reheat, and equipment should be changed every 24 hours (AARC 1993b). Prefilled sterile bottles reduce infection risk (Castel 1991). The more efficient the humidifier, the more easily can bacteria penetrate deep into the lung.
2. Bronchospasm can be caused in susceptible patients by:
   (a) dense ultrasonic mist,
   (b) an unheated nebulizer,
   (c) use of fluid other than isotonic saline (Church 1991).
3. For babies or people in acute renal failure, fluid overload can occur with the ultrasonic nebulizer, leading to inactivation of surfactant, airway blockage, ciliary damage and overwhelming of the mucociliary escalator (Shelly *et al* 1988).
4. Thermal injury can occur with heated humidifiers that are inadequately serviced.
5. Hypercapnic COPD patients may suffer loss of respiratory drive if uncontrolled oxygen is used as the driving gas. Most large nebulizers can be set up to run on 24% oxygen, but this often reduces the effectiveness of the mechanism.

Indications

A person's upper airway is his or her most efficient humidifying system. Humidification or nebulization is therefore necessary for people whose own humidifying system has been bypassed with a tracheal tube. Others who often benefit are:

• babies with respiratory problems whose small airways easily block with secretions,

• people on oxygen therapy who have hyperreactive airways (a heated system is necessary) or some who use a simple mask for prolonged periods with flow rates above 4 l/min (Fulmer 1984),
• patients using non-invasive mechanical aids, such as CPAP, which deliver high-flow dry gases (Conway 1992b),
• people with thick secretions, especially if infected,
• people who are mouth breathing, nil-by-mouth or have a dry mouth and find expectoration difficult.

Periodic administration of saline before physiotherapy, using a small jet nebulizer, only helps by wetting the mouth and aiding expectoration, but for some people with cystic fibrosis, 30 minutes of ultrasonic nebulization may deposit sufficient fluid in the airways to help shift secretions (Hodgkin 1993, p. 206).

Humidification is not necessary for the following:

• people using nasal cannulae because at low flow rates the patient's nose provides adequate humidification, and the moisture is lost by condensation in the narrow tubing (Campbell *et al* 1988),
• people with permanent tracheostomies because adaptation occurs (Shelly *et al* 1988),
• people using venturi masks because the entrained ambient air is not as dry as piped oxygen, water may condense in the entrainment ports and alter the F_1O_2, and attempts to humidify the oxygen and/or entrained air with a humidity adaptor are rarely effective (Gribbin 1993); it is better to set up a nebulizer to run on controlled oxygen.

Method

A mask or mouthpiece can be used. A mask is convenient for continuous treatment, and a mouthpiece is best for intermittent use or for people who feel smothered by a mask.

Lung deposition is enhanced by the upright sitting or side-lying position. Condensation is minimized by wide-bore tubing and avoidance of lengthy convolutions of tube. Pooled liquid should be emptied regularly into a separate container.

Production of a mist does not itself imply correct droplet size because the therapeutic range of 2–12 μm diameter is not visible, but regular checks for a visible mist show that at least there is no blockage in the system.

When small nebulizers are used for drug delivery, they are diluted with isotonic saline, but large nebulizers used for secretion clearance are usually filled with sterile water to prevent them becoming encrusted, although saline is theoretically more physiologically sound and should be used for people with hyperreactive airways. Sodium bicarbonate has been used in the past as the nebulizing fluid because it provides an alkaline environment that reduces mucus viscosity, but it disturbs pH and reduces resistance to bacteria (Sara 1965). Hypertonic saline increases the production rather than the clearance of sputum (Pavia *et al* 1978), and in the process can cause bronchospasm, coughing and desaturation, so is only used to induce sputum (p. 76) for diagnostic purposes.

5.4.3 Mobilization and breathing exercises

The simplest and most efficient way to clear secretions is to create an outward pull on the airway by increasing lung volume, so that trapped secretions can be released and coughed up (Andersen and Falk 1991). This aim is achieved by active exercise (Dodd 1991; Lannefors 1992) and deep breathing (Andersen *et al* 1979). Exercise shows the added benefit of increasing catecholamine secretion which speeds ciliary activity (Prasad 1993).

5.4.4 Postural drainage (PD)

For people whose clearance mechanism is defective, postural drainage is thought to use gravity to assist drainage of secretions, although the mechanism is unclear.

Method

PD should be avoided before and after meals to prevent loss of appetite or nausea and discomfort. If bronchodilators are prescribed, these should be taken 15 minutes beforehand.

Patients are positioned with the area to be drained uppermost (Appendix B), bearing in mind that these positions may need modification if lung architecture has been distorted by surgery, fibrosis, large abscess or bullae. The worst area is drained first in order to reduce the chance of infected secretions spilling into healthy lung. Patients on monitors should be checked for arrhythmias or desaturation before, during and after drainage.

Drainage times vary but ideally 10 minutes are needed in each position. If the disease affects the whole lung, each lobe requires drainage, but a maximum of three positions are preferable each time so that sessions do not become intolerably long. For localized bronchiectasis or an abscess, positioning for the exact segment is necessary. The procedure should be discontinued if the patient complains of headache, discomfort, dizziness, palpitations or breathlessness. Some patients benefit from sleeping in a modified postural drainage position (Verboon *et al* 1986), so long as this does not cause coughing during the night.

Effects

PD is effective if it provides symptomatic relief or long-term benefit. These benefits are offset in patients who find it uncomfortable or inconvenient. Long-term benefits are difficult to evaluate, especially as many studies have not isolated PD from other modalities. It is thought that PD increases mucus transport in the more distal airways, where coughing has less influence, but Mortensen *et al* (1991) have shown that total clearance is not changed several hours after treatment. This suggests that it might be less useful for affecting a disease process, e.g. interrupting the vicious cycle of CF, but appropriate for symptomatic management so that going to school is more amenable or going to the dentist more comfortable.

The direct effect of gravity on secretions may not be the only mechanism involved. Lannefors (1992) demonstrated how the lower lung showed the most clearance, the greater ventilation in dependent regions encouraging movement of secretions by high flows and mechanical squeezing. This argument is reinforced by the limited effectiveness of gravity with thick secretions as can be seen if a sputum pot containing a mucus plug is left upside down and the following morning the plug is still clinging to the side of the pot.

The head-down position increases the work of breathing (Marini *et al* 1984), tends to reduce tidal volume (Olséni 1994) and decreases FRC in people with normal lungs (Jenkins *et al* 1988). Before embarking on PD it is therefore advisable to balance the risks and benefits.

Indications

PD may be beneficial for people who show all three of the following criteria:

- production of more than 30 ml of sputum a day (Woodhead and Tattersfield 1987),
- difficulty in clearing it,
- patient preference, and greater effectiveness than other methods.

Without access to sophisticated equipment, 'greater effectiveness' can often only be judged by sputum volume and the patient's subjective report.

Those who benefit are people with lung abscess usually, bronchiectasis often and CF sometimes. PD is also beneficial for some patients with acute problems if they are too weak or tired for more active measures, but modified positions are usually required so that the work of breathing is not excessive.

For people with chronic conditions, poor compliance with this antisocial procedure is renowned (Currie *et al* 1986). A week's trial of PD should therefore include motivating patients to fit a programme into their daily routine, preferably with a home visit, so that results can be assessed accurately and decisions made on whether this and/or other measures are most suitable.

Precautions

It is unwise to tip a patient head down in the presence of:

- cerebral oedema, e.g. acute head injury or recent stroke,
- hypertension,
- subcutaneous emphysema,
- trauma, burns or recent surgery to the head or neck,
- recent pneumonectomy or surgery to the aorta, oesophagus or cardiac sphincter of the stomach,
- headache,
- breathlessness,
- symptomatic hiatus hernia,
- history of seizures,
- epistaxis or recent haemoptysis,
- abdominal distension, pregnancy, obesity,
- acute spinal cord lesion,
- pulmonary oedema, arrhythmias or cardio-vascular instability,
- undrained pneumothorax,
- bronchopleural fistula,
- risk of aspiration.

5.4.5 Manual techniques

Percussion or vibrations are performed in a postural drainage position. They aim to jar loose secretions from the airway walls.

Method

Percussion consists of rhythmic clapping on the chest with loose wrist and cupped hand, creating an energy wave that is transmitted to the airways. A sheet or pyjama top should cover the patient but thick covering dampens transmission through the chest wall.

Correct cupping of the hand ensures that the procedure is completely comfortable. Indeed, performed correctly, it can soothe frightened children and people with acute asthma. A slow single-handed technique is normally preferred because rapid percussion can cause breath-holding and occasionally increases airways obstruction (Wollmer *et al* 1985).

Vibrations consist of a fine oscillation of the hands directed inwards against the chest, performed on exhalation after a deep inhalation. **Shaking** is a coarser movement in which the chest wall is compressed.

Vibration, shaking and percussion should be interspersed with relaxed deep breathing to prevent airway closure, desaturation or bronchospasm.

Effects

Manual techniques reinforce patient dependency and have not been shown to improve lung function, oxygen saturation or, when performed independently, mucociliary transport (Sutton *et al* 1985). When combined with postural drainage they accelerate clearance from peripheral lung regions (Bateman *et al* 1981), but this study did not explain which modality was the effective one. Research on vibrations shows as many negative as positive outcomes (Rivington-Law 1981), and if performed on a squashy bed, much of the energy is absorbed by the mattress. Percussion has been seen to speed mucus clearance (Radford 1982), and produce moderate improvements in FEV_1 (Kang 1974). Self-percussion is ineffective and can cause desaturation (Carr 1994).

Studies are often unreliable and contradictory, so it is advisable that physiotherapists observe their endeavours by performing them if a patient with secretions is to have a

bronchoscopy, or by asking patients which techniques they find most comfortable and effective.

Indications

Manual techniques are suited to some people with large quantities of sputum who find these methods helpful. Patients with chronic problems usually prefer to choose an independent method, but those with acute problems may benefit. People with an acute sputum problem need extra time for relaxed abdominal breathing in order to prevent desaturation.

Precautions

Percussion and vibrations are to be avoided or modified in the presence of:

- rib fracture or potential rib fracture, e.g. metastatic carcinoma, osteoporosis,
- loss of skin integrity, e.g. surgery, burns or chest drains,
- recent or excessive haemoptysis, e.g. due to abscess or lung contusion,
- severe clotting disorder, e.g. ↑ PTT or PT, platelet count < 50 000 (see Glossary),
- subcutaneous emphysema,
- recent epidural infusion,
- unstable angina or arrhythmias.

5.4.6 Active cycle of breathing techniques (ACBT)

ACBT is a cycle of huffs from mid-to low lung volume interspersed with deep breathing and relaxed abdominal breathing (Webber and Pryor 1993). It has superseded the forced expiration technique (FET) which omitted the deep breathing and was often misinterpreted. The sequence is:

- abdominal breathing,
- three to four deep breaths,

- abdominal breathing,
- one or two huffs from mid- to low lung volume,
- abdominal breathing.

During huffing or forced expiration, the pleural pressure becomes positive and equals the alveolar pressure at a point along the airway called the equal pressure point (usually in the segmental bronchi). Towards the mouth from this point, the transmural pressure gradient is reversed so that pressure inside the airway is lower than outside. This squeezes the airways by a process known as dynamic compression, which limits airflow, but the squeezing of airways mouthwards of this point mobilizes secretions. The equal pressure point moves distally at low volumes, and it has been suggested that the lower the lung volume, the deeper the region from which secretions are cleared.

Effects

The depth of the mucus clearance has not yet been validated (AARC 1993c), and the effect is still thought to be in the larger airways (Conway 1992b), but ACBT may be working quietly in the small airways by 'milking' the mucus mouthwards. ACBT and coughing are equally effective (Hasani *et al* 1994) but correctly performed ACBT is less likely to cause bronchospasm or desaturation in at-risk patients. ACBT incorporates several components, and may include PD, so it is unclear which is the most effective element.

Method

Correct teaching is essential because huffing alone causes more airways obstruction than coughing (Fig. 5.7), mucus clearance can actually be impaired (David 1991), and incorrect technique can cause bronchospasm, paroxysms of coughing and desaturation (Steven *et al* 1992). Points to note are:

- avoid too forceful a huff,
- complete the full cycle,

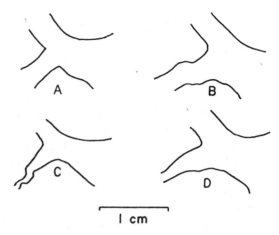

Figure 5.7 A section of the bronchial tree, (A) at FRC, (B) at full inspiration, (C) at full expiration, and (D) during coughing. (From Marshall, R. and Holden, W.S. (1963) Changes in calibre of the airways in man. *Thorax*, **18**, 54–8, with permission.)

- end with relaxed abdominal breathing.

Avoidance of high lung volumes is easier if patients take in only a half-breath before the huff. Higher lung volumes are used once secretions are mobilized. Teaching the huff is sometime helped by blowing through a peak flow mouthpiece, and for children by incorporating blowing games.

Treatment continues until the chest is subjectively or objectively clear, or until the patient tires. Technique must be checked regularly because patients tend to take in too deep a breath or skip the relaxed part of the cycle. ACBT gives patients independence and is usefully incorporated into the chest clearance routine of people with CF.

5.4.7 Autogenic drainage (AD)

AD is designed to produce the highest possible airflow in different generations of bronchi by a three-phase controlled breathing regime, clearing secretions from the small to large airways by gradually increasing lung volumes. It gives patients independence from ages four to five, but requires 30–45

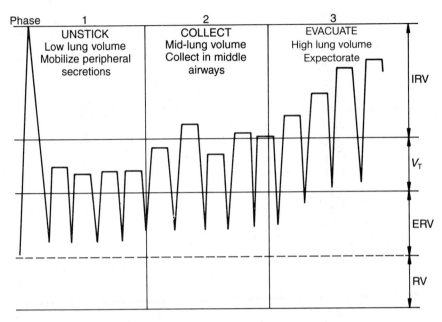

Figure 5.8 The three phases of autogenic drainage. (Reproduced with permission from Prasad, S.A. and Hussey, J. (1995) *Paediatric Respiratory Care*, Chapman & Hall, London.)

minutes to complete, and for people with CF is usually necessary twice a day. It can be incorporated into certain activities such as driving.

Effects

AD improves airflow in the small airways, clearing secretions that are not accessible with 'conventional physiotherapy' (usually defined as postural drainage, percussion and vibrations) (Hardy 1993). It improves SaO_2 (McIlwaine 1991) and shows greater mucus clearance than ACBT (Miller *et al* 1995).

Method

The patient sits upright and inhales slowly through the nose, pauses at end-inspiration, then exhales through the mouth. Breaths start from residual volume to unstick the mucus, then when when the patient feels the secretions moving, tidal volume breaths are taken to collect the mucus. Then when

crackles are felt, deep breathing clears the mucus (Fig. 5.8). Coughing is inhibited until secretions are accessible. Flow is controlled to achieve highest flows without airway collapse, aiming at a mucus rattle rather than a wheeze. Patients who find it difficult to breathe at low lung volumes can breathe at varying tidal volumes (Prasad 1993). Schöni (1989) describes details of the technique, but physiotherapists wanting to use AD require specialist training.

5.4.8   Mechanical aids

Positive expiratory pressure (PEP)

PEP is the application of positive pressure at the mouth via a face mask, one-way valve and expiratory resistance.

Effects   PEP incorporates the principle of maintaining lung volume so that secretion clearance is not hampered by collapsing airways. Breathing out against resistance

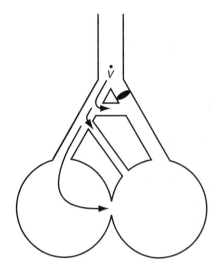

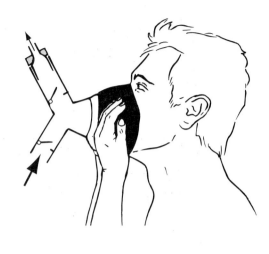

Figure 5.9 Collateral ventilation. Ventilation ($\dot{V}$) finds its way behind the mucus plug through collateral channels.

Figure 5.10 PEP mask in use. (From Oberwaldner, B. *et al*, (1986) Forced expirations against a variable resistance. *Ped. Pulmonol.*, **2**, 358–67. Redrawn by permission of John Wiley & Sons, Inc.)

opens up airways, evens the distribution of ventilation, forces air through collateral channels and pushes secretions from the lung periphery to the central airways, from where they can be coughed up (Fig. 5.9). PEP has the added advantage of counteracting airway closure caused by coughing. Its effects are more long-lasting than PD (Mortensen *et al* 1991).

Method A resistance is chosen so that the patient is able to breathe comfortably for two minutes into the mask and achieve a pressure of 10–20 cmH$_2$O during mid-expiration, using a manometer between the valve and resistance (Andersen and Falk 1991). The patient sits leaning forwards to protect the lungs from overdistension. With the PEP mask firmly over the nose and mouth, the patient inhales to tidal volume and then exhales actively, but not fully or forcefully, giving way to the resistance (Fig. 5.10). Ten PEP breaths are followed by ACB and coughing, each session continuing until the lungs

feel subjectively clear. During stable disease, most patients find that two 15-minute or three 10-minute sessions a day are adequate.

High pressure PEP creates pressures of 60 cmH$_2$O (Hardy 1993), using flow volume curves to gauge the correct pressure. This shows added benefits of reduced hyperinflation and improved lung function (Prasad 1993).

Indications PEP is mostly used by people with CF, especially adolescents and those seeking freedom from PD, but COPD patients who have difficulty clearing secretions also find it helpful (Christensen, Simonsen and Lange 1990). It is suited to people with moderate amounts of sputum and can be used by children as young as four years. Those with large amounts of sputum need the addition of other techniques, but PEP alone can be used as a stopgap, for example to enable a child with CF to go on a school outing. It is not advisable for people who wheeze.

Mechanical percussors, vibrators and oscillators

Various substitutes for manual techniques have been developed. They allow independence, but are expensive and need to be accompanied by other techniques such as deep breathing to discourage airway closure. The following are available:

- mechanical percussors and vibrators, some of which can feel quite violent, are preferred by some patients (Bauer *et al* 1994),
- high-frequency chest wall compressors, which are inflatable vests placed around the chest and show some potential (Arens *et al* 1994),
- oral high frequency oscillators or intrapulmonary percussors, described on p. 127; these shift mucus (Natale *et al* 1994) but not always in the right direction (Freitag *et al* 1989),
- small mechanical vibrators which are cheap and can be used gently over the chest of people with fractured ribs. They may help clearance from the lung periphery (Gross and King 1984).

Flutter

The combined effects of PEP and oscillation are exploited with the Flutter, a small device into which patients exhale to form a positive oscillatory pressure of 10–20 cmH$_2$O in the airways (Fig. 5.11). Oscillations are created by a steel ball in the device which vibrates as air passes through. Patients sit as if using the PEP mask and keep the cheeks taut. Pressure is controlled by the patient changing his or her inspiratory flow, and oscillations are controlled by tilting the angle of the device at the mouth. The aim is for maximum oscillation, which is assessed subjectively by the patient and objectively by the physiotherapist palpating the vibrations at the front and back of the chest.

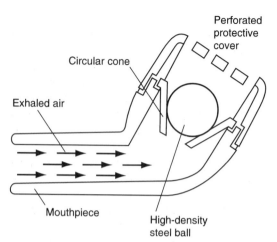

Figure 5.11 Flutter device. (Courtesy of VarioRaw.)

Konstan (1994) claims that CF patients produce three times more sputum with the Flutter than with conventional techniques. Other groups of people who appear to benefit are those with COPD (Callegari 1994) and those with productive asthma (Girard and Terki 1994). It may be found to be comfortable and even enjoyable.

Intermittent positive pressure breathing

Some weak or drowsy patients with sputum retention may respond to IPPB. If other interventions have been inadequate, this form of mechanical assistance can promote deep breaths in order to propel the secretions from behind, and/or maintain ventilation while other techniques are applied.

5.4.9 Cough

Coughing can occur voluntarily or be stimulated by irritants from inside or outside the lung.

Cough facilitation

Several problems may render a cough ineffective:

1. Poor coughing technique may be camouflaged by making loud but ineffectual noises in the throat. Patients need advice

to do a 'good belly cough', with a demonstration.

2. Pain following surgery inhibits coughing. Pain relief is discussed in Chapter 7.

3. Thick secretions reduce the effectiveness of coughing. Hydration is helpful over time, but an ultrasonic mist provides instant assistance.

4. A dry mouth inhibits expectoration. This can be overcome with a small saline nebulizer, hot steamy drink, mouthwash, or sucking ice or a piece of lemon.

5. Inhibition may be caused by embarrassment, disgust or anxiety. Patients may be anxious about stitches splitting, for which reassurance can be given because stitches rarely split unless the wound is infected or the patient is obese. Anxiety about stress incontinence can inhibit coughing, especially in elderly people. There may also be anxiety about nausea or setting off paroxysms of coughing.

6. If the upper airway is narrowed by a tumour, obstruction is sometimes relieved by the patient leaning in different directions to shift the position of the tumour before coughing.

7. Weakness due to neuromuscular or terminal disease demands a resourceful physiotherapist. All measures should first be taken to bring the secretions proximally. Good old IPPB, surprisingly, is sometimes helpful for this. Physical assistance can then be given by helping the patient sit over the edge of the bed if possible, then compressing the abdomen manually in co-ordination with expiratory effort. Some patients can assist themselves by sitting with a pillow pressed against the abdomen, then after a deep breath, bending forwards while exhaling. In semiconscious people who cannot cough, applying quick gentle pressure downwards and inwards over the trachea just above the suprasternal notch can sometimes elicit a cough. Bach (1993) claims that mechanically assisted coughing using a positive pressure blower with expulsive decompression can reduce the need for suction.

Precautions

Coughing should be avoided in the presence of recent pneumonectomy, aneurysm, subcutaneous emphysema, raised intracranial pressure or recent eye surgery.

Cough suppression

Coughing may need to be inhibited if patients have an irritating dry cough, paroxyms of coughing or when coughing is contraindicated, e.g. immediately after eye or cranial surgery or aneurysm repair. Multiple coughs or paroxysms of coughing can impair mucus transport and cause fatigue, bronchospasm and airway closure (Menkes and Britt 1980), and may lead to cough syncope from excessive intrathoracic pressure.

The first step when dealing with an unproductive cough is to identify the cause (p. 23). A cough caused by asthma, postnasal drip or GOR should disappear once the condition is controlled. A quarter of patients taking ACE inhibitor drugs develop a cough, which disappears on average four months after starting the drug. Other coughs usually disappear in time, but dry coughs can perpetuate themselves by irritating the airways. Factors which exacerbate coughing include change in air temperature and irritants such as perfumes and cigarette smoke. Cough suppression techniques include the following:

• for patients in whom it has become a habit, advice to inhibit the cough voluntarily,
• postural change, e.g. avoiding supine,
• swallowing,
• taking sips of cold water,
• nose-breathing,
• taking repeated short sniffs,

- taking slow shallow breaths,
- breathing through pursed lips,
- sucking lozenges,
- drugs as described on p. 102.

5.4.10   Nasopharyngeal suction

The worst part is the initial introduction of the catheter into the nostrils. Once past the turn at the back of the nose, it was not too unpleasant, until a cough is stimulated; then it feels like hours as the catheter is brought back up . . . it felt as if I was choking.

Ludwig 1984

These remarks come from a physiotherapist who found herself at the wrong end of a suction catheter, and they illustrate why most clinicians are, rightly, reluctant to put their patients through the ordeal of naso-pharyngeal suction, which is usually distress-ing and often painful. It is also dirty, risky and limited in effectiveness, but there are occasions when it is necessary.

Complications

Untoward effects of suction may be subclin-ical and go unrecognized. Common problems are the following:

1. Airway mucosa is exquisitely sensitive and can be damaged by passage of the catheter, poor technique or pull from the vacuum (Kleiber *et al* 1988). Damage can be tantamount to a crude biopsy, leading to bleeding and up to 50% reduction in mucociliary transport (Landa *et al* 1980).
2. Infective organisms find an easy target if the protective mucosa is damaged by repeated suction.
3. Suction vacuum can cause atelectasis.
4. Sustained hypoxia can be caused by atelectasis, sucking out oxygen, enforced apnoea (Petersen *et al* 1979) and increased oxygen demand due to stress.
5. Hypoxaemia or irritation of the vagus nerve can cause arrhythmias, brady-cardia and unstable BP. Stress can cause tachycardia.
6. Laryngospasm is a rare but dangerous complication. If the patient stops breath-ing and the catheter feels stuck, the crash team should be called and oxygen applied.

Indications

Suction is performed only if all of the following criteria are met:

- secretions are detrimental to the patient,
- secretions are accessible to the catheter, as indicated by crackles in the upper airway on auscultation,
- the patient is unable to clear the secretions by other means.

Weakness and semiconsciousness may be indications. Fatigue is not, because unless fatigue is extreme enough for the patient to need mechanical ventilation, coughing is still possible. Risks are increased in a combative patient, and those who need physical restraint for suction rarely need to undergo the procedure because they are usually strong enough to cough effectively, even though they may choose not to. Forcible suction is unethical, usually illegal and acceptable only in life-threatening situations.

Catheters

Catheters have an end-hole through which the mucus is suctioned, and side eyes to relieve vacuum if the end-hole touches the mucosa, because contact with the mucosa causes invagination. Both end-hole and side eyes are best slightly depressed to keep them at a distance from the mucosa (Lomholt 1982a). The side eyes should not be too large (Fig. 5.12(c)) or they reduce suction efficiency. The total size of the side eyes should be less than that of the end-hole so that they do not become the main suction channels and themselves damage mucosa. Catheters with multiple side eyes show

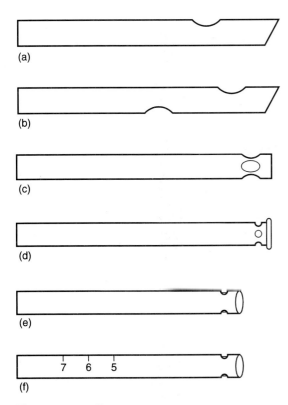

Figure 5.12 Different catheter tips.

reduced suction efficiency (Lomholt 1982b), but cause less invagination than those with one or two eyes (Link *et al* 1976). Catheters with one side eye (Fig. 5.12(a)) cause unnecessary trauma (Lomholt 1982b) and although cheap should not be used.

A beaded tip is designed to keep the eyes away from grabbing the mucosa, but does not always fulfil this objective (Jung and Gottleib 1976), and the bead makes it unsuited to nasal suction because of the enlarged tip (Fig. 5.12(d)). The ideal catheter is flexible, has a smooth, rounded tip and small, multiple, countersunk side eyes.

Method

A size 10 FG catheter is preferable, but some patients may need size 12. High suction pressures can be damaging, but low pressures can be less effective and cause pro-

longed suction time (Lomholt 1982b). Consensus indicates that adults require vacuum pressures at a minimum 70 mmHg and maximum 150 mmHg (Pilbeam 1992, p. 625), but there is no original research, so the lowest effective pressure should be used. The following steps are suggested:

1. Help the patient into side-lying in case of vomiting.
2. Preoxygenate for two minutes if this is not contraindicated. The oxygen mask should then be kept close to the patient's face throughout.
3. Explain to the patient how it will feel, how long it will last and that he or she may ask for a pause at any time, a request that must be responded to. Unconscious patients also need an explanation.
4. Connect the catheter to the apparatus and put gloves on both hands. The dominant hand needs a sterile glove, and both gloves should be non-powdered in case the powder finds its way into the lungs. Remove the catheter from the package and lubricate the tip with water-soluble or lignocaine jelly. Maintain the sterility of the catheter and gloves.
5. With the suction port open, slide the catheter gently into the nostril, aiming towards the occiput. If resistance is felt at the back of the pharynx, rotate the catheter slowly between the fingers and ease very gently forwards.
6. To reduce the risk of entering the oesophagus, ask the patient to tilt the head back, stick the tongue out and cough. If coughing is not possible, slide the catheter down during speech or inhalation, when the glottis is open. If the patient swallows, the catheter has slipped into the oesophagus, so slightly withdraw the catheter, reposition the head and proceed. The catheter is in the trachea if the patient coughs or expired air can be felt through the end of the catheter.

7. When the catheter stops, withdraw it slightly before applying vacuum pressure, in order to limit trauma. Note the length of catheter that has been inserted so that impaction can be avoided if further suction is necessary.
8. Apply suction and bring up the catheter slowly and smoothly, but avoid catheter rotation or sudden intermittent suction. Slow withdrawal reduces the need for a second attempt, but if the patient appears distressed, the catheter should be partially withdrawn until coughing or the distress stops, then the vacuum is removed and oxygen applied with the catheter still *in situ*, until the patient is ready to continue.

Rotation is unnecessary with multiple-eyed catheters, and ineffective with most other catheters (Emergency Care Research Institute 1977) because torsional stiffness prevents transmission of rotation to the catheter tip *in vivo*.

Intermittent suction has become enshrined in practice because authors quote each other in circular fashion without a research base. Intermittent suction involving the sudden on/off application of vacuum pressure has three disadvantages:

- it reduces effectiveness by decreasing flow from an average 18–20 l/min, to an average 8–9 l/min (Brown 1983),
- sudden release of pressure can damage mucosa (Frownfelter 1987),
- it is no less damaging than continuous suction (Czarnik *et al* 1991).

If suction pressure rises unacceptably, the rocking thumb technique should be used, which is the smooth and partial removal of the thumb from the control port of the catheter to reduce pressure gently. Protection of mucosa is best maintained by continuous movement without stopping even momentarily to change position of the dominant hand on the catheter.

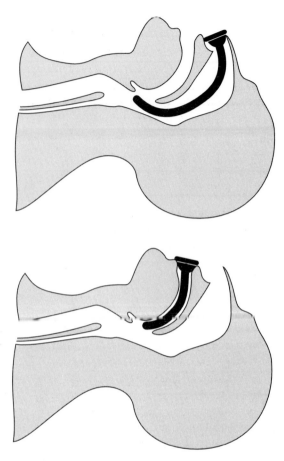

Figure 5.13 Oral airway and nasophrayngeal airway.

9. Afterwards, remove the gloves inside out over the catheter and discard them, give the patient oxygen and comfort and check the monitors.

If the nasal route is uncomfortable, the other nostril can be tried or the oral route used. For oral suction, the catheter is inserted into an oral airway, which is a plastic tube shaped to conform to the palate with a flange to prevent it slipping too far into the patient (Fig. 5.13). The catheter protrudes just beyond the end of the airway, then the airway and catheter are passed into the mouth, curve upwards, the patient is asked to breathe it in, then it is rotated and passed into the throat, curve downwards. During insertion it is held downwards so that it does not touch the soft palate and cause gagging. The patient is reassured that it will not prevent breathing. Passage of the catheter proceeds as described above. Introducing the airway is not painful but is often distressing.

Precautions

Nasopharyngeal suction should be avoided in patients with stridor because of the danger of total airway obstruction. It should be avoided if there is acute face, neck or head injury. If there is cerebrospinal fluid leak after basal skull fracture, an oral airway should be used because of the risk of infection. Bleeding may occur in patients who have clotting disorders (see Glossary) or who are receiving heparin or thrombolytic drugs. If the patient has pulmonary oedema, suction does not help the condition and will remove surfactant if performed repeatedly. Suction aggravates bronchospasm, but so too does excess mucus. Following recent pneumonectomy or lung transplant, the catheter should not be taken beyond the pharynx in case it impinges on the bronchial stump. Following recent oesophagectomy, the catheter should not be taken beyond the pharynx in case it misses the trachea and damages the oesophageal anastomosis.

It is advisable to wear a mask, goggles and gloves for self-protection. It is unlikely that blood-streaked sputum can find its way through any non-intact skin or mucous membranes, but it is theoretically possible.

Specimen collection

If a sputum specimen is needed, a sterile mucus trap is incorporated into the circuit. This should be kept upright during suction to prevent the specimen bypassing the system. If secretions are scant, either the catheter

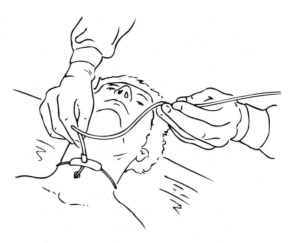

Figure 5.14 Minitracheostomy.

itself can be sent to the laboratory or the catheter swilled with a few drops of sterile saline to draw secretions into the mucus trap.

It is possible to obtain a deeper specimen that is less contaminated by pathogens lurking in the proximal airways. After preoxygenation, a catheter is inserted, 20 ml of saline is injected by syringe through the catheter over 10 seconds, the saline is withdrawn by the syringe (without suction), then the catheter is withdrawn.

Nasopharyngeal airway

A nasopharyngeal airway may be preferred by some patients who need frequent suction (Fig. 5.13). It is lubricated with lignocaine gel, inserted gently into the nose and left for 24 hours, with a safety pin across the top to prevent it disappearing into the patient.

5.4.11 Minitracheostomy

A relief for both physiotherapist and patient has been the advent of the minitracheostomy, which allows access for safe and comfortable suction and has consigned nasopharyngeal suction to the backwater of occasional use only. It is a simple procedure that not only treats sputum retention, but can also prevent the need for bronchoscopy or intubation (Preston *et al* 1986).

A minitracheostomy is performed under local anaesthesia on the ward. A narrow cannula is inserted surgically into the trachea, then left in place for as many days as necessary. Suction with a size 10 catheter can then be performed through the aperture, with saline instillation if necessary, and the patient can breathe normally throughout (Fig. 5.14). A spigot protects the airway when suction is not being performed.

A minitracheostomy preserves the function of the glottis so that coughing, speaking and eating are safeguarded, while spontaneous breathing and natural humidification continue.

Minitracheostomy is often performed later than indicated. The physiotherapist can act as instigator to ensure its appropriate and if necessary prophylactic use.

RECOMMENDED READING

Bach, J.R. (1994) Update and perspectives on noninvasive respiratory muscle aids. *Chest*, **105**, 1230–40.

Barnitt, R. and Fulton, C. (1994) Patient agreement to treatment: a framework for therapists. *Br. J. Ther. Rehab.*, **1**, 121–7.

Bott, J., Keilty, S.E.J. and Noone, L. (1992) Intermittent positive pressure breathing – a dying art? *Physiotherapy*, **78**, 656–60.

Hardy, K.A. (1994) A review of airway clearance techniques. *Resp. Care*, **39**, 440–55.

Ntoumenopoulos, G. (1995) Topical issues in cardiopulmonary physiotherapy. *Physiotherapy*, **81**, 92–4.

Starr, J.A. (1992) Manual techniques of chest physical therapy and airway clearance techniques, in *Pulmonary management in physical therapy* (ed. C. C. Zadai), Churchill Livingstone, London.

Williams, M.T. (1995) Chest physiotherapy and cystic fibrosis. *Chest*, **106**, 1872–82.

6. Management of breathlessness and pulmonary rehabilitation

6.1 DOES PULMONARY REHABILITATION WORK?

No patient is 'too sick' or 'too well' to benefit from a pulmonary rehabilitation program.
Menier 1994

Rehabilitation for people disabled by breathlessness is one of the most rewarding aspects of physiotherapy, yet it is one of the most neglected. It is rewarding because it can provide real improvement in the lives of people who have become entangled in a web of inactivity, low self-esteem and helplessness. It is neglected because of a widespread attitude that patients have reached a dead end. Physiotherapists themselves may feel helpless when faced with someone who has uncontrolled breathlessness, lungs like tissue paper, a pessimistic outlook, an unglamorous disease, and no nice straightforward problem such as excess sputum which can be dealt with by time-honoured techniques.

Rehabilitation has become widely accepted for people with neurological, musculoskeletal and cardiac conditions, but does it work for people with lung disease? Pulmonary rehabilitation does not reverse lung damage, but it modifies the disability that derives from it. Participants report a sense of well-being which is due to gaining control over symptoms, especially the fear of breathlessness. Other outcomes that have been demonstrated are (Brannon *et al* 1993; Murray 1993):

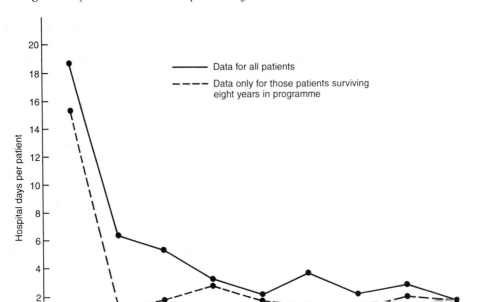

Figure 6.1 Analysis of hospital admissions after initiation of pulmonary rehabilitation. (From Hodgkin, J.E. (1993) *Pulmonary Rehabilitation: Guidelines to Success*, Butterworth, London, with permission.)

- ↑ exercise capacity,
- ↑ quality of life scores,
- ↑ survival,
- ↑ activities of daily living (ADL),
- ↑ return-to-work statistics, and work itself increases self-esteem and confidence,
- ↓ acute episodes,
- ↓ breathlessness,
- ↓ anxiety and depression,
- ↓ cost, especially by reduced hospitalization (Fig. 6.1).

Positive outcomes depend on realistic expectations, good teamwork and follow-up.

Chronic lung disease links physical and psychological factors by a potent blend of breathlessness and chronic disability, so the attitude and encouragement of the rehabilitation team play a major role. Potential team members should be involved at the planning stage so that they have a vested interest in its success. The team can include physiotherapist, occupational therapist, respiratory nurse, clinical psychologist, physician and dietitian. The contribution of the patient and family is central.

Rehabilitation benefits people with COPD, asthma, bronchiectasis, CF, those recovering from lung surgery, long-term institutionalized patients (Schleifer *et al* 1994), and even the very elderly (Couser 1995). Smokers should not be excluded because helping them to quit is part of the programme, nor should hypercapnic patients be excluded because exercise does not appear to precipitate diaphragm fatigue (Celli 1994).

Rehabilitation is especially needed after exacerbation of disease when patients are at their most teachable, and particularly to prevent the stepwise loss of function that follows hospitalization (Peach and Pathy 1981). Pulmonary rehabilitation should be a routine not optional service and is best considered a form of preventive therapy. It is more effective in the early stages of disease, but patients are often more motivated when the disease is advanced.

After patient selection, a typical sequence is the following:

- assessment of patient needs,
- goal setting,
- development of individual treatment plan, including home programme,
- on-going re-assessment of goals achieved and adjustment of plan,
- follow up.

The following are needed for a programme based in a hospital or day centre:

- room with easily-opened windows, free from dust-collecting furniture, and acoustics that can cope with choruses of coughing,
- comfortable upright chairs,
- steps,
- high walking frame,
- full-length mirror,
- placebo inhalers,
- oxygen,
- oximeter,
- refreshments,
- crash trolley and team members trained in basic life support.

Ideally, there would be a maximum of eight patients, with stratified programmes for mild, moderate and severe disease. Sessions are best arranged twice weekly for a minimum six to eight weeks. A typical structure is an hour's discussion, a break for socializing, and an exercise session. There is a choice of the following:

- an outpatient programme,
- an inpatient programme, which is expensive and fosters dependency but is useful for those too breathless to travel, or

when diagnosis is uncertain or disease unstable,
- a home-based programme, which misses out on support between patients, but facilitates adaptation to an individual's environment and is necessary for severely disabled people.

The present tendency is to favour a home-based programme because of patient preference, cheapness and the ability to identify problems at an early stage.

Many centres do not have the resources to provide a full programme, but even a three-day scheme has been shown to satisfy over 90% of participants (Flanigan 1991). All people with chronic lung disease should have at least basic education and advice on exercise and self-management. What should never happen is the not uncommon scenario in which patients are admitted to a medical ward for review of treatment, get undressed, climb into bed and, after a week, are so deconditioned they can no longer cope when discharged home.

6.2 THE CONCEPT OF BREATHLESSNESS

It's very difficult not to panic when you're fighting for breath . . . you feel as if a vacuum is sucking the air out of you . . . it threatens your very existence . . . you're quite literally fighting for your life.

Patient quoted by Williams 1993

Breathlessness is like pain in that it is subjective and includes individual reactions to the feeling as well as the feeling itself. But it is more intractable than pain and commonly goes untreated. It is difficult for outsiders to identify with the breathlessness that is associated with disease because self-inflicted breathlessness, such as results from running for a bus, is of known duration and under control.

Breathing is normally unconscious. **Breathlessness** can be defined as awareness of the intensity of breathing. **Dyspnoea** is breathlessness that is laboured, distressing and usually, but not always, associated with effort (Demediuk *et al* 1992). In practice, the terms breathlessness and dyspnoea tend to be used interchangeably. They should be distinguished from the objective terms:

- **tachypnoea**: rapid breathing,
- **hyperpnoea**: increased ventilation in response to increased metabolism,
- **hyperventilation**: ventilation in excess of metabolic requirements.

6.2.1   Mechanism

A respiratory physiologist offering a unitary explanation for breathlessness should arouse the same suspicion as a tattooed archbishop offering a free ticket to heaven.

Campbell and Howell 1963

The mechanism of breathlessness is obscure and fascinating. There is little relationship between blood gases and breathlessness, which makes sense of the limited effectiveness of oxygen therapy for breathlessness (p. 90). Although hypercapnia and hypoxaemia may force people to breathe more deeply, they are not directly related to the subjective experience of breathlessness. A patient can be severely hypoxaemic without feeling short of breath, and vice versa.

Breathlessness relates to mechanical abnormalities and work of breathing. It correlates with motor output as reflected in the pressure generated by the respiratory muscles, which can be consciously perceived as a sense of effort (O'Donnell 1994). It is caused by one or a combination of the following:

- ↑ airflow resistance, e.g. obstructive lung disease,
- ↑ elastic load, e.g. rigid chest, distended abdomen, fibrotic lungs,
- ↓ energy supply, e.g. malnutrition, shock states in which perfusion to the diaphragm is impaired,
- ↓ power, e.g. neuromuscular deficiency, fatigue, weakness,

- ↑ drive to breathe, e.g. parenchymal lung disorders such as pulmonary oedema, fibrosing alveolitis or pneumonia (which stimulate nerve impulses from interstitial receptors), acidosis, anaemia, thyrotoxicosis,
- ↓ alveolar surface tension, e.g. pulmonary oedema, acute respiratory distress syndrome.

These mechanisms are often interlinked, e.g. ↑ airflow resistance causes ↑ drive to breathe (Duranti 1995).

The result is an effort to breathe that is not satisfied by the breathing that results, creating a deluge of impulses from the respiratory centre. This is perceived as the sensation of breathlessness. Inspiratory muscle fatigue magnifies the perception of effort in the same way that a suitcase feels heavier the longer it is carried. The perception of breathlessness is heightened by uncertainty, distress, anxiety (Muers 1993), past life experiences, frustration and lack of social support (Reardon 1994). Hence the variation between breathlessness and the effect on a person's lifestyle.

Acute asthma shows typically how a combination of factors may cause breathlessness:

- bronchial irritant receptors stimulate an abnormal drive to breathe,
- airway obstruction and inefficient breathing at high lung volumes increase the workload,
- anxiety triggers and sustains breathlessness.

6.2.2   Effects on the patient

It's the worst feeling in the world, the worst way to die, it's like smothering to death . . . to lose control of your breathing.

DeVito 1990

The experience of breathlessness can vary from feeling that breathing is no longer automatic, to total preoccupation and unremitting fear. Fear itself makes breathing more difficult, and patients often find it difficult to communicate their feelings. It can be frightening just to watch a breathless patient.

A degree of imaginative skill is needed by those working with people who are breathless. Lung disease is not blessed with high social standing. Other conditions may elicit more empathetic responses: for example, paraplegics are seen as brave, heart attacks are assumed to afflict high achievers, and a white cane elicits instant sympathy. People labelled as 'only bronchitic', however, are often elderly and depressed, they spit and wheeze, and anyway 'have they not brought it on themselves?'. This attitude is shared by some health workers. Not everyone can identify with the experience of spending night after night in a chair unable to sleep, or dreading the effort of going to the toilet, or anticipating the cruel slowness of death.

6.3 ASSESSMENT FOR REHABILITATION

Assessment needs to take account of:

- respiratory impairment: ↓ lung function,
- respiratory disability: the effect of this impairment, e.g. ↓ exercise capacity or anxiety,
- respiratory handicap: social and other disadvantages resulting from the environmental effects of the disability.

In other words, one breathless person may be handicapped while another with a similar degree of disability is not handicapped.

Patients are assessed as described in Chapter 2, with extra attention to the factors described below.

The case notes should be scrutinized for evidence that exercise training is safe. Contraindications include unstable angina, recent embolism or myocardial infarct, 2nd or 3rd degree heart block and deep vein thrombosis. Relative contraindications include disabling stroke or arthritis, intermittent claudication, metastatic cancer, unstable asthma, resting pulse rate > 120 bpm, and resting systolic pressure > 200 mmHg or diastolic > 110 mmHg (AARC 1992). Steroid-induced osteoporosis is not a contraindication, indeed this condition benefits from exercise. A $PaCO_2$ above 8 kPa (60 mmHg) requires liaison with the physician. The drug history is relevant:

- certain drugs render the BP and pulse unreliable for monitoring purposes (p. 159),
- if prescribed, bronchodilators and anti-angina drugs should be taken before exercise,
- steroids should be at the lowest effective dose to minimize the risk of muscle weakness.

Patients with heart failure take longer to recover from activity. Right heart failure is compatible with reasonable exercise, but left heart failure requires a limited programme.

Oximetry (p. 233) is advisable because the response to exercise is unpredictable. The oximeter should be validated under exercise conditions, and an ear sensor used in preference to a finger probe which is less accurate on exercise. Small oximeters can be clipped to a belt. Transient desaturation is acceptable, but if the SaO_2 stays below 85%, oxygen is required (Brannon *et al* 1993, p. 295).

If oximetry is not available, it is worth checking the respiratory function tests because a value for TLCO (p. 49) above 55% predicted indicates that desaturation is unlikely during exercise (Mak *et al* 1993). This suggests that diffusion characteristics play a role in exercise-induced desaturation.

Changes in breathlessness for an individual can be measured (Fig. 6.2). Function can be measured by a quality of life scale (Curtis 1994), rating scale (Hodgkin 1993, p. 481) or home-made questionnaire (Table 6.1). These are more relevant to the patient's needs than physiological change, but some scales may be influenced by patients stopping 'wanting' to do what they cannot do. Scales

Visual analogue scale

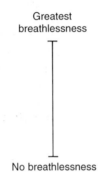

Greatest
breathlessness

No breathlessness

Breathlessness scale

1. Breathlessness with strenuous activity.

2. Breathlessness on stairs.

3. Breathlessness forcing patient to give up at least one activity.

4. Breathlessness forcing patient to abandon most activities or give up work.

5. Breathlessness on dressing, or preventing patient leaving home.

Figure 6.2 Measurements of breathlessness.

are most useful when they distinguish breathless and distress (Wilson and Jones 1991). Causes of distress include breathlessness itself, anxiety, fear, fatigue, weakness, embarrassment, frustration, dependency and loss of the capacity to be spontaneous.

It is helpful to ask patients how breathlessness affects their lives, and why they think they are breathless. Many patients are relieved when asked if their breathlessness is frightening, because they may not have heard this acknowledged before.

6.4   EDUCATION

Real education must entail emancipation: liberating people to make their own decisions on their own terms.

Fahrenfort 1987

Education is the most cost-effective aspect of a rehabilitation programme (Tougaard *et al* 1992), and its importance is underlined by current policies of early discharge from hospital. Education increases patients' confidence and reduces the uncertainty and fear that affects their quality of life (Small and Graydon 1992).

Education is not achieved by feeding information into an empty vessel and pressing the right buttons. It should encourage participation throughout. Age does not hinder intellectual ability, but elderly participants may need time for processing information. Hypoxaemia does not hinder mental speed but may impair memory. Retention of information is optimal if:

• the room is free of distractions,
• teaching sessions are brief,

Table 6.1 Questionnaire

How does your condition affect you?

Do you smoke?
If so, how many?
What do you understand about how smoking affects your health?

How often do you feel tired?
Do you find it exhausting to clear your chest?
How much exercise do you take?

How is your appetite?
What affects it?
What sort of food do you eat?

Do you get constipated sometimes?
If so, what do you do about it?

Which tablets or inhalers do you take?
What do you think each one does?

If you have oxygen at home, what flow rate do you use?
When do you use oxygen? (you can tick more than one):
• all the time
• at night
• at rest
• on exercise
• when you feel like it (describe what you feel)
• other (explain)

Does breathlessness make it difficult to do the following?
• dress
• wash/shower/bathe
• cook
• eat
• speak
• climb the stairs
• go to the toilet
• reach over your head
• go out, use public transport
• sleep
• other

How far can you walk?
Can you use stairs?
Do you use public transport?

How do you feel about your breathlessness?
Do you ever feel panic?
Do you ever feel:
• worried/frustrated/embarrassed/frightened/depressed/resentful?

What are you doing now to help your chest?
Do you know when you need to contact your GP?

• the teaching plan is set out clearly,
• the most important points are made first,
• language is simple, without jargon or abbreviations,
• advice for self-management is specific rather than general,
• information is reinforced regularly throughout the programme,
• booklets and handouts are included.

6.4.1 Motivation

The therapist–patient relationship can succeed or fail, depending on the care that the therapist takes in understanding the needs and circumstances of her patients.

Walker 1995

The essence of successful rehabilitation is motivation (Brannon *et al* 1993). Over 70% of patients with COPD do not comply with treatment (Mellins *et al* 1992) because of inadequate information, fear of breathlessness, depression or resentment.

It is natural for chronically disabled people to harbour resentment at their fate, which may be projected on to their family or any of the rehabilitation team. Allowing patients to talk gives them an opportunity to understand this process. If there is no appropriate outlet, the resentment turns inward and causes depression. People who are depressed usually respond to a receptive ear. Time is always needed when working with troubled people, but this is time well invested because little progress can otherwise be made.

Participants are unlikely to ignore their own beliefs and goals in order to follow a prescriptive approach. A hierarchical hospital environment tends to encourage passive obedience to authority, and some apparently compliant patients take up the sick role and assume that the experts know best. This is unhelpful in the rehabilitation process, and motivation is enhanced by participants taking responsibility for their own management.

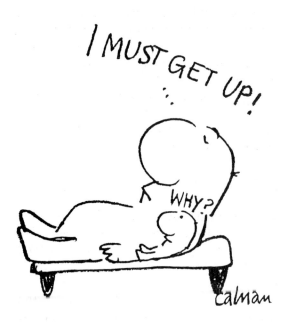

Factors that increase motivation are:

- realistic expectations,
- family involvement,
- verbal commitment from patients,
- praise, warmth, humour, honesty and responsiveness from the rehabilitation team,
- focus on health rather than disease,
- short simple regimes (Mellins *et al* 1992),
- active participation, e.g. invitations to question, comment, design programmes, contribute ideas,
- knowledge and understanding of the rationale of treatment,
- early success,
- access to notes (McLaren 1991),
- continuity of personnel,
- self-monitoring and autonomy, e.g. a written mutually-negotiated contract stating achievable and functional goals, the time to achieve them and the obligations of both patient and team.

Goals can be written into a large-print diary which logs daily exercise, symptoms, feelings, diet, drugs and side-effects, action

taken and the results. The achievement of the first goal gives a motivating boost.

Factors that decrease motivation are:

- fatigue,
- fear of failure,
- anxiety or depression,
- advice that is inconvenient or difficult to follow,
- embarrassment,
- boredom, e.g. repetitive exercise, 12-minute walking test, waiting for transport,
- coercion,
- lack of recognition of the individual as a whole.

Most participants are enthusiastic learners, and liberal use of teaching aids, using pictures rather then graphs, can explain the disease process in a way that is enjoyable. Enough detail is required only to understand symptoms and reduce anxiety.

6.4.2 Understanding reactions to the disease

Depression has been found in 63% of people with COPD (Hodgkin 1993, p. 280). It is so common that it is often accepted as a manifestation of the disease and not addressed, even though sleeplessness, poor appetite and low energy can sabotage rehabilitation. Anxiety is another frequent accompaniment to breathlessness and uncertainty.

Participants may not have considered the relevance of psychosocial factors to their disability, despite their myriad of feelings. Care should be taken in the use of language because the word 'psychological' may be interpreted as a psychiatric disorder, and the word 'disabled' is difficult for people who have not thought of themselves in this context. To use emotionally charged words without preparation is like using the word 'stump' to a new amputee.

It should be stressed that emotion is closely connected with breathing for all people including those with normal lungs, that it is natural for breathless people to feel depressed and anxious, and that it is an expression of humanity, not weakness.

Topics to discuss include:

- identification of stressors,
- recognition and management of depression (without taking comfort in smoking!)
- living with limitations,
- how to deal with panic during breathless attacks,
- the importance of activity and maintaining a social life,
- relationship with a partner, including concepts of guilt, dependence and resentment,
- relationships with others, coping with embarrassment or perceived stigma, e.g. how to explain about using oxygen or walking slowly, how to cope when the legitimacy of their 'invisible' condition if challenged.

Relationships may be affected by lack of spontaneity because breathless people often feel that they cannot waste breath in expressing anxiety, anger or happiness. Education and counselling for both partners can help prevent this emotional straight-jacket isolating them from those they need most.

The relevance of this topic is shown by evidence that attitudes and beliefs bear more relation to exercise tolerance than ventilatory capacity (Morgan *et al* 1983), and that denial reduces compliance (Borak *et al* 1991).

6.4.3 Sexuality

Sexuality and self-esteem are closely linked, and loss of sexual expression reinforces lack of confidence. Education can help discriminate between the effects of myth, illness and drugs on sexual activity. Myths perpetuated by society include the expectation that elderly people cannot have, do not want, or should not want sexual relations, and that disabled people are sexually neutered. Illness may cause deconditioning, breathlessness, fatigue

or poor self-image. Drugs such as some antihypertensives, antiulcer and cardiac drugs can affect sexual function, in which case a change in dose or type of drug may be indicated.

Many physiotherapists are comfortable to listen to patients talking about feelings, but patients can be referred for specialist help when appropriate.

6.4.4 Nutrition, fluids, drugs and oxygen

The role of the dietician is to identify individual nutrition problems, suggest six-meal-a-day menus, advise on healthy eating and explain which foods are mucus-forming, gas-forming, constipating or hard to digest.

Patients need to understand the effects and side-effects of drugs and oxygen therapy, the practicalities of equipment and the consequences of non-compliance. Further information is in Chapter 4.

6.4.5 Smoking withdrawal

There's nothing to giving up smoking. I've done it hundreds of times.

Mark Twain

Smoking cessation is the most important step in treating people with COPD, and 70% of smokers want to give up (Venables 1994). But their endeavours are hampered by the tenaciously addictive properties of nicotine, as well as less specific obstacles such as the comradeship enjoyed by smokers. Discussion is the most effective method (Clarke 1991), and physiotherapists are in an ideal position to contribute to the team effort, especially when hospitalization presents a 'teachable moment'.

Multiple reinforcements are more successful than relying on a single intervention, and every strategy for encouragement should be employed because failure drains the will. A

Stretching exercises are encouraged, e.g. trunk rotation, or pectoral stretch with the patient's hands on his or her lower back or standing in a doorway holding the door frame and leaning forwards. Other muscles that need stretching include the neck muscles, psoas, hamstrings and calf muscles.

Participants should be reminded of the following:

- avoid straining, pain or discomfort,
- keep movements relaxed and fluid, and allow the arms and legs to move independently of the body,
- be aware of the breathing pattern.

Music may be used for pleasure but not as a metronome. Participants should feel free to move at their own pace, or not join in if they wish. For severely breathless patients, the warm-up period is brief and may simply mean starting their modified exercise training slowly.

Exercise prescription

During activity, patients are discouraged from talking, rushing or breath-holding, which can disturb the breathing pattern and increase BP (Linsenbardt *et al* 1992). They are encouraged to take long comfortable strides and maintain a rhythmic quality of movement.

Four components make up the exercise prescription: mode, intensity, duration and frequency.

The **mode** of exercise should relate to the participants' lifestyles and be aerobic. Many choose walking or stair-climbing. Some prefer the stationary cycle or treadmill because they feel in control, have support for their shoulder girdle and can use oxygen easily. For treadmill walking, the speed is set at a minimum 0.9 mph and is increased by increments of 0.3 mph until participants feel they have reached their normal walking speed, then progression is by increasing treadmill elevation or speed. Others enjoy gym activities such as chair and floor exercises.

Arm exercises should be included in the programme for all participants (Celli 1994).

They help reduce the breathlessness associated with upper limb activities and have a carry-over effect on the respiratory muscles that can be equivalent to inspiratory muscle training (Hodgkin 1993, p. 275). Typically, patients lift a weight to shoulder level and down again for two minutes, in time with their breathing, followed by two minutes rest, the load being increased weekly.

A circuit of exercises, incorporating both mobility and strength, can be enjoyable and beneficial, including quadriceps and calf exercises, step-ups and wall press-ups.

Some patients enjoy exercising at the local leisure centre or swimming pool where the environment enhances compliance. Medical cover should be checked.

Three methods of prescribing **intensity** are used:

1. The predicted maximum HR can be estimated as either 220 minus age or as measured during an incremental stress test. Exercise is traditionally maintained at 70% of maximum HR, but this is often uncomfortable for respiratory patients, and a training effect can be achieved at 30–40% of maximum (Hellman 1994). HR is linearly related to $\dot{V}O_{2max}$ (p. 34), which can also be used to grade intensity. Multiples of $\dot{V}O_{2max}$ are sometimes expressed as METs (see Glossary), in which case prescription starts at 40% of maximal METs (Brannon *et al* 1993). These complicated methods are widely described, but are often considered invalid because:

   (a) many respiratory patients are too breathless to reach true maximal HR or $\dot{V}O_{2max}$,

   (b) HR is affected by cardiovascular drugs such as beta-blockers or digoxin,

   (c) even people with normal lungs show a wide variation in HR (Belman *et al* 1991).

Table 6.2 Perceived shortness of breath scale

1	Not breathless
2	Minimally breathless
3	Slightly breathless
4	Mildly breathless
5	Mildly to moderately breathless
6	Moderately breathless
7	Moderately to severely breathless
8	Severely breathless
9	Breathing not in control
10	Maximally breathless

As patients become familiar with the feelings associated with exercising at the appropriate target level, ratings from 4 (60% HR range) to 6 (85% HR range) define the appropriate level of exercise. Whichever of these the patient chooses, this is maintained while the level of exercise is gradually increased. (From Borg, G.A.V. (1982) Psychophysical bases of perceived exertion. *Med. Sci. Sport. Ex.*, **14**, 377–81, with permission.)

2. Exercise can be increased gradually by maintaining breathlessness at a constant tolerable level using a perceived shortness of breath scale (Table 6.2), while power output gradually increases. This is highly reproducible, correlates with physiological measures of exercise intensity, and even in people with normal lungs has been shown to result in greater improvement in endurance than using HR (Koltyn and Morgan 1992).

3. Patients can achieve a moderate training response if they are able simply to exercise briskly enough to increase breathlessness, again at a constant tolerable level, but avoid distress or desaturation.

The **duration** and **frequency** of training relate to the total amount of work done. Supervised training sessions usually last for 30 minutes, but for home practice sessions, respiratory patients find it more acceptable to exercise for one or more short sessions a day with brief warm up and cool down periods. Severely breathless people may prefer 'interval training', i.e. alternating periods of brief work and rest.

People who tend to rush at their exercise, in a fruitless attempt to get it over with, may find that counting with their steps helps them to pace themselves in the early stages, e.g. **in/ one**, **out/one**, or **in/one**, **out/one/two**. For others this disturbs their rhythm and distracts them from focusing on awareness of their breathing, level of effort and avoidance of fatigue.

Stair-climbing may be more efficient if performed by inhaling as the leg is raised, exhaling as the body is raised and interspersing every few steps with a rest. This may be slower than the patient's normal speed, but causes less distress and is compatible with exercise training if there is progression. Most patients find it best to exhale during the strenuous part of an activity.

Cool down

Patients are asked to slow down their activity for the cool-down period to prevent sudden pooling of blood in the lower extremities. They then rest, recheck their breathing pattern and fill out their exercise diary with a triumphant flourish. The diary includes the number of sessions per day, time taken per session, distance or number of steps and columns for suggested and actual programmes.

Progression

Patients progress by first increasing duration and then intensity (Brannon *et al* 1993, p. 291), usually in weekly increments. Daily practice sessions are preferable, e.g. a 20–30 minute walk, but success has been achieved with three low-intensity sessions a week lasting one to two hours each (Belman 1993). Improvement usually continues for four to six months, and when a plateau is reached, moderate exercise should be maintained for the rest of the patient's life at a minimum 15 minutes a day. An indoor programme is necessary when it is windy, rainy or smoggy.

Once a week, participants should put themselves back on the same programme as that of the final day of their training. If this is difficult, they have lost fitness and will need to increase their maintenance exercise. If training is interrupted by illness or holiday, the programme is restarted at a lower level. The difficult task of maintaining fitness needs follow-up from the rehabilitation team.

6.8   INSPIRATORY MUSCLE TRAINING

6.8.1   Rationale

There is conflicting evidence that respiratory disease can make inspiratory muscles either weaker or stronger than normal (Heidjra 1994), and that training can make the diaphragm either more or less susceptible to fatigue (Braun *et al* 1983).

Strong inspiratory muscles in respiratory disease are due to hypertrophy caused by working against the resistance of obstructed airways. Why therefore impose a further load?

Weak inspiratory muscles are due to:

- poor nutrition, which would respond better to dietary management, an intervention that can improve inspiratory muscle strength by 40% (Donahoe and Rogers 1990),
- inadequate oxygen delivery to the muscles due to heart failure and blood gas abnormalities, which respond better to fluid, drug and oxygen therapy.
- steroid induced weakness, which would respond better to drug review,
- mechanical disadvantage, which might be improved by breathing re-education (Martinez *et al* 1991).

A diaphragm that becomes more susceptible to fatigue after training is thought to have reached maximum adaptability and can improve performance no further. It is already chronically fatigued and is more likely to benefit from rest.

A diaphragm that becomes less susceptible to fatigue after training is in a fit state to adapt to the training stimulus and has achieved an optimum balance of supply and demand.

6.8.2   Effects

Having identified possible candidates for inspiratory muscle training (IMT), does this technique actually help them? There has been some debate over whether there is a purpose in improving inspiratory muscle endurance (Goldstein 1993), and there is limited evidence of clinically important benefit (Smith *et al* 1992). However, with rested and nourished patients, Weiner (1992) claims that IMT may improve exercise tolerance when combined with exercise training. With unsuitable patients, Jederlinic *et al* (1984) claim that IMT overrides the protective mechanism of fatigue and may cause exhaustion and desaturation.

6.8.3   Indications and contraindications

How can we select those patients with weak muscles for whom training might provide protection against chronic fatigue, and avoid overburdening those with fatigued muscles? The clinical symptoms of fatigue and weakness are similar, but the two states are distinguishable (p. 6). Fatigued muscles are unsuited to training, and overuse may split fibres, create 'use atrophy' (Braun *et al* 1983) and cause muscle damage (Anzueto 1992). Weak muscles may benefit from training, regardless of how breathless the patient is. Suitable candidates are:

- people who are fearful of any activity, because IMT can be used to desensitize them to breathlessness prior to venturing into exercise training,
- people who find breathing re-education difficult, in which case using the device might help to improve their breathing

pattern, before progressing to self-regulation of breathing.
• patients who enjoy it!

6.8.4   Method

Devices are cheap and simple. The principles are to increase the intensity of training, to alternate training with rest, and to avoid distressing levels of fatigue. For rested patients, a degree of acute fatigue is acceptable and, indeed, this itself can be a training stimulus. Intensity is increased by raising the resistance of the device and increasing the time.

Timing should increase from about five minutes twice a day to about 20 minutes three times a day. If the aim is to desensitize the patient to breathlessness, resistance should be at a level that leaves the patient slightly breathless. If the aim is to train the inspiratory muscles, resistance is set at 30% of maximum inspiratory pressure or MIP (p. 49) (Celli 1994), or a resistance is set that the patient can tolerate for 10 minutes (Brannon *et al* 1993, p. 391). For training, the programme should be maintained for life.

Patients should be relaxed but inhale with sufficient force to overcome the resistance. When patients have understood the technique, training can be combined with watching TV or reading. Compliance is reasonable when IMT fits into the patient's lifestyle and the resistance is not uncomfortably high. If oxygen is needed during training, nasal cannulae are used rather than entraining oxygen through the device, which upsets the resistance. Training diaries and further details of technique can be obtained from the manufacturers (Appendix C).

A **pressure-threshold** device incorporates a spring-loaded one-way valve which opens to permit airflow only when the preset inspiratory pressure has been reached. The load is independent of airflow and can be set at a percentage of MIP. This obliges the patient to generate a set inspiratory force with every

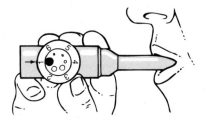

Figure 6.4 Pflex flow-dependent inspiratory muscle trainer.

breath and therefore creates a training effect. A **flow-dependent** device (Fig. 6.4) provides a resistance according to the size of various inspiratory orifices. The resistance can be altered by the flow rate, allowing patients to reduce the load with slow breaths. This is unlikely to produce a training effect so is best used for desensitization to breathlessness. Some PEP masks can be used as inspiratory muscle trainers by attaching a resistance to the inspiratory port.

Little work has been done on training the expiratory muscles, but for patients who actively recruit these muscles during expiration, benefit from blowing up balloons has been claimed (Chauhan *et al* 1992).

6.9   ENERGY CONSERVATION

Strategies to conserve energy tend to be used in the later stages of disease, but they are compatible with exercise training and, indeed, integral to it. Energy conservation gives patients greater control over how they achieve a balance of rest and exercise.

6.9.1   Activities of daily living

Occupational therapists are valuable allies in pulmonary rehabilitation. They assist patients to allocate selectively their diminishing energy by work simplification and appropriate aids such as trolleys, high walking frames and household gadgets.

If occupational therapy is not available, the physiotherapist can advise patients to:

- co-ordinate breathing with activity, e.g. inhale with pulling and exhale with pushing,
- move smoothly and eliminate unnecessary movement,
- plan in advance, allow time, pace activities and work in stages, organize the work space to reduce clutter and minimize reaching and bending,
- use a stool for kitchen work,
- rest elbows on the worktop for activities using the arms because even trivial upper limb tasks can cause distressing breathlessness,
- use non-iron clothes, an electric tooth-brush, casters under furniture, soap-on-a-rope, towelling bathrobes,
- develop economical lifting methods using leg power rather than the back and shoulders.

Advice needs to be individualized. Some people might find it more important to use their energy to get to the shops than to be independent with dressing. Some prefer to sleep downstairs rather than suffer the 'stigma' of a stairlift. Some find sitting in a shower easier than using a bath (Fig. 6.5), while others find that water on their face upsets their breathing. Some are not happy to have their spouse bath or dress them.

Participants share their own strategies, such as finding inconspicuous 'puffing stations' during shopping trips, e.g. by window shopping.

6.9.2 Stress reduction

Voluntary control of respiration is perhaps the oldest stress-reduction technique known. It has been used for thousands of years to reduce anxiety and promote a generalized state of relaxation.

Everly 1989

Breathing helps relaxation and relaxation helps breathing. People with chronic lung disease suffer muscle tension from stress,

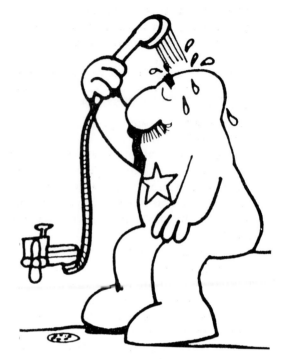

Figure 6.5 Energy conservation in the shower (Reproduced by permission from Moser, Kenneth M. *et al.* (1991) *Shortness of Breath: a Guide to Better Living and Breathing*, 4th edn, C.V. Mosby, St. Louis.)

breathlessness and the body positions needed to ease their breathing. The adverse physiological effects of stress are well-known (p. 216), and putting a tense person through a physical training programme without advice on stress reduction is silly.

Relaxation

Relaxation should be taught early in the programme so that it can be reinforced throughout. A variety of techniques are available (Payne 1995), and one should be chosen that does not encourage breath-holding, such as the physiological method (Mitchell 1987). Breathing itself can be used, e.g. by using the following suggestions:

1. Clear your chest if necessary to prevent disturbance by coughing.

2. Take up your preferred position (if this is sitting upright, it is advisable to supinate the forearms to discourage clinging to the chair arms).
3. Imagine that you are in a place that you find peaceful, such as a beach or sunny meadow.
4. Breathe abdominally (p. 114), if this is comfortable.
5. Feel where your body presses against the chair, allow the chair to do the work of your back muscles. As you breathe out, feel the tension leave your body. Feel your body melt into the chair as if you are meat without bone. Feel warm energy spreading through your body.
6. To help focus on your breathing and prevent your attention wandering, count silently as you follow your breath in: '1,2,3', and the same as you breathe out.
7. Check through your body for tension. Allow your mouth to fall slightly open. Re-check your breathing.

Rhythmic breathing and an adequate breathing rate should continue throughout.

Patients should be reassured that relaxation is not difficult to learn, that there is no right or wrong way of doing it, and that they can follow what feels right for them. Although it does not matter if they fall asleep, it is preferable to stay awake to enjoy the experience of alert tranquillity so that they can re-create it as desired.

The effects of this hypometabolic conscious state are decreased respiratory rate, oxygen consumption, heart rate and BP (Hodgkin and Petty 1987). Many find that it improves their breathing pattern without formal breathing re-education.

Daily practice is needed until the sensation is appreciated and the skill mastered, whereupon it is integrated into everyday life by identifying stressful situations and practising in different positions. In standing, patients can be asked to feel as if they have roots into the ground. Walking can become relaxed and comfortable. A few minutes at any time of day can be taken to check body tension. An illuminated aquarium is a blissful way of reducing stress at night.

Yoga

Yoga incorporates breathing techniques, meditation and postures that consume minimal energy. These induce physiological effects characteristic of deep relaxation, and one study shows them to improve lung function tests (Beck *et al* 1992).

Yogic breathing promotes breathing awareness, nose breathing and 'complete breathing', which begins with abdominal breathing, then expands the lower chest and finally the upper chest (Fried 1993, p. 239). Meditation reduces the respiratory rate, heart rate and BP (Fried 1993, p. 235).

Other therapies

It is useful to gain some knowledge of complementary therapies and local resources because patients sometimes request this information.

The Alexander technique uses inhibition of muscle tension to reduce the work of breathing and improve objective measures, such as peak flow and respiratory muscle strength (Austin and Ausubel 1992). Biofeedback gives auditory or visual feedback on, for example, muscle tension, so that participants can recognize the sensation and gain control over it (Hodgkin 1993, p. 404). Imagery uses visualization of peaceful scenes, which has been claimed to achieve the deeply relaxed alpha brain-wave state (Haas and Axen 1991, p. 285). Hypnotherapy reduces the metabolic rate through deep levels of relaxation (Sato *et al* 1986). Acupuncture works directly on reducing the perception of breathlessness and has been shown to increase exercise tolerance (Jobst *et al* 1986). According to Roth (1990) 'the best way to still the mind is to move the body', and activities such as circle dancing or t'ai Chi provide gentle exercise with a meditative effect. Many of these techniques also reduce hypertension (Stone and DeLeo 1976).

Mechanical rest

For chronically fatigued patients, nasal ventilation (p. 125) may be an integral component of rehabilitation.

6.10 HOME MANAGEMENT, SELF-HELP AND FOLLOW-UP

Follow-up plans should be set at the start of the programme. It takes a minimum of six weeks, and often longer, for participants to see an improvement in their condition. If expectations are not met, they may lose heart. Supervised training should be continued for a period after the initial programme to prevent detraining and demotivation (Swerts 1990), and follow-up in patients' homes, by telephone or newsletter, may be needed every two or three months, sometimes for years.

The home environment is where people feel most in control and are most responsive to advice, and home visits are especially useful for people who are elderly, anxious, forgetful, those using new equipment or those at the end-stage of disease. Home management is also supportive for the family. Spouses may be stressed, neglect their own health, feel guilty or be fearful of sleeping lest their partner die in the night. Children may lack attention and be caught up in conflicting emotions. Between visits, patients and their families should be offered a contact telephone number. Home visits also provide the opportunity to give advice on, for example:

- self-assessment, symptom management, recognition of the need for medical attention, e.g. a change in symptoms or new symptoms (Moser *et al* 1991, p. 98),

- prevention of infection, e.g. influenza vaccination, avoidance of people with respiratory infections,
- management of the environment, e.g. indoor exercise if the outside air is polluted, covering of nose and mouth when exercising in cold weather, bowls of water by radiators, prevention of dust,
- welfare rights (this needs corresponding advice to agencies on the needs of the unobtrusive respiratory patient),
- vocational guidance to improve self-esteem and social participation, while avoiding jobs with respiratory irritants or excess energy expenditure,
- tips such as a walking stick to advise motorists of a slow walking pace, advice to carers on simple massage techniques,
- advice for patients before visiting the doctor, e.g. write down questions to ask in advance, clarify points that are not understood,
- management of panic attacks, e.g. identification of trigger factors, strategies described in this chapter such as breathless management, breathing re-education and stress management, a reminder that rapid breathing is unnecessary during a panic attack and can be counterproductive, talking through helpful and unhelpful responses that the patient has developed, and physical rehearsals of the process of managing a breathless attack.

Mutual support between patients often begins spontaneously in waiting rooms, and may become one of the most constructive parts of the programme, providing practical assistance and reducing the social isolation into which many respiratory patients withdraw. This can be built into self-help groups in co-operation with organizations such as the British Lung Foundation (see Appendix C). Social outings, monthly lunches and annual celebrations may develop, which are

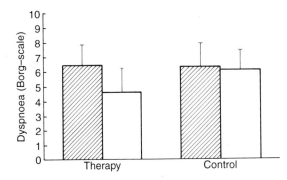

Figure 6.6 Pre- and postrehabilitation scores for dyspnoea, showing the effectiveness of breathing re-education, relaxation and exercise training. (Reproduced with permission from Strijbos, J.H. *et al.* (1989) Objective and subjective performance indicators in COPD. *Eur. Resp. J.*, **2**, 666.)

Improved lung function is not anticipated.

It is hoped that an abiding legacy of the programme is the friendship and courage that participants give each other. For those labouring under the double burden of disease and ageing, the outcome should be a more optimistic attitude towards a life that can be both active and fulfilling.

Western medicine has yet to make full adjustment to the increasing prevalence of chronic over acute disease, and tends to focus on illness rather than prevention and rehabilitation. Physiotherapists can play a part in educating others on the effectiveness of pulmonary rehabilitation by lecturing to medical and other students, initiating meetings with physicians and providing proof of cost-effectiveness to hospital managers (Figs 6.1 and 6.6 and Appendix E).

particularly supportive for people who do not like to be seen in public with their oxygen.

6.11 EVALUATION

Outcome measures include:

- comparison of questionnaires and breathlessness scores,
- number of participants completing the programme,
- diary review,
- medication, e.g. amount of antibiotics,
- GP visits or admissions to hospital,
- levels of anxiety and depression,
- independence in ADL,
- occupational performance,
- smoking,
- video evidence of improved flexibility, posture and gait,
- weight gain or loss as appropriate,
- specifically in relation to exercise training, ↑ walking distance, improved shuttle test, ↑ $\dot{V}O_{2max}$, ↓ exercise heart rate, ↓ blood lactate levels (Mohsenifar *et al.* 1983).

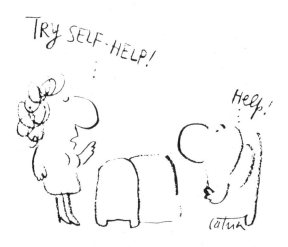

RECOMMENDED READING

(See also Appendix E)

Belman, M.J. (1993) Exercise in patients with COPD. *Thorax*, **48**, 936–46.
Carrieri-Kohlman, V., Douglas, M.K., Gormley, J.M. *et al.* (1993) Desensitization and guided mastery: treatment approaches for the management of dyspnea. *Heart Lung*, **22**, 226–34.

Celli, B.R. (1994) Physical reconditioning of patients with respiratory diseases: legs, arms and breathing retraining. *Respir. Care*, **39**, 481–99.

Chatham, K. (1995) Respiratory muscle training. *Br. J. Ther. Rehab.*, **2**(1), 31–6.

Clark, C.J. (1994) Setting up a pulmonary rehabilitation programme. *Thorax*, **49**, 270–8.

DeVito, A.J. (1990) Dyspnea during hospitalization for acute phase of illness as recalled by patients with COPD. *Heart Lung*, **19**, 186–91.

Gaskin, L. and Thomas, J. (1995) Pulse oximetry and exercise. *Physiotherapy*, **81**, 254–61.

Mellins, R.B., Zimmerman, B. and Clark, N.M. (1992) Patient compliance. *Am. Rev. Resp. Dis.*, **146**, 1376–7.

Nisell, O. (1992) Causes and mechanisms of breathlessness. *Clin. Physiol.*, **12**, 1–17.

O'Donell (1994) Breathlessness in patients with chronic airflow limitation. *Chest*, **106**, 904–12.

Peel, C. and Mossberg, K.A. (1995) Effects of cardiovascular medications on exercise responses. *Phys. Ther.*, **75**, 387–96.

Royal College of Physicians (1981) Disabling chest disease: prevention and care. *J. R. Coll. Physicians*, **15**, 69–86.

7. Physiotherapy for specific groups of people

7.1 PEOPLE UNDERGOING SURGERY

Keyhole technology has facilitated bedside surgery in the intensive care unit, and opened up surgery for those previously denied it because of disease or debility. It has also altered patients' requirements for physiotherapy. Physiotherapists working on a surgical ward need acumen in order to identify patients who need treatment, and empathy for the individual because what is routine for the physiotherapist is a unique event for each patient.

Everyone who has surgery could doubtless benefit from physiotherapy advice and care, but most physiotherapists select for treatment only those patients deemed to be at risk because of:

- pre-existing lung disease,
- surgery to the upper abdomen or chest,
- smoking history,
- advanced age,
- obesity,
- malnourishment,
- excess anxiety,
- prolonged preoperative stay,
- lengthy anaesthetic.

People who undergo lower abdominal surgery or who are otherwise not in a high-risk category gain from physiotherapy input into the team management of pain, positioning and handling.

7.1.1 Respiratory complications of surgery

The effect of an upper abdominal incision seems to strike at the root of normal respiration.

Bevan 1964

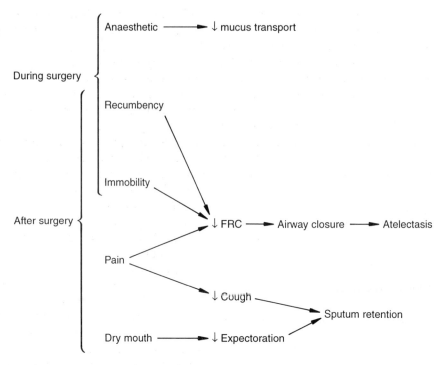

Figure 7.1 Interrelation of factors affecting postoperative lung function.

The respiratory system bears the brunt of the after-effects of surgery, the cause being mechanical rather than infective. Postoperative complications are described below.

Atelectasis is the commonest respiratory complication and is caused largely by pain (Simpson *et al* 1992). Following chest or abdominal surgery, pain leads to guarding spasm of the trunk muscles, inhibition of breathing; tidal breathing falling into the closing volume range, airway closure and atelectasis (Fig. 7.1).

Other causes of atelectasis are:

- prolonged recumbency, which affects the amount and distribution of ventilation and causes intrathoracic pooling of blood which further displaces air from the lung,
- loss of oscillations in tidal volume and occasional sighs which normally punc-

tuate breathing and stimulate surfactant production.

Mucus plugs are usually caused by atelectasis rather than the other way round, so their removal rarely leads to recruitment of collapsed alveoli (Susini *et al* 1992).

Atelectasis creates a restrictive lung defect and reduces lung compliance. A degree of atelectasis occurs in 95% of postoperative patients (Westbrook and Sykes 1992) and is clinically significant when there are X-ray changes and reduced breath sounds. It can be prevented by measures to increase lung volume. Greater efforts are needed to inflate collapsed alveoli than to inflate those that are partially open. Prevention is therefore better than cure.

Hypoxaemia is caused by the shunting of blood through airless lung. When present for a few hours it is related to the anaesthetic. When present for several days, it is related to the operation and the patient (Hudes 1989). High-risk patients may suffer nocturnal hypoxaemia for up to five nights after surgery due to rebound intense REM sleep to make up for earlier disrupted sleep (Roberts *et al* 1993). Patients who have had major surgery, or those with respiratory or cardiovascular disease, should be monitored for nocturnal oxygen desaturation to prevent premature cessation of oxygen therapy. Postoperative hypoxaemia impairs healing, promotes infection and contributes to postoperative confusion (Hanning 1992).

Chest infection may occur several days after surgery. Atelectasis can predispose to chest infection, but has different risk factors and the two are distinct (Dilworth and White 1992). Fever indicates infection but is not associated with atelectasis (Brooks-Brunn 1995).

Respiratory depression can be caused by toxic levels of opioids (p. 175).

Postoperative deterioration in lung function reaches a maximum within 48 hours of surgery. However, it may not be significant and many patients leave hospital happily ignorant that they still have a degree of hypoxaemia.

7.1.2 Other complications of surgery

Fatigue, usually related to the degree of trauma, is more severe and prolonged than expected by most patients. It can be minimized by encouraging frequent short walks rather than infrequent long ones, and by negotiating with patients rather than imposing a programme on them.

Some drugs contribute to the 'big little problem' of postoperative **nausea**. This is experienced by 30% of patients and is most common after lengthy surgery, if there is pain or dizziness and for patients who are anxious or obese or female. Nausea inhibits deep breathing. It can be relieved by drug review (Watcha and White 1992), powdered ginger (Phillips 1993), hydration, pain relief, or acupressure to P.6 located two thumbs'

width above the distal crease on the inner wrist in line with the middle finger (McMillan 1994).

Anxiety increases diaphragmatic splinting and stimulates metabolic and hormonal stress responses which delay healing and promote infection (Salmon 1992). Anxiety is reduced by giving preoperative information and granting postoperative autonomy.

Depression may occur if surgery causes mutilation or altered body image, e.g. colostomy, head and neck surgery or mastectomy. An understanding ear or referral to a self-help group (Appendix C) may prevent a sense of loss degenerating into long-term depression.

Paralytic ileus is loss of gut activity and bowel sounds. It is normal for the first day or two, but may last longer after abdominal surgery, leading to restricted diaphragmatic movement, a nasogastric tube and nil-by-mouth requirements.

Fluid imbalance can lead to hypovolaemia or fluid overload. Hypovolaemia is due to pre- and postoperative fluid restriction, the drying effect of premedication and unhumidified anaesthetic gases. It can cause desaturation even if gas exchange is not impaired (Westbrook and Sykes 1992). Fluid overload is due to overenthusiastic fluid replacement.

Postural hypotension may be a sign of unrecognized hypovolaemia. Such patients should avoid sudden motion or position change.

Urine retention, **flatulence** or **constipation** impair excursion of the diaphragm. Urine retention can be helped by acupressure to Ki.1 in the hollow proximal to the mid-transverse arch of each foot. Flatulence can be relieved by pelvic tilting and knee rolling in crook-lying.

Hypoxaemia increases the risk of **wound infection** (Whitney 1989), which is suspected if there is increased pain, pyrexia and erythema.

Incessant **hiccups**, due to irritation of the diaphragm, cause sharp pain at the wound site. They may be inhibited by metoclopramide, chlorpromazine, sugar, acupressure to CV.17 (on the sternum at mid-nipple level), an array of techniques to raise $PaCO_2$ (breath-holding, rebreathing, drinking a glass of water from the wrong side), dropping a piece of ice down the back to hyperextend the neck, or prayers to St Jude, the patron saint of lost causes.

Deep vein thrombosis (DVT) is a blood clot that develops surreptitiously in the lower limb, often during surgery, due to calf compression, immobility and impaired blood flow. It complicates one-fifth of major operations (Ashby 1995), but is notoriously under-diagnosed, being clinically silent in 50% of patients (Forbes 1994). It may become evident as tenderness, swelling and warmth of the calf, generalized fever and sometimes pain on dorsiflexion (Homan's sign). Diagnosis can be confirmed by ultrasound or Doppler imaging (Goldhaber and Morpurgo 1992). The clot may break free and cause **pulmonary embolism** by lodging in the pulmonary vascular bed (p. 86).

Postoperative **haemorrhage** leads to any of the following signs:

- obvious bleeding,
- rapid filling of drainage bottles,
- signs of hypovolaemic shock, which suggest internal bleeding.

7.1.3 Preoperative management

Stress increases postoperative complications, lengthens hospital stay (Liu 1994) and is thought to contribute to muscle breakdown, delayed healing and immunosuppression (Salmon 1992). Preoperative instruction is aimed at reducing this stress and enhancing co-operation for postoperative care. Instruction has been shown to lessen postoperative complications (Cupples 1991), increase ability to deep breathe and cough (Lindeman 1971), reduce analgesic requirements by half and lead to discharge nearly three days earlier (Egbert *et al* 1964). It is especially important

for children and those expecting to wake up in the intensive care unit, where they will feel relieved at the sight of a familiar face. For anxious patients facing major surgery, it should be carried out early because anxiety at impending surgery inhibits receptivity (Cupples 1991).

Some patients find it beneficial to have relatives present for the preoperative visit. The visit is mainly educational and can be brief. It includes:

1. Patient assessment.
2. Explanations, i.e:
    (a) inactivity leads to inadequate lung expansion, so that mobilization and sometimes deep breathing are needed after the operation,
    (b) if there is extra sputum, coughing may be necessary,
    (c) prevention forms the basis of management.
3. Advice to ask for adequate pain relief.
4. Information specific to the operation. Most patients like to know everything about the wound, drips, drains and what it will feel like, while a few make it clear that they want to know little. People undergoing complex procedures may benefit from visits by patients who have had similar surgery.
5. Advice to keep active before surgery and, if applicable, to stop smoking. Just 24 hours' abstinence from smoking improves the patient's cardiovascular status (Munday *et al* 1993), and this includes no passive smoking in the ward day room (Dennis 1994).
6. For high-risk or anxious patients, practice in how to roll, deep breathe, use the incentive spirometer, sit up and cough with minimum pain.
7. Any questions?

People with lung disease may need attention to sputum clearance and an exercise regime to compensate for the inactivity of hospitalization.

Anxious people benefit from relaxation (Mogan *et al* 1985), but mindless reassurance does not engender trust, and can impair the 'work of worry', which is a natural and necessary part of adjusting to the operation and its outcome. Postoperative distress is related to lack of accurate anticipation and knowledge (Salmon 1992).

The tradition of prolonged preoperative fluid restriction is now considered unjustified. Clear oral fluids up to two hours before surgery improves comfort, reduces dehydration and makes it easier to expectorate postoperatively without compromising safety (Phillips *et al* 1993).

Before surgery, pre-emptive analgesia reduces postoperative pain by preventing noxious impulses gaining entry into the central nervous system, where they 'wind up' the response to subsequent afferent inputs. This memory of pain can be prevented by adding, for example, anti-inflammatory drugs to the premedication or using preoperative nerve blocks. Drug dosage to prevent pain is significantly less than that required to abolish pain after it has occurred (Katz *et al* 1994). A notable illustration of this is the elimination of postamputation pain syndromes by epidural analgesia up to three days preoperatively (Cousins 1989).

Postoperative recovery can be facilitated by factors as diverse as a leafy view through the window (Ulrich 1984) and positive suggestions under anaesthesia (Williams *et al* 1994).

7.1.4 Pain management

What is so surprising is that this deplorable state of affairs has persisted and continues to persist in many hospitals, despite considerable advances in the pharmacology of analgesic drugs.

Smith 1991

Postoperative pain is notorious for being widespread and unnecessarily severe. Possible reasons for this 'deplorable state of affairs' are the following:

1. Inexperience, tradition and overwork (Justins and Richardson 1991).
2. Ignorance of the fact that addiction occurs in less than 1 in 3000 people who take analgesic drugs (Lavies 1992).
3. Wide and unpredictable variations in patients' perception of pain and response to drugs.
4. An attitude that pain is unimportant, inevitable and to be borne with fortitude, especially in cultures which see stoicism as a virtue and distress as a weakness. Patients' own low expectations have allowed this situation to continue without an outcry (Lavies 1992).
5. Rudimentary pain assessment.

Pain is what the patient says hurts, but some staff have a limited understanding of the subjective nature of pain and may disbelieve patients. McCaffery and Ferrell (1992) found that 50% of nurses doubted patients' reports, and it is common to hear criticism of patients for having a 'low pain threshold' or being 'naughty' for complaining of pain. Pain is more than a sensation, it is the reaction to that sensation. It is a personal experience. It may be difficult for us to accept the reality of a patient's distress because it is frustrating to feel helpless and easier to deny it by assuming that patients are making a fuss. But we do not serve our patients well if we allow ourselves to lose our sensitivity and become part of a system that can actually shame patients who express pain.

Whose pain should the physician control? The patient's? That of the relatives? Or his own, generated by his inability to help the patient?

Szasz 1968

Pain and breathing

The relationship between pain and atelectasis (Fig. 7.2) can be understood readily by

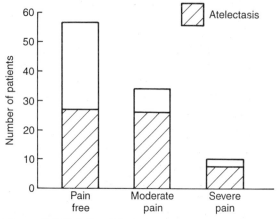

Figure 7.2 Relationship between postoperative pain and atelectasis. (From Embling, S.A. (1985) Incidence, aetiology and implications of atelectasis following cardiopulmonary bypass surgery, MSc dissertation, University of Southampton, with permission.)

anyone trying to take a deep breath when in the dentist's chair. Pain not only inhibits breathing, it also increases oxygen consumption and risk of infection, delays healing and postpones mobilization and hospital discharge (Carron 1989).

Assessment

Accurate assessment of patients in relation to both pain and respiration allows logical decisions to be made about management, with the help of the patient who will have his or her preferences. It also prevents unnecessary interventions, such as asking a patient with no secretions to cough.

Postoperative pain should be assessed and recorded on the patient's chart like any other vital sign in consultation with the nursing team. A visual analogue scale or flow chart (Gould *et al* 1992) can be used to assess pain at rest and, more importantly, during activity. Interactive computer animation (Swanston 1993) assesses pain for computer buffs.

If pain cannot be assessed by the patient, objective signs are pallor, sweating, shallow breathing, breath-holding and ↑ pulse, BP and respiratory rate. Severe pain causes nausea, vomiting and ↓ pulse and BP.

Pain assessment is also a right for people who are cognitively impaired or do not speak English, not just those who can complain in a way that is easy to understand. Family members can be involved in assessment if appropriate. Elderly people tend to be stoic about reporting pain and are at risk of undertreatment. Pain assessment for children and infants is on p. 291.

Reduction in the perception of pain

There are many things that make pain worse, such as the spirit in which it is inflicted. You are indeed acutely vulnerable to the attitude of people surrounding you.

Donald 1977

Perception of pain varies with some factors that physiotherapists cannot modify, such as type of incision, operative technique, discomforts such as drainage tubes and nasogastric tubes, and the patient's upbringing and previous experiences. Perception of pain also varies with factors that physiotherapists can modify, such as:

- anxiety or fear,
- discomfort,
- physical tension,
- lack of autonomy or privacy,
- depression,
- sleep fragmentation (McIntosh 1989).

This is fertile ground for the physiotherapist. Physical tension can be eased by simple relaxation (Miller and Perry 1990). Anxiety can be reduced by keeping patients informed. Autonomy can be enhanced by including them in decisions. Above all, patients need reassurance in words and actions that they will be heard and responded to. 'Tell me if it hurts and I'll stop' is music to their ears.

Handling patients in pain

. . . pain works subversively, undermining one's self-confidence and self-control, worn dismayingly fragile. The sense of anticipation is honed, to hysteria almost, and one quickly learns to be thoroughly suspicious of the well-meant: 'this won't hurt'.

Brooks 1990

Physiotherapists should be seen as experts in the relief of pain rather than its perpetrators. The essence of physiotherapy is skilful handling, and there are few rewards greater than relief on the face of a patient whose pain we have alleviated. Guidelines are the following:

1. Most importantly, patients must be assured that they are in control.
2. Analgesia should be given automatically before physiotherapy, instead of first 'checking' to see if treatment causes pain, a strategy known as shutting the stable door after the horse has bolted.
3. Unnecessary handling should be avoided.
4. The patient should be informed of why, how and when each movement will take place. Words to avoid are 'just relax', which signals to any seasoned patient that they are about to be hurt, or 'sorry' after an unexpected movement instead of clear explanations before the movement. The 'wince-sorry' scenario is familiar to those who have witnessed patients being hurt and then routinely apologized to.

The principles of handling patients in pain are to offer them advice and support, but allow them to move themselves as much as possible, for example:

Long-sitting to lying (Fig. 7.3). Patients are asked to push back against the physiotherapist's hand and forearm so that they are actively using their back extensors and therefore reciprocally relaxing their abdominal muscles. Reassurance is needed so that patients push back hard enough to eliminate eccentric abdominal muscle work. Physiotherapists need the support of their knee and fist on the bed to protect their own back. This principle can also be used for helping a long-sitting patient to lie back on to the pillow after he or she has leant forwards for auscultation.

Rolling (Fig. 7.4). Patients are asked first to bend their knees, then remain in supine but shift away from the physiotherapist to make room to roll. They then hold on to the physiotherapist's arm or a bed rail, push with their knees and roll towards the physiotherapist in one piece. They are encouraged to emphasize pushing with their legs rather than pulling with their arms in order to inhibit abdominal muscle work. Again the physiotherapist uses a fist on the bed for support.

Medication

It is an ethical obligation at the core of a health professional's commitment to ensure that patients have access to the best level of pain relief that can safely be provided.

Carson 1994

Physiotherapists must be active team members to ensure that analgesics are based on the principle that prevention is better than cure. Lack of teamwork and understanding have led to patients receiving one-quarter of the dose prescribed (Rosenberg 1992), male doctors assuming that patients feel less pain than female doctors, and senior nursing staff allowing patients less medication than juniors (Pitts and Healey 1989). An acute pain team is invaluable (Gould *et al* 1992).

Morphine remains the favourite opioid analgesic. Side-effects include nausea, constipation, hypotension and elimination of spontaneous sighs. An exaggerated fear of the side-effects of respiratory depression and dependence often leads to inadequate dosage. Large doses of morphine depress respiration, but sedation is not synonymous

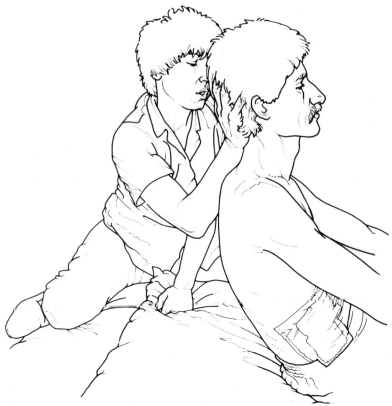

Figure 7.3 Helping a patient from long-sitting to lying. The helper needs the support of her knee and fist on the bed.

with respiratory depression (Pasero 1994), and hypoventilation is an unreliable and late sign. However, if breathing is shallow, irregular or less than 10 breaths/minute, the doctor should be informed. Oximetry is helpful. Depression of respiration is reversible by the opiate antagonist naloxone without loss of analgesia. Opioid dependence is rare unless administration is continuous in a patient who has no pain (Aitkenhead 1989). Well-managed narcotic drugs improve ventilation and gas exchange when breathing is made easier by relief of pain (Harcus 1977). Vickers (1992) claims that the opioid tramadol does not depress respiration. Non-steroidal anti-inflammatory drugs engage the peripheral as well as the central nervous system and can reduce opioid requirements by over 20% (Cashman 1993).

Intramuscular route Use of the time-honoured 'p.r.n.' intramuscular injection is widespread despite being the least effective mode of pain relief. This 'as required' analgesia has no rational basis, is usually interpreted as 'give as little as possible', produces wide fluctuations in serum levels, leaves pain unrelieved in half the recipients (Jacox *et al* 1992) and augments a vicious cycle of anxiety and pain, especially in patients who do not want to appear demanding. P.r.n. analgesia is berated in the literature, but popular because it is considered, mistakenly, to be the safest regime. Uncomfortable patients also use more staff time.

Regular, intermittent dosage is more effective than the p.r.n. regime because it takes less time to prevent pain than to subdue it,

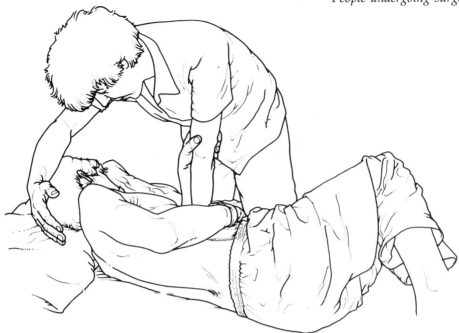

Figure 7.4 Helping a patient to roll into side-lying. The patient is given control, rather than being manoeuvred into position.

but dosage may still be inadequate and lead to 'spectacularly ineffective' outcomes because of wide variations in uptake, distribution and elimination of an intramuscular drug (Hull 1988). Blood concentration varies by at least a factor of five, and even if this variable is overcome, the concentration at which each individual becomes pain free varies by a factor of three or four (Justins and Richardson, 1991).

Intravenous route The intravenous route gives superior pain relief, works immediately and provides either a continuous infusion or bolus doses. Patient-controlled analgesia (PCA) delivers a preset dose of drug by a syringe pump when the patient presses a button. This accommodates to individual need, reduces anxiety, encourages mobility, reduces sleep disturbance, is preferred by patients for the autonomy it allows, requires less drug to achieve the same pain control and leads to earlier discharge (Thomas, 1995). A programmed lock-out interval ensures that each dose achieves peak effect before the next

dose is released. Respiratory depression is rare, although oximetry is advisable if the patient has limited understanding and staffing levels are low. PCA does not reduce the incidence of nausea, which can be avoided by adding antiemetics to the PCA (Barrow *et al* 1994). Relatives should be warned not to press the button.

Regional analgesia Transmission within the peripheral nervous system can be blocked by regional techniques. These act locally, do not befuddle the entire central nervous system and cause less nausea.

Intercostal nerve blocks are used after unilateral abdominal incisions, thoracotomy or rib fractures. They are administered by repeated injections into multiple nerves or, more comfortably, by continuous infusion or extrapleural infusion (Majid 1992). Respiration is not depressed, but pneumothorax is a risk and the X-ray should be scrutinized if any positive pressure techniques are anticipated.

The **epidural** route alters spinal processing by delivering drugs to the epidural space, the catheter being left *in situ*. Opiates, local anaesthetic or both work directly on the opiate receptors along the spinal cord, and can control pain originating anywhere below the cranial nerves. In increasing order of efficacy, administration is by intermittent blockade, continuous infusion or PCA (Owen *et al* 1993).

Advantages of epidurals are legion: prolonged pain relief, improved lung function, ↓ oxygen consumption, ↓ incidence of DVT and infection, hospital stay shortened by an average of a week (Smedstad 1992), and an increase in graft blood flow after vascular surgery (Cousins 1989). Disadvantages are partial sensory or motor loss, and blockade of sympathetic outflow which is especially noticeable in hypovolaemic patients. Patients should, therefore, lie flat for 30 minutes after a top-up to avoid hypotension. High blocks are mainly associated with hypotension, while blocks further down the spinal cord may cause urine retention. Respiratory depression is found in fewer than 1% of cases, usually occuring within ½–1 hour of a top-up or 6–12 hours later (Jacques 1994), and is reversible with naloxone. Other epidural side-effects are nausea and paralytic ileus.

The **intrathecal** route delivers opioids to the subarachnoid space (Grace and Orr 1993), producing profound analgesia without motor, sensory or sympathetic block. Complications include 'spinal headache' due to CSF leakage through a punctured dura and loss of the intracranial CSF 'cushion'. If this occurs during mobilization, the patient should be returned to bed.

Further measures for one-sided surgery include the **paravertebral** route, which combines the effects of epidural and intercostal analgesia, **intrapleural**, which provides a continuous intrapleural infusion of local anaesthetic (Kavanagh 1994), **extrapleural** or **extradural** routes. Pneumothorax is a risk.

Oral drugs can be used several days after surgery if acute pain has subsided, but the effect is variable.

The **transdermal** route uses skin patches for trauma-free, safe, but slow-acting analgesia (Arts 1994) or antiemesis (Biddle 1992). EMLA (eutetic mixture of local anaesthetics) cream causes skin anaesthesia when applied to the skin an hour before a painful procedure, and no child should now be submitted to venepuncture, lumbar puncture or any injection without prior application of this 'magic cream'. Needle-phobic adults also benefit. It is considered risky for neonates.

Non-invasive sophistication is taken further by **iontophoresis** of local anaesthetics, which penetrates deeper than EMLA cream and is effective within 10 minutes (Irsfeld *et al* 1993).

The **transmucosal** route uses the mucous membranes, which impose less of a barrier than skin and allow speedy drug absorption (Striebel 1993), as cocaine abusers have discovered. Sublingual administration has meant that children now delightedly anticipate their postoperative fentanyl 'lollipops' (Yaster 1995).

Cryoanalgesia

Pain after thoracotomy or rib fracture can be eliminated by cryoanalgesia, an open procedure which freezes the intercostal nerves and then allows them to thaw, creating total pain relief by rendering the area anaesthetic. The nerve regenerates and sensation returns after a period of between two weeks and several months, but 20% of patients develop neuralgias (Kavanagh 1994).

Entonox

Short-lived analgesia can be achieved within 60 seconds of inhaling a 50% mix of nitrous oxide and oxygen (Entonox), delivered from a cylinder via face mask and demand valve. It is not metabolized and is eliminated unchanged by the lungs. Side-effects on the cardiovascular and respiratory systems are minimal (Sacchetti 1994), but the patient may feel light-headed, drowsy or nauseous. A gratifying side-effect is the maintenance of a normal FRC, which would otherwise be reduced by an average of 22% in narcotic-treated patients (Kripke *et al* 1983). It is suitable for children as well as adults (Lawler 1995).

If used continuously for over 12 hours, minor bone marrow changes occur (Austin 1993), but this is not a problem with physio-therapy because only a few minutes' inhalation is necessary. Despite its 175-year history, Entonox is still not utilized for the many minor but distressing hospital procedures for which it is ideal. Depending on local policy, it may or may not need medical prescription, but medical staff must sanction its use (Lawler 1995). The initiative usually comes from the physiotherapist. Contraindications are:

1. Acute head injury or low cardiac output, because of peripheral vasodilation.
2. Sealed pockets of air (e.g. subcutaneous emphysema, bullae, pneumothorax, bowel obstruction, ear surgery or balloon-tipped catheters), because nitrous oxide is 32 times more soluble than air and readily diffuses into gas-collecting areas. The X-ray of a patient with fractured ribs should be checked before using Entonox in case of pneumothorax.

Other precautions relate to the 50% oxygen content, so that Entonox is unsuited to patients who need more than 50% oxygen, or hypercapnic COPD patients dependent on a hypoxic drive to breathe. They require a different mix, to be re-prescribed.

Transcutaneous nerve stimulation (TNS)

TNS is underused in postoperative care. It does not depress the respiratory system, is non-invasive, non-toxic, cheap and produces mobile and happy patients. It is best used as prevention rather than as a last resort, and high-risk patients should be identified early.

Effects Effectiveness varies between patients, and TNS is normally used as an adjunct to analgesic drugs, but one study has reported 95% of postoperative patients needing no narcotics when using TNS (Bayindir 1991). Agreeable side-effects include reduction in nausea and paralytic ileus (Akyüz 1993).

Mechanism TNS is thought to reduce pain by:

- at high frequencies, closure of the pain gate by stimulating large nerve fibres to override pain input from small fibres,
- at low frequencies, the release of endorphins (Han *et al* 1991).

Other theories are that peripheral nerves are fatigued by repeated stimulation or that sympathetic overactivity is suppressed (Marshall 1991).

Method The skin is washed to minimize irritation. It is then checked for sensation because anaesthetic areas do not respond to TNS, while stimulating areas of hyperaesthesia worsens pain. Gel is applied evenly and electrodes fixed securely. Two or four electrodes are applied, close to each corner of the incision, as soon as possible after surgery. Acupuncture points can be stimulated instead of local areas. If sterile electrodes are used, two long electrodes are applied in theatre alongside the wound and under the dressing, with the controls set at a level that has been determined before surgery.

When adjusting the controls, individual needs vary, but most patients find the following sequence successful:

1. Increase output (amplitude) slowly until a mild thumping is felt.
2. Move the rate (frequency) dial around its full extent to find the most comfortable adjustment. If more than half the full

extent is achieved without any sensation, a pulse width adjustment is needed.
3. Readjust output for maximum relief of pain and optimum comfort of the sensation.

No motor contraction should be felt, and patients need a reminder that a stronger stimulus does not mean stronger pain relief. Readjustment is necessary as the patient adapts to the sensation or becomes more awake. Some machines provide a pulsed or boost mode to reduce accomodation, and the patient can use this when moving or coughing, or the connector pins on the machine can be changed at intervals to reverse polarity. Patients can adjust their own controls, decide how many days to continue using the machine, and whether to use it at night. Liaison with nursing staff and daily skin washes are needed.

Problems

1. Gel or adhesive tape can irritate the skin. This is dealt with by using self-adherent electrodes, a stockinette-type bandage instead of tape, changing the electrode position frequently or using different gel.
2. TNS near the chest is contraindicated for people using a demand or synchronous pacemaker.
3. Stimulation should not be applied over a pregnant uterus or damaged skin.
4. TNS electrodes should be placed as far as possible from ECG electrodes to minimize interference.

7.1.5 Postoperative care

Details of techniques to increase lung volume are covered in Chapter 5, but points specific to surgery are discussed below.

Aspects of assessment

Assessment is particularly relevant in this area because many patients will need no treatment other than a reminder to keep mobile. As well as the assessment described in Chapter 2, a few other points should be noted.

The temperature chart will normally show a slight pyrexia following surgery as a reaction to tissue trauma, but fever beyond 48 hours raises suspicions of a chest infection.

Is oxygen titrated to the patient's needs? Does the mask stay on and, if not, does the patient need explanations, adjustment for comfort or replacement with a nasal cannula?

Nasogastric tubes are often present for feeding or to prevent vomiting and gastric distension, and although necessary, they indicate that coughing will be more difficult and the protective oesophagogastric sphincter will be disabled so that the lung may be colonized with bacteria from the stomach.

Mobilization

Bed mobility and independence are encouraged by a rope attached to the end of the bed, by which patients pull themselves up. As soon as possible they can be encouraged to sit with legs dangling over the edge of the bed.

If early mobilization is surgically or medically acceptable, this should be on the first postoperative day. Extra care is needed during the first walk because of postural hypotension associated with fluid shift to the thorax during recumbency. For catheterized patients, leg bags are more convenient and dignified than loose catheter bags. Posture correction is incorporated as soon as discomfort has eased.

Positioning

If pain, surgical procedure or instability delay mobilization, emphasis should be on accurate and comfortable positioning, alternating from side to side and, if possible, sitting out of bed. Positioning itself can re-expand atelectatic lung (Westbrook and Sykes 1992), but regular position change is needed to prevent atelectasis reappearing in dependent zones.

Breathing exercises

Breathing exercises are not usually necessary even after major surgery (Stiller *et al* 1994), but if mobilization is delayed, positioning limited, or respiratory complications develop, deep breathing may be required. This should be done in a position that achieves a balance between comfort and optimal ventilation. For patients who can neither mobilize nor lie well forwards on their side, incentive spirometry in upright sitting is advisable. A transmural pressure close to $20 \, cmH_2O$ is needed to open atelectatic areas, which corresponds to inspiration near TLC (Andersen *et al* 1979).

Cilia are immobilized by general anaesthesia, but accumulated secretions are usually cleared by mucociliary transport in the immediate postoperative period. Superficial secretions in the throat may be the only problem, which are easily removed by throat-clearing. Stronger expiratory manoeuvres should not be routine, because expiration beyond FRC causes airway closure, which is not easily reversible in patients who are weak and in pain (Craig 1981). Forced expiration, unnecessary coughing, percussion and vibrations cause pain and splinting, and may simply produce the lesion that they are supposed to cure.

If there is subjective or objective evidence of accessible secretions and coughing is necessary, patients may prefer to remain in side-lying, but if they are willing, sitting over the edge of the bed is mechanically efficient and allows for maximum support (Fig. 7.5). Pressing on the incision with a pillow is less effective than sensitive and accurately-timed manual support, but when patients are alone, they may find a pillow, towel or cough belt helpful.

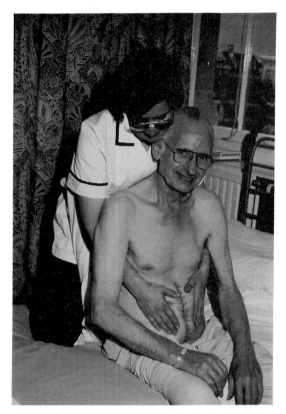

Figure 7.5 Manual support for postoperative coughing after laparotomy. Gentle firm pressure is directed at holding the wound edges together.

If patients are too weak, fatigued or drowsy to co-operate, mechanical aids may be indicated.

Prevention of deep vein thrombosis (DVT)

Patients most at risk of DVT are the following:

- those who are elderly or obese, or have malignancy, blood clotting or vascular disorders,
- those undergoing lengthy surgery, especially of the hip or knee,
- those with a previous history of DVT.

Half the deaths from pulmonary embolism could be avoided by following prophylactic guidelines for DVT prevention (Forbes 1994). Some examples are:

- intermittent or sequential pneumatic leg compression devices during and after surgery (Bright 1994),
- leg elevation before, during and after surgery (Ashby 1995),
- for high-risk patients, drugs such as dextran or heparin,
- graduated anti-embolism (TED) stockings, usually prescribed for continuous use until discharge, which constrict vessels and supposedly increase the velocity of blood flow.

The rationale of TED stockings is questionable, especially as epidural analgesia reduces the incidence of DVTs by causing the opposite effect, i.e. vasodilation (p. 178). If there is benefit, the wrinkles to which they usually succumb can create a counterproductive tourniquet.

But whither physiotherapy? The theory that postoperative leg exercises have any place in prevention has been relegated to the realms of fantasy unless someone can be found to set up camp beside patients and prod them into near-continuous ankle exercises both during and after surgery. The fact that sluggish circulation is a predisposing factor for DVT does not mean that occasional ankle wiggling after the operation will have any effect. There is also no evidence that getting a patient out of bed several times a day prevents DVT formation, especially as the thrombus often forms during surgery and the risk continues for six to eight weeks after discharge when most patients have been fully mobile for some time (Forbes 1994).

Limb exercises are necessary if bed rest is prolonged, in order to prevent joint stiffness and muscle weakness, but if a DVT has been confirmed, leg exercises and mobilization are usually contraindicated until several days after anticoagulation therapy has been established, or after discussion with medical staff.

Discharge

With the present early discharge policies, advice on self-management is becoming more important. In the light of evidence that early discharge leads to more complications and readmission rates (Moore 1994), physiotherapists need to ensure that their voice is heard when discharge decisions are taken.

7.1.6   Abdominal surgery

Almost every abdominal organ is now amenable to laparoscopic surgery, which, compared with laparotomy, causes less pain, lung dysfunction and mood depression, discharges patients in one to three days and returns them to work sooner (Freeman and Armstrong 1994). However, when procedures such as pumping air into the peritoneum and tilting the patient head down are used to facilitate exploration, diaphragmatic function can be significantly disturbed (Baxter 1995).

For laparotomy, analgesia tends to be taken less seriously than after chest surgery, even though it often causes more pain than sternotomy because most physical movements require abdominal muscle contraction. Upper abdominal surgery also causes reflex inhibition of the diaphragm and is associated with more pulmonary complications than chest surgery (Luce *et al* 1984 p. 300). It is followed by a 20–40% incidence of chest complications compared with a 2–5% incidence with lower abdominal surgery (Celli 1993). A small pleural effusion is common after abdominal surgery and is related to fluid overload or atelectasis. Malnourishment is also common after abdominal surgery and is due to:

- malabsorption associated with pre-existing gut pathology,
- the catabolic effects of surgery,
- preoperative fasting,
- postoperative nausea and precarious appetite,
- institutional food.

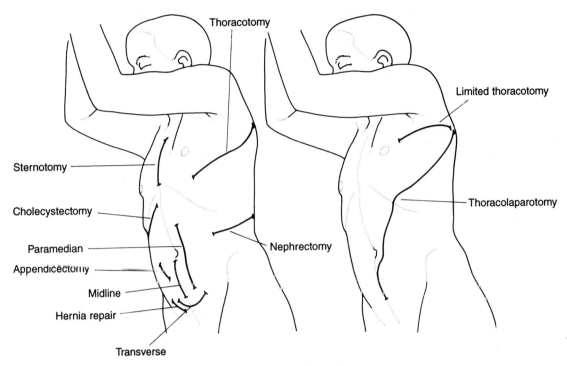

Figure 7.6 Surgical incisions.

Poor nutrition delays wound healing and causes weakness of inspiratory and expiratory muscles, leading to impaired cough and increased incidence of pneumonia (Windsor and Hill 1988). To facilitate rehabilitation, preoperative fasting in excess of six hours should be avoided (Thomas 1987). For patients who are malnourished or who are not expected to eat orally in the days following surgery, especially if they undergo major surgery, enteral feeding should start as soon as the gut is functioning (Mainous and Deitch 1994).

7.1.7 Lung surgery

Incisions

The pain was everywhere. I couldn't get across what I felt. I wanted to move myself but they were insistent on moving me. I lost the ability to control the situation. I felt very alone. The whole thing was one of the most personal experiences of my life. It took a long time to be able to talk about it.

> Katie, a nursing sister,
> following thoracotomy

A full thoracotomy involves rib resection and transection of major chest wall muscles, leading to restricted shoulder movement and 'one of the most intense postoperative pain experiences known' (Kavanagh 1994). Pain should be controlled by local anaesthetic infiltration of intercostal nerves before closure, epidural or other potent technique. A degree of atelectasis is inevitable after thoracotomy because of loss of lung tissue, pain and interference with pleural function.

A full thoracotomy or limited thoracotomy (Fig. 7.6) may be needed to resect part of all of a lung, but video thoracoscopy has led to reduced pain and disability, shorter hospital stays and return to work within one to two weeks (Wood 1993a). Thoracoscopy leaves only 1.5 cm scars, spares muscles and can now be used for 70% of thoracic procedures (Nicholson 1993), including major pulmonary, pleural, cardiac and oesophageal surgery.

Procedures

A small, localized tumour can be removed by **wedge resection**. For a larger lesion, a lung segment can be removed by **segmentectomy**. More commonly, a **lobectomy** is performed to remove a lobe, the vacated space being accommodated by expansion of the rest of the lung.

A **sleeve resection** is removal of the T-junction of a bronchus with its lobe, which often leads to oedema around the anastomosis and ciliary impairment from nerve damage. Postural drainage may be needed. Positive pressure techniques are risky in the immediate postoperative period.

A complete lung is removed by **pneumonectomy**. The lung space is filled with air, blood and fibrin, the quantity of which is regulated by the surgeon judiciously and briefly unclamping a chest drain, sometimes every two to four hours, as judged by X-ray evidence of mediastinal deviation. Drainage of the vacated space should be sufficient to prevent the bronchial stump becoming soggy, but not so enthusiastic that the remaining lung is pulled into the space, risking a tension pneumothorax. The physiotherapist must not touch the clamp. In the days following removal of the chest drain, the pneumonectomy space fills with fluid and inflammatory exudate and, in the ensuing months, this organizes into fibrous tissue. The space also shrinks by upward shift of the hemidiaphragm, lateral shift of the mediastinum and approximation of the ribs.

Effects and complications

1. Following lobectomy, contusion in adjacent lung causes short-term $\dot{V}_A/\dot{Q}$ mismatch and hypoxaemia. Following pneumonectomy, hypoxaemia often occurs on exercise. The average drop in vital capacity is 15% after lobectomy and 35–40% after pneumonectomy (Van Mieghem 1989).

2. Escape of air into the pleura is to be expected because the pleura has been entered. The air leak manifests as bubbling in the drainage bottle.

3. Escape of air into subcutaneous tissue may occur, causing subcutaneous emphysema. If this is severe, patients will need reassurance that it is temporary, ACBT in preference to coughing, and sometimes massage of swollen eyelids to allow temporary vision (which can also be taught to relatives).

4. Problems associated with malignancy (the usual reason for lung surgery) include a smoking history and malnutrition.

5. Damage to the recurrent laryngeal nerve, especially following left pneumonectomy or upper lobectomy, may affect speech and cough.

6. Bronchopleural fistula, which is a communication between a major airway and the pleura, is a serious complication caused by infection and breakdown of the bronchial stump. This is suspected if there is X-ray evidence of an air/fluid level in the pleura and signs of infection, such as a spiking temperature. If the patient lies down with the fistula upwards, there will be excessive coughing and production of quantities of bloody-brown secretions. Empyema may ensue. Small fistulae close naturally with antibiotics, but large defects need chest drainage, glueing via bronchoscopy (York *et al* 1990) or surgery to resuture the bronchial stump. Spread of infected material is minimized by asking the patient to sit upright and/or lean towards the thoracotomy side.

Physiotherapy

Physiotherapists may be involved in the preoperative evaluation of fitness for surgery (p. 34).

Following uncomplicated thoracoscopic surgery, patients can sit out in a chair four to six hours after surgery (Nicholson 1993). Despite early mobility, chest assessment should continue for several days because of surgical interference with lung function.

Physiotherapy after thoracotomy includes shoulder and postural exercises once pain allows. This maintains range of movement and is sometimes seen to improve saturation.

Some patients suffer pain from overstretching of the thoracic joints during surgery, and this may be eased by mobilizations of the joints at the spine.

Points to note in relation to pneumonectomy are the following:

- if sputum clearance is necessary, ACBT is preferred to coughing, to protect the stump,
- some surgeons request no side-lying on the **non-operative** side for several days following a normal pneumonectomy, to prevent fluid spilling on to the anastomosis,
- some surgeons request no full side-lying on **either** side for several days following radical pneumonectomy, which entails entering the pericardium, in case of cardiac herniation,
- no head-down tip and, for some surgeons, no lying flat,
- normally, the remaining lung is able to accommodate the entire resting pulmonary blood flow but, during rehabilitation, pulmonary hypertension may occur on exercise.

7.1.8 Pleural surgery

The indication for pleural surgery is, most commonly, pneumothoraces that are recurrent, bilateral or persist over a week (Parry 1992). First, through the thoracoscope, bullae or blebs are identified and resected, sutured, stapled or ablated. Then a **pleurodesis** may be performed, which is the thoracoscopic introduction of irritant chemicals, fibrin glue or laser pulses into the pleura. This sets up a sterile inflammation, which leads to fibrosis and adherence of the two layers of the pleura. Kindly surgeons add local anaesthetic to the irritant agent.

Alternatively, a **pleurectomy** strips off the parietal pleura so that a raw surface is left at the chest wall, to which the visceral pleura adheres. This can require a thoracotomy, but may be less painful than the acute pleurisy set up by a pleurodesis.

Other indications for pleural surgery are certain pleural effusions and persistant bronchopleural fistulas (Kennedy 1994).

Pleural surgery leaves a long-term, mild restrictive defect.

Chronic empyema may require **decortication** via thoracotomy, which removes pus and fibrous tissue from the visceral pleura. The parietal pleura is spared unless long-standing empyema and deformity mean that it will impair lung expansion (Odell 1994).

7.1.9 Heart surgery

Incision

Access to the heart is usually by median sternotomy (Fig. 7.6), which requires cutting the sternum and dividing the aponeurosis of pectoralis major.

Procedures

Open heart surgery involves cardiopulmonary bypass, which allows surgeons to operate on a quiescent heart in a bloodless field. This involves stopping the heart, removing circulating blood from the right atrium, filtering and oxygenating it outside the body, then pumping it back into the ascending aorta. Neither heart nor lungs function during this period, and the lungs are either kept slightly inflated or completely collapsed.

Some surgeons fill the pericardial sac with crushed ice or chilled saline to reduce the metabolic rate and protect the brain, myocardium and other vital organs from hypoxia. This is no longer considered essential, but moderate cooling to 30° may be retained to provide a safety margin. After surgery, the pericardium is either closed, using pericardial chest tubes for drainage, or left open and drainage allowed through mediastical chest tubes.

For coronary artery bypass grafting (CABG), the saphenous veins and/or internal mammary artery (IMA) are used to replace diseased coronary arteries. The IMA shows improved patency rates and survival times, but has to be harvested from the chest wall, puncturing the pleura and leading to postoperative shoulder girdle pain and greater impairment in lung function than when using the saphenous veins (Rolla 1994).

Complications

1. Postoperative cardiovascular instability may restrict turning or other physiotherapy techniques.
2. Lower lobe atelectasis, mainly of the left, occurs in 30–88% of patients (Jindani 1993), due to compression of the left lower lobe and/or trauma or cold injury to the phrenic nerve. This is so common as to be hardly considered a complication unless it progresses and, indeed, many patients leave hospital with radiological changes not yet resolved.
3. Phrenic nerve injury may lead to diaphragmatic paralysis, occasionally bilaterally.
4. Aggressive fluid replacement may cause pulmonary oedema (Lowell 1990), and excess fluids or pericardial inflammation may cause pleural effusion (Jindani 1993). Pleural effusion is usually left-sided and not significant.
5. Disorientation is due to the alien environment in which the patient wakes up,

sleep deprivation and impaired cerebral perfusion during bypass. It is common in elderly people. Permanent neurological defects occur in 11–57% of patients and stroke in 2% (Harris *et al* 1993).
6. Retraction of the sternum and ribs may cause diaphragm dysfunction (Dickey 1989), and 1st rib fractures have been found in 50% of patients following sternal retraction (Weiner 1992).
7. Impaired renal perfusion during bypass may cause acute kidney failure (Jindani 1993).
8. In the following years, gradual occlusion of the grafted vessels limits the life of the operation.

Physiotherapy

After CABG, blood pressure should be observed before, during and after treatment because hypertension exerts pressure on grafted vessels. A raised diastolic pressure is more relevant than raised systolic pressure because coronary artery perfusion is highest during diastole. The operation notes may indicate the limits within which the BP should be maintained.

Patients are ventilated until haemodynamically stable. If hypoxaemia persists after extubation, CPAP may be helpful (Thomas *et al* 1992). Until the patient can mobilize, regular positioning on alternate sides reduces postoperative complications (Tidwell 1990), so long as this can be achieved with comfort and safety. Right-side-lying tends to cause less BP instability and better gas exchange than left-side-lying (Tidwell 1990).

A proportion of patients will appear euphoric on the first day on realizing that they have survived, then sink into depression for some days afterwards. They should be encouraged to take things gently on the first day to avoid debilitating mood swings which interfere with rehabilitation.

If breathing exercises or incentive spirometry are necessary for respiratory complications, manual support of the wound on inspiration improves comfort and allows greater excursion in some patients.

Bed exercises provide the opportunity to check for neurological damage and, for those confined to bed because of complications, are necessary for joint range and muscle strength.

When pain permits shoulder joint elevation, it should be performed bilaterally to avoid a shearing stress on the sternum. After IMA grafting, many surgeons ask for left shoulder elevation to be limited to 90° for the first 24 hours, and some request that the patient not be turned immediately after surgery.

Within the limits of fatigue, patients should aim at:

- gentle walking on the 2nd postoperative day, and stair-climbing on the 4th or 5th day, gradually increasing thereafter,
- postural correction in front of a mirror,
- immediate embarkation on a comprehensive exercise programme such as that described by Ungeman-deMent *et al* (1986).

If the sternum is heard or felt to click on movement, a cough belt is needed for support. One handle is passed through the other and both are pulled on coughing.

Patients with continuing chest wall pain benefit from joint mobilizations (Dickey 1989). Patients are often ready for discharge in a week, and it is useful to check the breathing pattern and posture to make sure that there are no lingering signs of tension which could become a habit.

CABG is effective in reducing angina, but functional impairment often continues after surgery (Allen 1990), and coronary artery disease is not eliminated. The patient and family are well advised to cultivate a lifestyle that retards the disease process in the grafted vessels. Table 7.1 gives basic information to take home, which should be tailored indi-

Table 7.1 Home advice for people following heart surgery

1. Take some form of enjoyable exercise for about half-an-hour daily, increasing the level gradually so that you aim to produce a rise in pulse rate to over 100 per minute (unless you are on beta-blockers). Find some regular exercise that you enjoy and can maintain indefinitely, e.g. a daily two-mile brisk walk. Very strenuous activities such as squash are not recommended. Avoid fatigue.

2. Take a rest in the afternoon for the next six weeks.

3. Do not lift, push or pull anything heavy for two to three months. This allows the breast bone to heal.

4. Sexual activity can be started when you feel well enough.

5. Avoid driving for six weeks. Check your insurance policy.

6. Work can be resumed from between 6–12 weeks, depending on the level of exertion.

7. Expect a degree of breathlessness, tiredness, poor concentration, memory loss and aches and pains across the shoulders and chest. These are normal and should improve over the next six weeks.

8. Make a list of questions to ask the doctor at your follow-up appointment.

9. No smoking.

10. Keep happy!

vidually to each patient, but a cardiac rehabilitation programme is advisable.

7.1.10 Overview of cardiac rehabilitation

An integrated rehabilition programme is necessary to gain optimum benefit from heart surgery. Cardiac rehabilitation after surgery or myocardial infarct (MI) has led to reduced BP, medication and smoking (Hedbäck *et al* 1990), earlier return to work, and decreased angina, depression and anxiety (Hertanu 1986). Carson (1989) claims a 20% reduction in mortality. Cost-effectiveness itself is usually a sufficient incentive for managers to set up a programme: Huang *et al* (1990) showed a 38% reduction in hospital readmission rates, and Lavie *et al* (1992) showed a 20–25% reduction in major cardiac events. Elderly patients, too, achieve significant benefits (Hellman 1994).

Rehabilitation can be started two to three weeks after surgery and four to six weeks after MI. The basics of education, exercise and relaxation are similar to pulmonary rehabilitation (Chapter 6), but some differences are outlined here.

Education

Morbidity and mortality caused by angina are not proportional to the number of vessels involved (King and Nixon 1988), suggesting that factors outside the coronary system govern the impact on the patient's life. Education is therefore a central component of the programme, especially as fear is frequently associated with disorders of the heart and depression is a common outcome of heart surgery or an MI. Many patients fear a repeat heart attack, and symptoms need to be explained clearly.

Other feelings, such as guilt and shame, are not uncommon because of the association of heart disease with lifestyle. These can be defused in group discussion. Groups also allow participants to swap practical suggestions, watch each other recover, boost morale and enjoy learning relaxation by massaging each other's necks.

Hyperventilation syndrome is common after a cardiac event, but once identified is easily manageable (Chapter 8) because it has not had time to become entrenched. Fatigue is also common, but if accepted does not provoke anxiety.

Preparation for return to work is individualized, but all participants benefit from advice on lifting techniques that do not strain the sternum

Exercise training

Exercise training enables people to perform higher workloads for longer periods (Brannon *et al* 1993, p. 94). Exercise increases coronary perfusion, but has not been proved to increase collateral coronary circulation (Brannon *et al* 1993, p. 71).

Assessment includes identifying the characteristics of each patient's angina and the feel of their individual pulse. Normal protocol is for participants to exercise to 75% of their maximum heart rate, but improvements have been shown at intensities as low as 40% maximum (Lavie *et al* 1992). Excessive heart rates are inadvisable because although blood is forced into the coronary arteries during systole, it cannot enter the muscle fibres to supply oxygen to the tissue until diastole. Patients on beta-blockers can achieve a training effect (Hertanu 1986) using a perceived exertion scale (Brannon *et al* 1993, p. 288) rather than their pulse. Type A personalities (Ferguson 1992) tend to underestimate their degree of perceived exertion.

Exercise should include warm up, cool down, stretching exercises and fitness exercises as described in Chapter 6. Hydrotherapy is popular because it includes the above components, is relaxing and facilitates shoulder and trunk mobility. Patients take their own pulse before, immediately after, and five minutes after exercise, noting the time it takes to return to normal. Exercise should not place a shearing stress on the sternum because union takes 8–12 weeks. Sessions last about 30 minutes, preferably three times a week, with less intensive exercise being encouraged between sessions. Details of exercise specific to cardiac patients can be found in Broad (1991) or Brannon *et al* (1993).

Improvement normally levels off in about three months, after which maintenance exercise continues. When continuing the programme at home, the precautions described on p. 189 should be followed and patients reminded not to take exercise after a large meal.

If resources are limited or patients do not enjoy the intensity of exercise training, improvements in quality of life have been shown with more gentle exercise in which the risks of training do not need to be comprehensively assessed (Worcester *et al* 1993).

Safety

Participants must have been medically assessed, have had an exercise test and take the precautions described on p. 159 and below.

Participants should bring their antiangina medication.

Systolic BP should not rise more than 20 mmHg or fall more than 10–20 mmHg during exercise, and pulse pressure should be below 20 mmHg (Brannon *et al* 1993, p. 3).

Participants should not be pushed beyond what is comfortable, nor exercise through angina or breathlessness of suspected cardiac origin. Excessive breathlessness is unsafe and reduces compliance. If a patient gets angina during exercise, he or she should stop exercising and take his or her medication. If symptoms are unrelieved after 15 minutes of repeated medication, the doctor should be called. It is also useful to ask patients if they forgot to take their regular tablets. One oft-forgotten precaution is to listen to patients because they often detect that something is amiss before it becomes obvious.

A check ECG should be requested if the pulse behaves abnormally, if exercise tolerance declines over two or three sessions, or if patients feel that their heart is not 'right'. A drug review should be requested if angina occurs, side-effects increase or if exercise tolerance is reduced by pulmonary oedema.

If patients say they do not feel well or feel unusually tired, they should be advised to sit down, have a drink if they feel like it, and stop exercising. If patients develop dizziness or palpitations, change colour or develop an irregular pulse which takes more than one minute to recover, they should lie down. Observation of their breathing should be maintained. When one participant feels unwell and is being attended to, it is advisable to keep chatting to the rest of the class in order to avoid anxiety.

Unsupervised exercise training is unsafe for patients who have complex arrhythmias, exercise-induced hypotension, exertional angina uncontrolled by drugs and those unable to self-monitor (Brannon *et al* 1993, p. 3).

Relaxation

Relaxation is an essential component of the programme. When compared with exercise training alone, it has led to lower readmission rates, mortality, recurrent infarctions and the need for surgery (Van Dixhoorn *et al* 1987). Stress management should be included, especially as many patients have a background of tolerating stress without being aware of it. Angina provoked by stress is thought to last longer than exertional angina (Brannon *et al* 1993, p. 83).

7.1.11 Heart and lung transplantation

Each new day is welcomed with open arms come sun, rain or snow. Gone are the excuses for putting off activities until the weather is better or the time more opportune.

Marsh (transplant patient) 1986

Receiving a transplanted heart, lung or both can cause profound change in a patient's attitude to life. Postoperative feelings of resurrection are common and the patient's mood may swing between depression and euphoria (Ellis 1995).

The indication for transplantation is end-stage heart or lung disease. Examples are cardiac myopathy for heart transplant, bullous emphysema or pulmonary fibrosis for single lung transplant, cystic fibrosis for heart–lung transplant, and CF or pulmonary vascular disease for both lungs. Relative contraindications are the side-effects of heavy steroid use and sometimes previous thoracic surgery. Recipients are matched with donors for factors such as blood type and organ size, but a smaller donor organ is usually acceptable. Rigid criteria are applied to donor and recipient (Corley 1994).

Procedures

The operations are no longer technically awesome, and now that immunosuppressive therapy is better able to prevent organ rejection, the main limiting factor is lack of donor organs. A quarter of CF patients die while waiting (Piper *et al* 1992).

Cardiopulmonary bypass is used for heart transplants and some lung transplants. For single lung transplants, a thoracotomy incision is used. For bilateral lung transplants, a massive trans-sternal bilateral thoracotomy (clamshell incision) allows sequential single-lung procedures, which create two separate bronchial anastomoses and preserve the coronary-to-bronchial collateral circulation. A sternotomy is used for other procedures.

A heart-lung transplant (HLT) transplants heart and lungs *en bloc* and retains the collateral circulation. HLT may incorporate a domino procedure, in which the recipient's healthy heart is used as a donor for a second recipient.

Complications

All transplants are complicated by the side-effects of long-term immunosuppressive drugs. Cyclosporin can cause renal damage, and steroids can cause opportunist infection and altered body image due to extra body hair or a cushinoid appearance.

Some transplants are complicated by rejection. Acute heart rejection is suspected if there are temperature or ECG changes, confirmed by biopsy. Chronic heart rejection narrows coronary arteries, and annual angio-

graphy is required to identify this. Treatment is only by retransplantation.

Transplanting the lung has proved more difficult than other organs. It is the only organ in contact with the atmosphere and has evolved a strong immunity to anything foreign. Complications following lung transplant are the following:

1. Infection is caused by denervation of the lung, which impairs mucociliary transport and the patient's awareness of the presence of secretions, an awareness that people with CF have developed to a fine art. Patients are reminded to expect some secretions in the immediate postoperative period because it takes a few days for the debris to clear. Some secretions continue to be produced from the native airway above the anastomosis. A further hindrance in the short term is postoperative oedema around the anastomosis.

2. Pulmonary oedema may be caused by the ischaemic insult of surgery followed by reperfusion. Diuretics may thicken secretions.

3. People with preoperative CO_2 retention find that the new normal oxygenation may suppress their hypoxic respiratory drive. The resulting hypercapnia usually normalizes within a week.

4. Acute or chronic lung rejection can occur from a few days to several years postoperatively. FVC and FEV_1 should reach a plateau several months after surgery and then remain stable, but a reduction of 10–15% is a warning of possible rejection, and suspicions are confirmed if there is fever, breathlessness, hypoxaemia and fine crackles on auscultation. X–ray signs are similar for both rejection and opportunistic infection, and gentle bronchoscopy or biopsy is needed to distinguish the two. Patients are given a diary in which to record spirometry readings, weight and medication. Treat-

ment of rejection is by increased steroids. Confirmation of rejection indicates that physiotherapy should be modified as follows:

(a) suction should be minimal because it may damage the anastomosis and exacerbate oedema from surgery and erythema from rejection,

(b) exercise training is temporarily ceased or modified.

5. Obliterative bronchiolitis is a devastating complication that occurs in about 40% of recipients (Kramer 1994) usually 6–18 months after surgery, following repeated rejection of a transplanted lung. It is a combined obstructive and restrictive disorder, the small airways becoming obstructed by inflammation and then obliterated by granulation tissue, which then fibroses. PEP or CPAP gives symptomatic relief, and augmented immunosuppression is attempted, but retransplantation is the only treatment and carries a high mortality.

6. Stenosis may occur at the anastomosis site. Treatment is by balloon dilation or insertion of a silastic stent, but the condition is usually associated with obliterative bronchiolitis.

Physiotherapy

Preoperative education and preparation takes place when the patient attends the surgeon's assessment clinic because there is little time once a donor has been found. An exercise programme should be adhered to for those who are not deteriorating rapidly. For patients needing mechanical assistance while awaiting surgery, nasal ventilation is usually more successful than CPAP.

Postoperative respiratory care is similar to that given for other chest surgery, with scrupulous attention to prevention of infection, and other considerations described below.

Following lung transplant or HLT, suction if needed should be undertaken without the catheter damaging the anastomosis, which in ventilated patients is just below the end of the endotracheal tube. Intensive humidification and sometimes postural drainage may be needed because of impaired mucociliary clearance. It is thought that some innervation occurs over time (Mihm 1989), and long-term chest clearance is not needed. Bag-squeezing and IPPB should be used with caution because of the risk of pneumothorax.

Many patients are debilitated and need extensive rehabilitation. In the early stages, the following is a guide to a progressive exercise regime:

- day 1 – bed exercises and dangling legs over the edge of the bed,
- day 2 – sitting out in a chair,
- day 3 – walking on the spot, upper limb exercises, walking round the room,
- day 4 – walking outside the room,
- day 5 – exercise bicycle, stairs.

After discharge, patients pursue an exercise programme at home or in the gym, with the following precautions:

1. Transplanted hearts can show a training effect, but are denervated so that the transmission of angina is impaired, the pulse is not a reliable monitoring tool and there is a delayed heart rate response to exercise, requiring ample warm-up and cool-down periods. After 6–12 months of exercise, responses may become near-normal although the intensity and duration of exercise is limited.

2. Corticosteroids may cause osteoporosis, myopathy or delayed healing.

3. Nutritional support is needed for people with CF.

7.1.12 Repair of coarctation of the aorta

Stricture of the aorta causes hypertension in the upper body and hypotension in the lower body. Patients may be symptomless, with the

condition having been picked up on routine
X-ray, but surgery is advisable before hypertension wreaks damage in later life. Repair is
by resection of the narrowed segment and
anastomosis or insertion of a dacron graft.

The following precautions are needed postoperatively to avoid any sudden rise in BP
that might strain the anastomosis:

1. The head-down tip should be avoided.
    Some surgeons prefer the patient not to
    lie flat.
2. Mobilization should be slow and fatigue
    avoided. Extra care is needed during the
    2nd postoperative week when patients
    are beginning to feel well enough to exert
    themselves.
3. Vigorous exercise should be discouraged
    for several months.

7.1.13   Oesophagectomy

Surgery to resect a carcinoma of the oesophagus carries a high mortality, but can relieve
the distressing symptom of dysphagia and
occasionally effects a cure. A two-incision
laparotomy and thoracotomy is less disruptive to diaphragmatic function than a single
thoracolaparotomy (Craig 1981).

As well as the usual postoperative complications, those specific to oesophagectomy are:

*   leakage from the anastomosis,
*   pleural effusion and sometimes empyema,
*   weakness after protracted preoperative
    malnourishment.

Complications are reduced with early extubation, along with adequate pain control
and preoperative preparation (Caldwell
1993). Postoperative precautions are:

*   avoid the head-down tilt in case reflux of
    gastric contents damages the anastom-
    osis (some surgeons prefer patients to
    maintain head elevation),
*   avoid naso- or oropharyngeal suction,
    which might accidentally enter the oeso-
    phagus and impinge on the anastomosis,

*   (for some surgeons) avoid neck move-
    ments that might stretch the anastomosis.

Discharge advice is detailed by Savage
(1992).

7.1.14   Chest drains

Simple wound drains are adequate to remove
blood from the affected site after most forms
of surgery, but if the operation has interfered
with pleural pressures, underwater seal chest
drains are needed. This airtight system
allows air and blood to escape from the
pleural space while preventing their re-entry.
It also restores normal negative pleural pressures and allows lung re-expansion. Chest
drains are also used after heart surgery,
although some cardiac surgeons find that
simple wound drains are sufficient.

Indications

After heart surgery, one drain is usually
placed inside the pericardium to prevent
cardiac tamponade (blood accumulating in
the pericardium), and one outside the pericardium to drain blood from the mediastinum.

After lung, pleural or oesophageal surgery,
two drains are placed in the pleura, one in
the apex to remove air and the other in the
base to remove blood. Pleural drains may
also be required after heart, kidney or upper
abdominal surgery if the pleura has been cut.

After pneumonectomy, a single drain is left
in the vacated space. This remains clamped
except when there is X-ray evidence of a
mediastinal shift (p. 184).

A pneumothorax breaks the seal between
the two layers of pleura, and a single chest
drain in the pleura is needed to restore
negative pressure and reinflate the lung.

Mechanism

The underwater seal, consisting of the distal
end of the drainage tube submerged in 2 cm
of sterile water or saline, acts as a one-way

valve. Fluid drains by gravity and air is expelled through the water into the atmosphere. Fluid cannot return so long as the bottle is below the level of the patient's chest. Air cannot be sucked back because the water acts as a seal while offering minimal resistance to drainage. The length of tube under the liquid determines the pressure required to expel the unwanted contents in the chest, so is kept short without breaking the underwater seal. The underwater seal also produces a siphon effect which enhances drainage.

Drainage depends on gravity or suction. Free drainage occurs when the exit tube is open to the atmosphere. This allows the water level in the underwater seal tube to swing (if it is a pleural drain), reflecting the change in pleural pressure with breathing. If gravity is inadequate for drainage, for example, with excess fluid drainage or air leak, suction is applied, typically at pressures of minus 10–20 cmH$_2$O, with more negative pressures for large air leaks (Kam *et al* 1993).

One bottle is used if little drainage is expected. This acts as both underwater seal chamber and collection chamber. Two bottles may be used individually or in series (Fig. 7.7). There is sometimes a third chamber in series to regulate the negative pressure at a preset value. Integrated devices with several chambers avoid the floor becoming littered with bottles and tubing.

Management

Any patient with a chest drain needs to be seen by a physiotherapist for advice on mobility, posture correction and shoulder movement. Some also need respiratory care.

The principles of safe handling of chest drains are the following:

1. Before treating any patient who has a chest drain, the location of the clamps should be checked so that they can be found instantly if required.
2. Bottles should be kept below the level of the patient's chest to prevent their contents being sucked back into the patient. If the bottle needs to be lifted above the patient for turning, the tubing should be clamped near its exit from the chest for the duration of the manoeuvre.
3. Except when lifting the bottle above the patient, it is preferable to avoid clamping during moving, deep breathing, coughing or mobilization, because drainage is encouraged by these manoeuvres. Care should be taken to avoid disconnection during any activity.
4. When handling patients, the tubing should be held against and in alignment with the patient's chest, to minimize discomfort.
5. The tubing should be kept exposed throughout treatment to avoid accidental kinking.
6. The bottle should be observed before and after physiotherapy to check for any change in drainage, air leak or swing in the water level. Extra drainage is expected after treatment, but excessive loss suggests haemorrhage and should be reported.
7. If the system is on suction but the patient needs to mobilize, the surgeon's permission is first obtained to temporarily disconnect the suction, then the suction tube is disconnected from the exit tube so that the patient can walk while connected to an open system. If the suction apparatus is simply unplugged from the wall socket, the system would then be closed and allow no exit of air, so that a pneumothorax could develop.

If air is bubbling through the water, there is a hole in the visceral pleura, allowing air to escape from the lung at each breath. This hole should seal in time, but positive pressure techniques would hinder this process and are to be avoided unless essential. An air leak is also a sign to avoid clamping because this would allow a pneumothorax to develop.

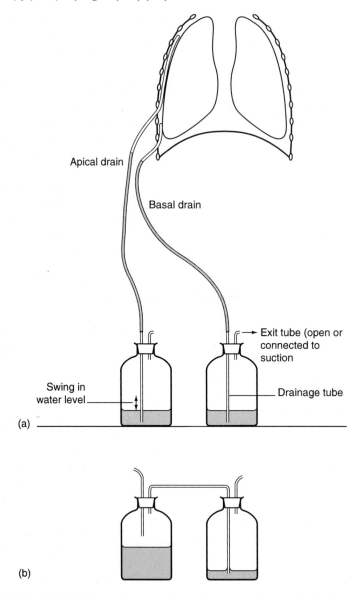

Apical drain

Basal drain

Exit tube (open or connected to suction

Swing in water level

Drainage tube

(a)

(b)

Figure 7.7 Underwater seal chest drains. (a) Two individual bottles allow separate drainage of air via an apical drain and fluid via a basal drain. (b) Two bottles in series provide underwater seal and collection chambers. This prevents the fluid level in the underwater seal chamber rising and needing regular emptying.

If clamping is essential, this should be momentary only, and if both drainage bottles show bubbling, they should not be clamped at the same time. If there is any change in the air leak after treatment, this should be reported.

If there is no pressure swing, this means that:

- the tube is kinked or blocked (sudden),
- the lung has successfully re-expanded, thereby occluding the pleural end of the tube (gradual),
- the system contains a collection bottle, which tends to obliterate the swing, or is on suction, which overrides pleural pressure changes.

The procedure of 'milking' chest drains to dislodge clots and maintain patency can cause pulmonary trauma. Gentle hand squeezing is now recommended (Kam *et al* 1993).

Chest drains are removed by nursing staff after the lung has fully expanded and drainage is complete. The distress of the procedure is often unrecognized, despite being described as their worst memory by nearly half the patients in one survey (Carson 1994). Entonox analgesia is an essential requirement, unless surgeons have preplaced minicatheters for local anaesthetic infusion (Carson 1994). The patient is asked to take and hold a deep breath during removal to avoid air being drawn into the chest.

Problems

If any junction in the system becomes disconnected, or the bottle breaks, the following steps should be taken:

- immediately clamp the tubing close to the patient's chest,
- clean and reconnect the tubing,
- unclamp to restore drainage,
- report the incident.

If the tubing becomes disconnected from the patient, the following steps should be taken:

- ask the patient to exhale and, at the same time, press gauze, sheeting or a hand against the wound at end-exhalation, speed taking precedence over sterility,
- ask the patient to breathe normally,
- notify the doctor, but stay with the patient and maintain pressure on the wound,

- observe breathing rate and chest symmetry,
- if the patient is distressed, give reassurance and oxygen.

7.1.15 Head and neck surgery

Major head and neck surgery can lead to respiratory dysfunction that is equal to upper abdominal surgery (Campbell *et al* 1987). Partial or total laryngectomy is undertaken to remove a tumour of the larynx. Partial or radical neck dissection is required for malignant invasion of other tissues. A more extensive commando procedure resects part of the mandible, tongue, neck structures or floor of the mouth. The combination of mutilation, loss of speech and limited ability to express feelings can be a devastating experience for the patient. Speech therapy is essential and comprehensive multidisciplinary support helps to limit the frustration and grief that can lead to isolation and hinder rehabilitation.

Tracheostomy

A tracheostomy is formed temporarily during some operations in order to protect the airway from aspiration or swelling. It is permanent if a laryngectomy is performed. For the first few days the tube has an inflated cuff, which encircles the tube within the trachea to prevent aspiration.

For non-laryngectomy patients, the cuff is deflated as soon as there is a cough reflex. For those who have had a laryngectomy, the cuffed tube is removed after about 48 hours, when haemorrhage is no longer a risk, and replaced with a permanent uncuffed tube. This incorporates an inner cannula to prevent trauma from repeated tube changes. The inner cannula is removed and cleaned twice a day to prevent obstruction by secretions.

Some people without laryngectomies require a long-term tracheostomy, in which case speech is possible with a fenestrated tube. This has inner and outer cannulae with matching openings in their outer curves allowing air to pass through the larynx. It may be cuffed or cuffless. Another device has an inner cannula with a flange that closes on expiration, thus forcing air through the vocal cords for speech.

Complications of tracheostomy

Complications of tracheostomy include the following:

1. Obstruction due to thick secretions or blood clot.
2. Displacement of the tracheostomy tube, especially if there is excessive movement in the immediate postoperative period.
3. Haemorrhage. This may be obvious or indicated by pulsation of the tracheostomy tube synchronously with the patient's pulse. If suspected, the airway should be suctioned and the cuff inflated. This will temporarily inhibit aspiration until medical attention arrives. The head-down position inhibits aspiration of blood into the lungs.
4. Fistula formation, which is suspected if suctioned secretions contain swallowed food and drink.
5. Infection, partly because the oral pharynx is teeming with bacteria, and partly because poor suction technique is widespread.
6. Erosion of the trachea due to excessive movement of the tracheostomy tube, and late onset stricture due to granulation tissue as eroded areas heal.

Management

It takes about a week for a tract to be established following tracheostomy, so tracheal dilators are on hand in case the tube becomes dislodged. Continuous humidification is needed, but if the tracheostomy is permanent, this is discontinued when the airway has adapted to its new exposure to the environment. Patients will then need to maintain adequate fluid intake, and are supplied with a spray with which to moisten

the stoma regularly using sterile saline. People with chronic lung disease may need on-going intermittent humidification.

If the sternomastoid muscle has been excised, the patient's head will need manual support during postoperative movement. If the spinal accessory nerve has been transected, there might be shoulder pain and limited abduction, and patients should adhere scrupulously to an exercise regime, postural correction and advice such as avoiding traction to the brachial plexus. Connecting tubes need to be supported during movement so that they do not drag on the wound. Swallowing may be problematic. Mouthwashes should be offered liberally.

The greatest fear of tracheostomy patients during their early postoperative days is the inability to summon help, and a bell must always be within reach. They will need time for lip-reading and deciphering written requests in order to reduce frustration. They may need questions that require only a yes or no answer. They do not need a raised voice.

For disfiguring surgery, a mirror should be given to patients only if someone is available to be with them for their first view. Visitors need preparation before their first visit. Self-esteem often improves when patients are encouraged in activities ranging from cleaning their own inner tube to helping other patients. With a long-term tracheostomy, patients or carers will need to be taught to do their own suction, although many patients can huff out their secretions.

Major head and neck surgery requires a comprehensive exercise programme such as that described by Herring *et al* (1987). Advice includes protecting the stoma from water and dust, instructions to carers on mouth-to-stoma resuscitation, and who to contact if there are problems. Assistance with swallowing difficulties will be given by the speech and language therapist. Self-care is emphasized throughout rehabilitation.

Voice restoration is by laryngeal devices held at the neck, oesophageal speech or the artificial creation of a tracheo-oesophageal puncture and valve through which patients can generate a more fluent form of oesophageal speech. Women may have more difficulty adapting to their new self-image because of the low-pitched voice and cosmetic changes.

7.1.16 Mastectomy

Postmastectomy patients require advice on full shoulder girdle movements and posture correction. At first, functional shoulder joint movements are encouraged below 90° elevation to avoid wound tension (Philip 1987). On discharge, verbal or written instructions should be given to ensure that the patient achieves full range of movement.

7.2 ELDERLY PEOPLE

The majority of respiratory patients on medical wards are elderly, and much can be done to reduce the dependency, anxiety and depersonalization to which they are susceptible in this environment.

Ageing is often considered to be what is left when other factors have been accounted for, but old age is becoming less accepted as an explanation for ill-health, so it is useful to clarify which changes are due to ageing and which to avoidable factors. Some examples are the following:

1. Confusion can be caused by hypoxaemia, dehydration, infection, pain, overmedication, disturbed sleep, depression or the disorientation created by admission to hospital. It should not be accepted as normal unless dementia has been diagnosed.
2. Depression, often unrecognized, is a common outcome of the helplessness associated with hospitalization, especially in people who have got out of the habit of asserting themselves. This underlines the importance of consulting patients throughout treatment. Depres-

sion should also be suspected if staff comment that 'she's forgetful, she's a wanderer, she's beginning to dement'.
3. Postural hypotension is related to vascular insufficiency, dehydration or the side-effects of certain drugs.
4. Impaired absorption, distribution, metabolism and elimination of drugs is common in the elderly. Adverse drug reactions are often missed. Sixty per cent of serious adverse drug reactions in elderly people have been blamed on diuretics, which are often given for oedema even though oedema in the elderly is usually caused by immobility (Valacio and Lie 1994).
5. Regulation of body temperature may be unstable, causing impaired response to a cold environment or inability to develop a pyrexia in response to pneumonia.
6. Silent aspiration of stomach contents may occur, especially at night.
7. Aches and pains are pathological and not to be accepted as part of normal ageing.
8. Some reduction in exercise tolerance is to be expected, and a linear reduction in $\dot{V}O_2max$ (see Glossary) has been demonstrated (Paterson 1992), but needless immobility can be due to unobtrusive and treatable conditions such as anaemia or painful feet.
9. An assumption that incontinence is inevitable may lead to mopping-up taking precedence over preventive action such as maintenance of mobility and ensuring access to the bathroom.
10. Constipation may be due to medication, dehydration, change of diet or the immobility of illness and hospitalization. Exercise and abdominal massage reduce the incidence of constipation (Resende and O'Neill 1992). Massage has the added benefit of reducing anxiety and restoring the benefits of touch, which are often lost to the elderly (Fraser and Kerr 1993).

11. Reversible respiratory disease is often missed, or may not be treated even if the diagnosis is made (Sherman *et al* 1992).

12. Misery is not an inevitable accompaniment to old age.

Practical ways to help maintain orientation in elderly people are to:

- encourage dressing whenever possible,
- avoid using patients' first names uninvited (Gordon 1994),
- ensure that patients are kept fully informed,
- encourage them to bring to hospital their budgerigars and as much clutter of personal possessions as practical and allowable.

Autonomy can be maintained by respecting patients' senior status, experience and wishes regarding management. This means, for example, allowing them to return to bed when they request, rather than enforcing unhappy hours slumped in uncomfortable hospital chairs. Discomfort reduces the depth of breathing, and the zeal with which patients are hauled out of bed has led to 'chairsores' becoming more prevalent than bedsores in some hospitals (Mulley 1993). Respiratory health is best maintained by a personally tailored programme of mobility and a return to a home environment as soon as possible.

7.3   PEOPLE WHO ARE DYING

It begins with an easy voice saying,
Just a routine examination;
as October sunlight
pierces the heavy velvet curtains.
Later it is the friends who write but do not
*   visit . . .*
it is boiled fish . . .
it is doctors who no longer stop by your
*   bed . . .*
it is terror every minute of conscious night and
*   day to a background of pop music.*

Wilkes 1980

Physiotherapists are suited to working with people who are dying because of their use of physical contact, which can often communicate what words cannot, and their experience with disabled people, who have similar needs to people who are dying (Purtilo, 1976). An area as subjective as death requires more of us as humans than as 'experts', and working with dying people can be both enriching and painful. End-stage disease is not a time to withdraw physiotherapy, because there is much that can be done to ease the passage towards a good death.

7.3.1   Reactions of patients

Now and then the whole thing becomes unreal.
Out of the middle of the night's darkness, or
bringing me to a sudden, chilling halt during
the day, the thought comes: this can't be
happening to me. Me with only a few months to
live? Nonsense. And I stare up at the darkness,
or out at the sunlit street, and try to encompass
it, to feel it. But it stays unreal.

Bell 1961

When told that they are dying, most people feel overwhelmed and experience a variety of reactions. Fear of dying is often greater than the fear of death. There is fear of isolation, fear of an agonizing disintegration, fear of the unknown. 'Will it hurt? Will I suffocate? Will I drown in phlegm? Will it be disgusting?' If fears remain unspoken, they become distorted or concealed by anger.

Guilt is an extra burden that is common in people dying from smoking-related disorders. Anger is another ever-ready emotion that may arise from feelings of helplessness, or act as a defence against experiencing grief. Grief is a normal response to an abnormal situation, but if suppressed it can develop into a psychiatric disorder. Patients should not be treated with antidepressants for their grief (Stewart and Shields 1985), but allowed to express sorrow, anger, guilt, unusual humour or any natural feeling, for which they should not have to apologize.

Many patients deny reality in order to avoid the pain of grief or fear, and they act and talk as if they expect to get better. These defence mechanisms are natural and to be respected. When and if patients are ready to confront the truth, they may sink into a depression that can paradoxically be a creative process by which they begin to take responsibility for the way they respond to change. Only then can they accept their loss and allow fear to dissolve.

These reactions are not stages that occur in logical order and with defined boundaries, but they weave in and out of a patient's awareness, so that a moment of anger may open into acceptance, followed by the mind curling back into the darkness of fear. These mechanisms take time to work. Cancer and emphysema give patients time, which with support can be used wisely.

7.3.2 Reactions of relatives

When someone you love dies, you pay for the sin of outliving them with a thousand piercing regrets.

Simone de Beauvoir 1966

Bereavement carries its own burden of morbidity and mortality (Timmons and Ley 1994, p. 244), and living near to death arouses a kaleidoscope of emotions. Relatives may experience similar reactions to the patient, as well as feeling impotence and a variety of responses, including relief or remorse. They, too, need the opportunity to express their feelings, and this includes sharing the truth with the person who is dying. Unfortunately, patients and their relatives are sometimes out of step, either because the patient is given a falsely optimistic forecast, or because one or both parties try to 'protect' the other, sometimes with the collusion of health staff. Just when they need each other the most, they are separated by a conspiracy of silence.

The health problems suffered by bereaved people are reduced if talking is encouraged (Timmons and Ley 1994, p. 246). Children also benefit from open communication and need the opportunity to be close to their dying relative. They know their own limitations and may simply want to pop in and out of the sick room. Children often fantasize that they are to blame for the death of a parent or sibling, or they may feel they must avoid distressing their parent and therefore avoid talking about it. Siblings of dying children are often the forgotten mourners, and McGowan (1994) found that 50% develop fears of getting cancer themselves. Free discussion should be allowed and, as appropriate, encouraged.

7.3.3 Reactions of staff

The sister was very cross with me and told me to pull myself together because the consultant was coming.

Blanckenhagen (cancer patient) 1986

Once a patient's condition is known to preclude recovery, this is sometimes interpreted as failure by health staff. Reactions may manifest as avoidance, heroic measures to prolong life, dishonest reassurance, unsuitable bonhomie or the use of drugs to suppress patients' expression of emotion. Health staff working with people at the end of their life need support themselves in order to support patients appropriately. They need access to their own feelings because expression of feelings by staff, when appropriate, has been found to be therapeutic for patients, who find professional detachment unhelpful and even offensive (Fallowfield 1993).

7.3.4 Communicating with dying people

His yellow eyes watched us being taught at the bedside of each patient and when we came to his bed we all walked directly past him to the patient on his other side. Not a word was said. Not a greeting. Not even a nod . . . Dismay turned to guilt with the thought that I, too, had no idea how to approach or comfort a dying patient.

Carmichael 1981

It is not easy to find the right words to say to people who are facing death. The key is to listen. Patients find relief if they feel that it is acceptable to talk, and the astute listener can pick up indirect questions. Patients may drop hints that they would like to talk by ploys such as mentioning other people who have died, joking about their future or asking how long their illness will last. We can indicate a willingness to listen by asking if we can sit on the bed, maintaining eye contact and asking non-threatening questions such as 'how do you feel in yourself?' While patients are talking, they can be encouraged by prompts such as, 'go on' or simply 'mm?'.

During and after talking, patients need time to process their thoughts, and we should develop the art of using silence constructively. It is not helpful to rationalize patients out of their feelings, tell them what to do, or say that we know how they feel (we do not). It is, however, helpful to provide information that reduces anxiety, and discussion itself helps to divest death of its power. Uncertainty is one of the hardest things to bear (Bortoluzzi 1994), and patients who are left in ignorance feel a loss of control that shackles their coping strategies.

We might also find it useful to ponder our own reactions: 'Am I feeling uncomfortable? Am I helping or hindering her flow of thought? Am I responding to his needs or mine? Am I frightened of death myself?'

Honesty is essential in this form of communication. The overwhelming majority of patients want to be told their diagnosis (Sell *et al* 1993). Fear of the unknown is a heavier burden than the truth. Most realize eventually that they are dying, and are then alone to face the truth from which they were being sheltered. When patients ask questions about their prognosis, however indirect, to avoid giving information is unethical and keeps patients in a subordinate position. Lying to patients may be due to a false assumption that distress equals harm, or uncertainty about who should take the initiative, but physiotherapists have as much right and responsibility to inform patients as other health staff (Sim 1986), and can act to bridge the gap that sometimes exists between patients and their physicians. Honesty should be tempered by sensitivity, with an emphasis on what medical science has to offer, and a check that patients do not associate emotive words such as 'cancer' with misconceptions about an inevitable and distressing death.

Important exchanges with the patient should be communicated to the doctor and head nurse. If it is difficult to talk with the patient, an appropriate member of the health team should be asked.

To reveal the diagnosis to the family without the patient's knowledge creates tension and mistrust between all involved and is unethical. Family requests should be respected, but have no legal standing and should not take precedence over the rights of the patient (Snider 1995).

Reaction to bad news is varied and sometimes irrational, including regression to childlike behaviour, projection of hostility, relief, or despair at the loss of fulfilment. Patients may choose to face in a different direction from that which we intend, but no defence mechanism is maladaptive unless continued use causes undue distress. Patients should be left with some realistic hope, even if this is directed towards a minor everyday achievement. And it is always worth casting a backward glance when leaving the bedside, because it is sometimes necessary to return and pick up the pieces.

7.3.5 Management of symptoms

As soon as it is known that patients are in need of care rather than cure, the emphasis is on allowing them to choose both the method and timing of treatment.

Breathlessness

Breathlessness is the most dreaded accompaniment to advanced lung disease and is present in 60% of people with any advanced cancer (Clarke 1993). The pharmacological and physical management of breathlessness is discussed in Chapters 4 and 6, but further measures can be taken for people who are dying.

Specific causes of breathlessness should be identified and treated, e.g. pleural effusion, ascites, anxiety or anaemia. Steroids relieve breathlessness associated with diffuse malignant lung involvement, and increase appetite and well-being. The normal constraints on using these drugs are unnecessary at the end of life. Nebulized morphine with lignocaine can relieve breathlessness, and the cannabinoids can be used for their bronchodilator and tranquillizing effects (Ahmedzai 1988). Patients being managed at home often feel relieved if they can self-administer nebulized morphine because of its many symptom-relieving properties. Its reassuring presence may reduce the incidence of respiratory panic.

Patients vary in their response to oxygen. It is usually of no value and simply sets up a barrier between patient and family (Burford and Barton 1993), but it is worth a trial in those with hypoxaemia (Bruera *et al* 1993), so long as care is taken to prevent a dry mouth.

Cough

Cough occurs in 30% of people with all cancers and 80% of people with lung cancer (Twycross and Lack 1984). Pulmonary oedema, infection or bronchospasm can contribute to a cough, and these can be dealt with pharmacologically. Smoking cessation will ease the cough, but not for two to four weeks, so the patient may decide that it is not worth it. Nebulized lignocaine (Trochtenberg 1994) is useful for a terminal cough caused by pooling of saliva; it can be given several times a day but is especially useful at night. Physical management depends on whether the cough is productive or not (see Chapter 5).

Death rattle

People who are too weak to expectorate may collect excessive secretions in their throat. The resulting 'death rattle' is distressing for visitors and neighbouring patients. Repositioning the patient may reduce the noise, but secretion formation can be prevented by administration of hyoscine using a patch or syringe pump at the first indication of moist breath sounds (Ahmedzai 1988). Suction is not indicated.

Difficulty in swallowing

Hyoscine is also useful for patients who cannot swallow easily. A speech therapist provides valuable support.

Dehydration

When it comes to dying, arms are for hugging not for intravenous infusions.
                                                          Potts 1994

People who are dying often escape symptoms associated with dehydration, such as headache, nausea and cramps. The troublesome symptoms of dry mouth and halitosis can usually be relieved by sucking crushed ice or lemon slices (Main 1993).

Pain

Seventy per cent of patients with advanced malignancy experience pain, and fear of pain often exceeds fear of death (Main 1993). If pain is allowed to fill the patient's field of consciousness, it can lead not only to distress, but also to withdrawal, indifference to personal appearance or degeneration of personality.

potassium, excitable neuromuscular junctions and the sensory aberrations characteristic of HVS. Sympathetic dominance leads to symptoms such as palpitations, dry throat, tremors and sweating, and autonomic instability of blood vessels and nerves causes symptoms in almost any system of the body, sometimes one-sided (O'Sullivan *et al* 1992).

Cerebral vasoconstriction can cause dizziness, faintness, headache, visual disturbance, epilepsy (Fried 1993, p. 187) and blackouts in children. Coronary vasoconstriction, compounded by decreased oxygen yield to the tissues due to leftward shift of the oxygen dissociation curve, may cause angina (Magarian, 1982) or atypical chest pain. Up to 90% of non-cardiac chest pain is thought to be associated with HVS (DeGuire *et al* 1992), but misdiagnosis of heart disease is frequent especially as patients often have tachycardia, arrhythmias and adrenaline-induced ECG changes. Despite its independent existence, HVS is thought to be both a risk factor and a complication of ischaemic heart disease (Weiner 1991).

A misdiagnosis of asthma is also common, and there may be some overlap because both hypocapnia and rapid breathing can cause bronchospasm, but the breathlessness of HVS is distinctive because it is poorly correlated with exercise and tends to increase in, for example, enclosed or crowded spaces. 'Air hunger' is a more specific description of the quality of breathlessness and is highly suggestive of HVS. The patient feels a need to take a deep satisfying breath, but also feels difficulty in inflating the lungs.

Hyperventilation causes respiratory alkalosis, which shifts the dissociation curve to the left, depressing phosphate levels and leading to disturbed glucose metabolism, paraesthesia, fatigue and disorientation. The kidneys attempt to offset the alkalosis by excreting bicarbonate. The respiratory centre is reset in order to maintain a normal pH, increasing the drive to breathe and obliging the patient to continue hyperventilating despite a persistently low $PaCO_2$. Activity may relieve symptoms, but sometimes loss of fine tuning means that breathing may not adjust to activity. Symptoms may worsen when driving or watching TV, which can heighten arousal without an accompanying increase in activity.

Other symptoms are shown in Table 8.1.

8.4   ASSESSMENT

People with HVS should arrive for physiotherapy after screening to exclude organic disease. By this time they may also have been given a selection of diagnoses from multiple sclerosis and peripheral neuropathy to myocardial infarction and psychosis. Some have been dismissed as malingerers or told that it is all in their mind. Others have been told that it is 'only hyperventilation', somehow disqualifying further consideration. The first priority, therefore, is to ensure that patients feel welcome and know that their problem is taken seriously. They need space, time, privacy and an attentive ear.

The case notes should be checked for other disorders that cause breathlessness, such as heart disease, asthma, interstitial lung disease, pulmonary embolus or neuromuscular disorder. Anaemia should be identified because low haemoglobin may mean that breathing retraining exacerbates symptoms. Patients are sometimes mistakenly put on beta-blockers, which can cause bronchospasm and exacerbate HVS. If patients are being weaned off sedatives, relaxation will be difficult unless treatment coincides with peak effect of the drug. The history from the notes needs to be supplemented by questions about social background, factors that precede symptoms and the patient's interpretation of them.

8.4.1   Subjective

Feelings of flying apart, absolute terror, falling down through the world, spinning through the universe

Patient quoted by Bradley 1994

Table 8.1 A selection of the signs and symptoms associated with hyperventilation syndrome

System	Manifestation
Neurological	Tingling and numbness (especially extremities/around mouth)
	Faintness
	Blurred vision, migraine
	Poor memory and concentration
	Tremor and tetany
Psychiatric	Panic attacks
	Phobias (especially claustrophobia/agoraphobia)
	Anxiety, clammy hands, flushed face
	Suppression of emotion
	Depression
	Mood swings
	Depersonalization
Gastrointestinal	Oesophageal reflux
	Difficulty swallowing
	Nausea
	Abdominal pain, indigestion, wind
	Irritable bowel
Musculoskeletal	Myalgia
	Stiffness, cramps
	Tetany in severe cases
General	Difficulty in breathing, talking, swallowing
	Air hunger
	Weakness
	Insomnia
	Hypoglycaemia
	Blurred body awareness
	Difficulty concentrating

Feelings vary from anxiety to fears of impending madness. Medical phobias and fear of dying are common (Timmons and Ley 1994, p. 142). Patients may complain of an inability to take a satisfying breath, or may in fact be unaware of any breathing abnormality. If symptoms have worsened while they are on a waiting list, this may be because a common response to receiving a diagnosis of a breathing disorder is to practise deep breathing exercises.

Patients are often puzzled at why symptoms affecting so many parts of the body can be caused by a breathing disorder, and may not report 'irrelevant' symptoms. Acceptance of the diagnosis is easier when they are asked specific questions about symptoms that are likely to correspond to their experience. We also need to find out the patient's opinion of the cause of their problem.

Patients should say all they want at this stage because it relieves tension and reduces their need to talk during treatment, which upsets the breathing pattern.

8.4.2 Observation

It is normal to sigh when sad, breath-hold when frightened, say 'phew' when relieved and breathe fast when stressed, but people who chronically hyperventilate often have a habitually labile breathing pattern, with disturbance continuing long after the stress is withdrawn. The breathing rate may be excessive, and the breathing rhythm erratic with a variety of patterns:

- shallow, fast and apical,
- sighing and yawning,
- irregular, with numerous hesitations,
- prolonged inspiration and curtailed expiration,
- excessive thoracic movement, sometimes with abdominal paradox,
- 'cogwheel' breathing, as if the patient dare not let the air out,
- 'statue' breathing, as if the patient has momentarily forgotten to breathe,
- audible hissing in florid cases.

Conversely, changes in breathing may be subtle and hardly evident on observation because the breathing required to maintain hypocapnia is less than that required to induce it.

Other signs are a stiff posture and gait, excessive hand movements or other indication of tension, speech uncoordinated with breathing, rapid speech, as if the patient is trying to cram several sentences into one, and strategies to sneak in more air such as a dry cough, throat clearing or chest heaving before answering questions. Belching may be caused by air swallowing, cold hands by vasoconstriction and licking of the lips by a dry mouth.

8.4.3   Questionnaire

Any person who demonstrates an unusual mix of clinical features which include some of the above should raise suspicions of HVS. The diagnosis can be confirmed by the Nijmejen questionnaire (Fig. 8.2), which has been validated by Vansteenkiste *et al* (1991).

8.4.4   Tests

Objective tests can be distressing and are limited in accuracy because of the absence of normal precipitating factors, but the following are available:

The provocation test entails rapid breathing for one minute, which in patients with a chronically low $PaCO_2$ brings on familiar symptoms speedily (not just dizziness which is normal). It consists of the following:

- advice that the test may bring on a dry mouth and be tiring (but patients are not told to anticipate their symptoms),
- advice to report any feelings that occur,
- instruction to take fast deep breaths for one minute 'as if you're climbing a hill'.

The test reassures patients of the validity of their symptoms and shows them that they have some control, but it is also considered hazardous (Fried 1993, p. 42), and for patients with chest pain it should be performed under medical guidance and with

ECG monitoring because there is a danger of arrhythmias or ischaemia if overbreathing is prolonged. Cerebral vascular disease and epilepsy are contraindications.

Voluntary overbreathing is an established technique in psychotherapy to enable people to gain access to their feelings, and the provocation test sometimes brings out emotions. Some patients need the opportunity to discuss these, and proffering a box of tissues lets them know that tears are acceptable.

A low $PaCO_2$ is not itself diagnostic, because the syndrome is intermittent, but a value below 4.3 kPa (32 mmHg) would raise suspicions. A more specific test is to use capnography to measure expired CO_2 at the mouth. End-tidal CO_2 is close to the arterial value when lung function is normal. If the resting level is erratic, or if after a provocation test of voluntary hyperventilation it has not normalized within five minutes, HVS is implicated (Timmons and Ley 1994, p. 109). Capnography is not distressing and can be used to provide feedback for patients and outcome measures for physiotherapists (Fig. 8.3).

8.5   EDUCATION

Before launching into explanations, it is worth checking the patient's expectations. Goals can then be agreed, e.g. in the short term to cope with panic attacks and in the long term to integrate a normal breathing pattern into everyday life. The mechanism of HVS can be explained using the vicious cycle (Fig. 8.1) and this by itself often improves symptoms. The explanation should include reassurance that HVS is a normal response to stress, not a psychiatric illness, and stems from chemical reactions to certain events that have become a habit. Bradley (1994) provides a book full of patient-friendly education.

Patients should gain an understanding of the following:

- physiotherapy will not eliminate the cause nor remove precipitating factors, but the aim is for a collaborative approach so

	Never 0	Rare 1	Sometimes 2	Often 3	Very often 4
Chest pain					
Feeling tense					
Blurred vision					
Dizzy spells					
Feeling confused					
Faster or deeper breathing					
Short of breath					
Tight feelings in chest					
Bloated feeling in stomach					
Tingling fingers					
Unable to breathe deeply					
Stiff fingers or arms					
Tight feelings round mouth					
Cold hands or feet					
Palpitations					
Feelings of anxiety					

Total: /64

Figure 8.2 Nijmejen questionnaire. Patients mark with a tick how often they suffer from the symptoms listed. A score above 23/64 is diagnostic of hyperventilation syndrome.

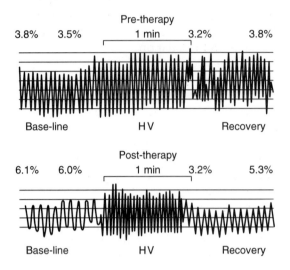

Pre-therapy

3.8%   3.5%   1 min   3.2%   3.8%

Base-line   HV   Recovery

Post-therapy

6.1%   6.0%   1 min   3.2%   5.3%

Base-line   HV   Recovery

Figure 8.3 End-tidal CO_2 trace (%) before and after physiotherapy. HV = voluntary hyperventilation. (From Rowbottom, I. (1992) and Lothian Respiratory Function Service, City Hospital, Edinburgh, with permission.)

that patients can identify precipitating factors and break out of the vicious cycle by methods that they can control,
- commitment is required, especially in incorporating practice into everyday life,
- benefit is achieved from a small but fundamental shift in attitude and lifestyle that allows time for relaxation and reflection,
- a nice deep breath does not help relaxation,
- relearning the new lower level of breathing involves experiencing the discomfort of air hunger, but after practice the respiratory centre will become retuned to registering normal as normal.

Some patients respond to the 'good' and 'bad' approach. 'Bad' breathlessness is the distressing symptom that they complain of. 'Good' breathlessness is the feeling of air hunger that they initiate and control as part of their breathing re-education. Although 'good', it is not comfortable, and patients who find it distressing will appreciate acknowledgment of this.

8.6   BREATHING RE-EDUCATION

After preliminary discussion and explanation, the patient settles comfortably into half-lying or lying, with a pillow under the knees.

8.6.1   Awareness of breathing

Suggestions to facilitate patients' awareness of their breathing include the following:

- rest one hand on the upper chest and one on the abdomen to distinguish upper chest and abdominal breathing,
- experiment with slight alterations in the depth of breathing, then the rate of breathing, to distinguish the two concepts,
- try alternate nose and mouth breathing to feel the difference,
- feel the passage of your breath, feel it pass through your nose, down your windpipe and into your lungs, then gently turning back along the same route,
- feel the cool air on the in-breath and warm air on the out-breath,
- what is the size of your breath, what is the shape of your breath?
- try a pause between the out-breath and the in-breath,
- take a deep breath followed by a breath-hold (which should be short to avoid tension, but long enough to bring awareness of the sensation of air hunger),
- try breathing out as far as you can,
- what is the difference with your eyes open and closed?
- what is the rest of your body doing?
- what do your neck muscles feel like?

8.6.2   Relaxation

Breathing cannot be re-educated in a stressed person, and most patients need a session of relaxation (p. 164). Some people find that the thought of being obliged to relax itself causes tension, and prefer to do relaxation after breathing re-education.

Tense people often find relaxation an alien concept, and it may be easier after back or neck massage, during which they are advised to focus on the experience and not feel that they have to talk or 'do' anything. Even the old infra-red lamp has been found helpful for relaxation, usually to the back with the patient prone. Some patients find that lying prone for relaxation makes them feel less vulnerable.

Focusing on the breath itself helps relaxation, especially if patients are encouraged to gently 'breathe in the good air' and 'breathe out the tension', as if freeing the breath. A relaxed state should be maintained by bringing the patient's attention to areas of tension throughout treatment, especially the jaw and throat. Physiotherapists should ensure that they themselves are relaxed.

It is not unusual for symptoms to appear in the early stages of treatment because of a paradoxical, but transient, increase in hyperventilation. Relaxation lets down a wall of tension and may release buried feelings, and breathing re-education may feel subconsciously threatening because of interference with such a basic need. If this occurs, an explanation is all that is required.

8.6.3 Abdominal breathing

Patients are then taught abdominal breathing (p. 114), taking care to maintain small gentle breaths. In lying, abdominal breathing may be facilitated with the hands behind the head.

8.6.4 Slowing the breath

The combination of education, relaxation and abdominal breathing has shown improvement in 94% of patients (Pinney *et al* 1987). If further treatment is required, patients should practise 'breathing less' – but gently, gently – avoiding tension and exacerbation of abnormal breathing patterns. 'Breathing less' means reducing the rate or depth of breathing, or both. Patients usually understand this

concept, but may need a reminder that slow breathing does not mean deep breathing. 'Low and slow' is the key. Some need only a pause at end-exhalation.

If patients tense up, the emphasis should be on smooth, gentle, rhythmic breathing. To help patients maintain their rhythm, it is best not to ask for verbal feedback during the practice, but rather to observe the patient's breathing pattern. When a session of breathing practice is finished, it is best for the patient to stop smoothly and avoid gasping.

If patients still find this difficult, more structured support can be given by pacing the patient's breathing to the physiotherapist's voice. The patient's breathing pattern is first observed closely, then he or she is asked to breathe in time with the physiotherapist's words, the rate of which is slightly slower than the patient's breathing. Suggestions for instructions are:

'In-and-out, in-and-out . . .'
'In-and-out-two-three, in-and-out-two-three . . .'
'In-and-relax-out, in-and-relax-out . . .'
'In-and-let-it-out, in-and-let-it-out . . .'

Words and timing should be flexible to suit the patient, but they need to be repeated rhythmically. Some patients find that pacing brings a sense of security in the early stages, the words acting as a 'breathing pacemaker'. Progression is aimed at independent control without the physiotherapist's voice.

Patients should experience a modicum of discomfort from air hunger, but not enough to develop tension. If they feel an irresistible need, they can take a conscious and controlled deeper breath, then get back gently into rhythm again, sometimes with a preliminary breath-hold as compensation (but not if this causes tension).

Advice can be given at appropriate intervals:

- keep it smooth, shallow and abdominal,
- swallow if you need to suppress a deep breath,

without food for more than three hours. This should be emphasized for patients who eat heavily at night, which can produce night-time or early-morning symptoms. Meals should be slow and enjoyable, and patients should avoid excessive coffee, cola or chocolate. If they must smoke, deep drags are to be avoided.

Much encouragement is needed to help patients integrate their new breathing pattern and attitude into the distractions of everyday life. If progress is slow, more attention should be given to identifying individual fears and precipitating factors. Reassessment of the abnormally high demands to which patients often subject themselves may be fruitful. Family and friends can be enlisted as extra sources of encouragement.

A handout helps to correlate this mass of information. A tape can be made of each physiotherapy session and be given to the patient; the educational component of the session acts as a reminder, which may be useful because poor concentration is a frequent symptom, and the relaxation component can assist practice at home. Some patients ask for a tape of the physiotherapist's voice counting at three levels of fast, medium and slow. They can use this to pace themselves at the correct level, to the point of feeling air hunger but not distress. Relaxation tapes are also available commercially, but patients must be reminded to ignore instructions to breathe deeply.

Practice in breathing re-education should take place if possible little and often, usually about two to three times a day for 15 minutes. In addition, spot checks throughout the day can be integrated so that they fit in with regular events, such as coffee breaks, queues, coming home from work, or television advertisements. Timers jog the memory, as will stickers on toothbrushes, telephones and other strategic locations. Breathing should be checked every day before getting out of bed.

Although disruption to daily life should be minimal, many patients find it worthwhile to set aside 20 minutes a day for relaxation. Others find individual ways of relaxing, such as a rocking chair or personal stereo. A hot bath is often unhelpful because excessive heat stimulates the respiratory centre. Many people need reassurance to overcome guilt at allowing themselves time to relax.

Despite the plethora of potential advice, it is important not to burden patients with excessive homework because they tend to become preoccupied with their daily programme. It is often best to use education as the basis for individuals to make their own decisions.

Physiotherapy is needed weekly until self-management is stabilized, then sometimes monthly for adjustment and encouragement, followed by occasional top-up visits. Three to 14 weeks of treatment have shown positive outcomes, i.e. improvement in questionnaire scores, capnography, anxiety and depression (Tweeddale *et al* 1994). Once learned and reinforced, the new breathing pattern can be maintained automatically because there is no structural damage. Self-awareness and stress management, however, must last a lifetime. Patients often report that HVS has given them the opportunity to rethink their lifestyle.

The physiotherapist's most useful assets are warmth, humour and acute observational skills. Patience and commitment are needed, but the reward can be a dramatic restoration of enjoyment to a life that has sometimes become a shambles.

RECOMMENDED READING

Grossman, P. (1985) A controlled study of a breathing therapy treatment of HVS. *J. Psychosom. Res.*, **29**, 49–58.

Howell, J.B.L. (1990) Behavioural breathlessness. *Thorax*, **45**, 287–92.

Innocenti, D.M. (1993) Hyperventilation, *Physiotherapy for Respiratory and Cardiac Problems*, (eds B.A. Webber and J.A. Pryor), Churchill Livingstone, Edinburgh, pp. 377–97.

Rowbottom, I. (1992) The physiotherapy management of chronic hyperventilation. ACPRC J., **21**, 9–12.

9. *Intensive care*

9.1 INTRODUCTION

Patients are admitted to an intensive care unit (ICU) if they require intensive therapy, intensive monitoring or both. They are not necessarily critically ill, but are at risk of failure of one or more major organs. Their needs range from observation of vital signs after major surgery, to total support of physiological systems. Admission usually depends on expectation of recovery, and the majority of patients return to their previous health status (Rustom 1993).

9.2 THE ENVIRONMENT

9.2.1 Effects on the patient

He may cry out for rest, peace, dignity, but he will get infusions, transfusions, a heart machine
. . . he will get a dozen people around the clock, all busily preoccupied with his heart rate, pulse, secretions or excretions, but not with him as a human being.

Kübler–Ross 1973

It is ironic that seriously ill people find themselves in an environment that itself causes stress and fatigue, factors which are major contributors to hindering a patient's recovery (Swann 1989). It is not an optional extra to give attention to this aspect of patient management, but an integral part of physiotherapy. The effects of stress are the following (Brannon *et al* 1993):

- ↑ respiratory rate, heart rate and BP,
- perceptual distortion and impairment of judgement, causing poor response to advice and education,

- ↑ metabolic rate and protein breakdown in patients who are already catabolic and nutritionally depleted, thus consuming energy that should be used for healing,
- release of thyroid hormones (which increase oxygen consumption), and ADH (which retains fluid),
- sleep disruption, which augments stress,
- tendency to infection, gastric ulceration, muscle tension and blood clotting abnormalities,
- depression,
- exhaustion.

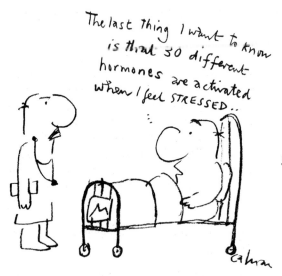

The severity of the stress response varies with patients' ability to control their situation. The causes of stress are the following:

1. **Communication.** Inability to communicate has been found to be the most stressful experience in the ICU (Pennock 1994; Villaire 1995).
2. **Sleep fragmentation.** It is claimed that lack of sleep leads to death faster than lack of food (Wood 1993b). A full 90-minute cycle is needed to achieve the restorative benefits of sleep, yet this is

rarely achieved in the ICU (Wood 1993b). The more ill the patient, the more sleep he or she needs and the less is got. Disruption is due to noise, interruptions, anxiety, pain, difficulty finding a comfortable position and the fear of some patients that falling asleep means not waking up again.

3. **Fear.** Patients face unknown and previously unmet fears which may compromise their coping mechanisms. Fear is compounded if patients are unable to communicate.
4. **Sensory deprivation.** Despite being outlawed by the International Court of Human Rights, sensory deprivation is found in the ICU, albeit unintentionally, due to social isolation, loss of touch, immobilization, certain drugs, taped eyelids, sometimes no windows and often removal of hearing aid or glasses. This leads to a form of emotional solitary confinement that can leave patients feeling intense loneliness despite constant attention.
5. **Sensory overload.** Patients find themselves lost in a sea of electronic wizardry and bombarded by unfamiliar beeping, constant overhead lights, telephones, confining equipment, painful procedures, tubes in every orifice and incomprehensible conversations over their heads. Most conversations are between staff, not with the patient (Wood 1993b). ICU noise is consistently above internationally recommended levels and leads to adverse physiological effects (Kam 1994). The combination of sensory deprivation and overload causes disorientation and sometimes delusions.
6. **Helplessness, dependency and depression.** The less patients are able to do for themselves, the more frustrated they feel, and this may deteriorate into depression, especially for long-stay patients. Depression can become internalized as anger, which is difficult for patients to

express when they are dependent on the goodwill of those who care for them.

7. **Discomfort**. Immobility, gagging on the endotracheal tube, dribbling and sweating, a dry mouth and unscratchable itches all cause discomfort, especially in people who are paralysed or otherwise restrained. Physical restraint is one of the commonest stressors in experimental medicine and has been shown to cause gastric ulcers (MacKellaig, 1990).

8. **Loss of time sense**. Patients struggle to keep track of time through a tranquillized haze, especially when there is no day–night sequence in lighting or routine. Many become disoriented, and the more alert become bored. Occasionally patients find that this empty time gives them an opportunity to reassess their values, especially if they have been close to death, and they emerge with a sharpened perception of what is and is not important in their life.

9. Loss of privacy, dignity and identity. It is easy for us to forget how people feel when they lose their autonomy, clothes, teeth, personal space and surname. Patients who are elderly or from a different culture are particularly vulnerable to this form of depersonalization.

Day and night, morning and evening disappear. Consciousness, beautiful dreams, cruel nightmares and a sometimes even crueler reality are lost, or so it seems, confused and intertwined. And all around . . . there is a whole world of people who do not realize that one's ears hear.

Ruiz 1993

9.2.2   Effects on relatives

Relatives can do much to ease a patient's stress, so long as they in turn are given support. They may feel bewildered, daunted by the environment and reluctant to voice their concerns. Enforced passivity leads to frustration and resentment. Visitors need:

- encouragement to become involved in their relative's management, e.g. mouth care, physical comforts and certain passive movements,
- information about equipment, the patient's condition and the reason for physiotherapy,
- the opportunity to say what they are thinking or feeling,
- reassurance that touch and conversation are welcomed by most patients.

9.2.3   Effects on staff

Emotional responses can become dulled by the frequency with which they are elicited. People working in an ICU need some psychological defences, but not those that are incompatible with sensitive patient care.

If we become stressed, we are not only less able to identify with the experience of the patient, but we also make mistakes. Reactions to working in the ICU include anxiety because of the responsibility, frustration at communication difficulties or inability to relieve suffering, overdetachment, guilt at wishing a long-term patient would die, and inappropriate joking with other staff, which can be misunderstood by patients and relatives.

Strategies to reduce staff stress include the following:

1. Involvement of all staff in decision-making.
2. In-service training to increase knowledge and confidence.
3. Staff support, e.g. feedback, sharing of ideas, debriefing after traumatic incidents and recognition that doubts are acceptable. Once staff can accept their own reactions, they better understand those of their patients. This support helps modify the tendency for health workers to focus all their energy on looking after patients at the expense of themselves, which does not benefit patients in the long run.

9.2.4   Patients' rights

Legal rights

A competent adult is entitled to refuse treatment, even if this treatment is life-saving (Everhart and Pearlman 1990). It is illegal to force physiotherapy on patients who resist, or who are unable to resist but have made their wishes clear. If patients do not know that they have these rights, they should be informed. If they are not lucid, the physiotherapist makes the decision.

Moral rights

Patients have a right to the truth, to participate in decision-making, to refuse to be used for teaching, and to be given full care even when their choice differs from ours. These rights should not be violated if a patient is young or has learning difficulties.

Ethics

If a patient is unable to make choices, and continued treatment is extending death rather than prolonging life, discontinuation of treatment should be a team decision, and include consideration of the relatives' views. Some countries acknowledge 'living wills' (advance directives) as legal documents, which allow individuals, when competent, to express a wish to be spared life-sustaining treatment in case of intractable or terminal illness (Snider 1995). 'Do not resuscitate' orders should be discussed with patients when possible (Wagg 1995).

9.2.5   Teamwork

Interpersonal factors are the main cause of stress in high-dependency areas (Biley, 1989), and poor communication is a significant cause of mistakes (Donchin 1995). Success depends on mutual respect and assertiveness, mutual teaching and learning, shared coffee breaks, flexibility and, above all, good communication.

Problems may arise over boundaries and autonomy. If physiotherapists would like to ask for review of a therapy that is not their direct responsibility, they can raise the subject diplomatically by asking for advice, or by making a connection between medical management and rehabilitation. If physiotherapy is medically prescribed, physiotherapists can thank the doctor for his or her advice, and clarify that the patient will be assessed and treated as appropriate. Results are likely to be positive when communicating in a way that makes it easy for others to agree.

Communication between physiotherapists and nurses is facilitated by the physiotherapist offering to help change sheets when it fits in with turning the patient during treatment, and the nurse incorporating regimes such as hourly incentive spirometry into the nursing plan. Turning for physiotherapy should be co-ordinated with turning for pressure area care.

9.2.6   Infection control

Hospitals are curious places and ICUs even more curious. Immunocompromised patients are crowded together and bombarded with ICU-hardened bacteria which flourish among the invasive technology. Widespread broad-spectrum antibiotic therapy is then added to encourage superinfection by resistant organisms (Kollef 1994).

Loss of upper airway defences in mechanically ventilated patients leaves them vulnerable to colonization from equipment, staff and the bacteria swarming in their own gut. Nosocomial pneumonia afflicts 20% of intubated patients.

Measures to prevent infection include:

- most importantly, handwashing between patients,
- plastic aprons changed between patients (Gill and Slater 1991),
- meticulous attention to sterile suction technique,

- respect for tracheostomies as the surgical wounds that they are,
- not allowing an open catheter mount to touch the sheets,
- minimizing the time that patients spend supine, which risks aspiration of gastric contents (Torres 1992).

More elaborate procedures include selective digestive decontamination and continuous aspiration of subglottic secretions to reduce microaspirations through the cuff (Vallés 1995).

9.3 MECHANICAL VENTILATION

Intermittent positive pressure ventilation (IPPV) replaces or augments the function of the inspiratory muscles by delivering gas under positive pressure to the lungs.

9.3.1 Indications

Most ventilated patients do not have respiratory disease but are in established or impending respiratory failure. The following people need IPPV:

1. Patients who are unable to ventilate adequately, oxygenate adequately, or both. Examples are respiratory depression due to anaesthesia or drug overdose, inspiratory muscle fatigue due to exacerbation of COPD, and severe hypoxaemia due to lung parenchymal disease.
2. Patients who are able to breathe adequately but for whom this is deemed inadvisable, e.g. acute head injury.

Mechanical ventilation should not be used so that pain relief can be given. Analgesia can be administered by methods that do not inhibit respiration (Chapter 7), and fractured ribs or the aftermath of major surgery are not by themselves indications for continued IPPV.

9.3.2 Airway

The connection between ventilator and patient is through a sealed tracheal tube (Fig. 9.1). An endotracheal tube (ETT) through the mouth or nose can be used for up to two weeks, but is uncomfortable, may damage the larynx and creates more resistance than the patient's own airway, especially with high gas flows (Slutsky 1993). A nasal tube is marginally better tolerated than an oral tube, but causes more resistance. A tracheostomy tube is more comfortable, causes less resistance and is used if longer-term ventilation is required. If a patient has a newly-created tracheostomy, extra care is needed to avoid disturbing the tube.

A cuff prevents escape of the ventilating gas and reduces, but does not eliminate, the risk of aspiration. It is inflated until an airtight seal is achieved, using a manometer to ensure that cuff pressure does not exceed 25 mmHg and risk airway damage.

The problems of tracheal tubes are:

- interference with communication,
- risk of chest infection because of loss of defence mechanisms, damage to the mucociliary escalator and a welcoming environment for bacteria in the pool of secretions above the cuff,
- with an endotracheal tube: discomfort, gagging, retching, oversalivation and bronchospasm,
- with a tracheostomy: mucosal damage, especially if the tube is mishandled, and the complications described on p. 196.

The frustration of being unable to speak can be relieved by a speaking tracheostomy tube (Manzano 1993; Tucker 1991), and advice from a speech and language therapist.

Humidification is supplied by a hot-water bath, which is the most effective device, or a heat–moisture exchanger (HME), which is adequate for short-term use in well-hydrated patients who do not have excessive or thick secretions. HMEs bring less risk of infection, and some devices incorporate antibacterial

(a)

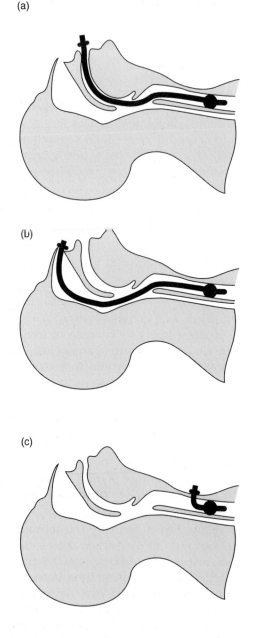

(b)

(c)

Figure 9.1 Tracheal tubes: (a) oral endotracheal tube, (b) nasal endotracheal tube, (c) tracheostomy tube.

properties, but the non-hygroscopic variety can lead to tracheal tube occlusion from thick secretions (Branson *et al* 1993).

HMEs should be removed during aerosol treatment via the ventilator circuit, and their use should be limited to five days (Branson *et al* 1993), but the physiotherapist may request an earlier change to a hot-water bath if sputum clearance is a problem.

Both hot-water humidifiers and HMEs increase airflow resistance, but less so than bubble-through systems, which are unsuitable (Hirsch 1991).

9.3.3   Principles

A bewildering array of all-singing, all dancing ventilators are flooding the market, leading to a 'terminology soup' which complicates classification. A ventilator breath can, however, still be classified according to how it is triggered into inspiration, controlled (generated) during inspiration and cycled into expiration.

Either the patient or ventilator can **trigger** inspiration. Patient triggering is usually according to the patient's flow or pressure (typically minus 1 to minus 2 cmH$_2$O). If the ventilator initiates inspiration automatically, it is triggered according to time.

The **control** mechanism is the factor which remains constant despite changes in ventilatory load. Volume control means that the ventilator delivers a specific minute volume according to preset variables such as respiratory rate, tidal volume and I:E ratio. Airway pressure depends on these variables and lung compliance, but a pressure limit is set for safety. Pressure control delivers gas under a preset constant pressure. The delivered tidal volume is influenced by lung compliance and fluctuations in patient effort, so volume monitoring is advisable.

Volume control is commonly used for adults because it can be relied on to deliver a consistent minute volume regardless of lung compliance. Pressure control is safer for patients with stiff lungs (peak airway pressure $> 60\, cmH_2O$) and babies because it limits alveolar distension.

Inspiration **cycles** into expiration according to a preset time, pressure, volume or flow. Pressure cycling means that if the lungs are stiff or airway resistance high, the machine cycles prematurely.

Pressure control is different from pressure cycling. A pressure-controlled breath will not necessarily cycle at a preset pressure, for example inspiration might continue until a preset time.

Alveolar pressure is not equal to that measured at the airway opening, unless there is zero flow, because of resistance to gas flow in the airways. Alveolar pressure is more negative during patient triggering and more positive during a positive pressure breath.

9.3.4 Effects and complications

1. An advantage of IPPV is rest for the inspiratory muscles. This rest is hindered by, e.g. a narrow ETT, obstructed airways, stiff lungs, poor trigger sensitivity or inappropriate settings so that patient and machine are not synchronous. Excess workload becomes evident by accessory muscle activity. The disadvantage of resting the muscles is atrophy, one study showing a 50% loss of strength in only 11 days of controlled ventilation (Anzueto *et al* 1987).

2. Mechanical ventilation allows complete control of inspired gas and can deliver up to 100% oxygen. Gas exchange also depends on mean airway pressure, which includes the effects of PEEP.

3. Positive pressure accentuates the perfusion gradient from upper to lower regions, leaving the top virtually without blood flow (Fig. 9.2). It also displaces blood away from the thorax and

reduces renal, hepatic and splanchnic blood flow (Beale *et al* 1993).

4. While spontaneous breathing draws ventilation down to dependent lung regions (p. 7), IPPV reverses this gradient because:
   (a) the diaphragm is passive,
   (b) positive pressure gas takes the path of least resistance, which is the more open upper region,
   (c) the lower region is compressed by the increased perfusion.
   Dependent areas receive the least ventilation and are vulnerable to progressive atelectasis.

5. Disturbed ventilation and perfusion gradients result in $\dot{V}_A/\dot{Q}$ mismatch, which would lead to hypoxaemia if not offset by the inspiratory pause, supplemental oxygen at a minimum 35% and a generous minute volume.

6. Dead space increases because of reduced overall perfusion, and to a lesser extent because of positive pressure distending tubing and the patient's airways.

7. IPPV with overinflation depletes surfactant (Heulitt 1995).

8. Positive pressure in the chest impedes venous return to the heart, leading to a drop in cardiac output of typically 25% (Ponte 1990). Compensation is by peripheral vasoconstriction, which maintains filling pressures to the heart. This mechanism may not be viable in patients who are elderly, hypovolaemic (either absolutely or implied by peripheral dilatation, e.g. in septic shock), suffer autonomic neuropathy such as in Guillain–Barré syndrome, or who already have a raised right atrial pressure from COPD. These patients may drop their BP, especially when first put on the ventilator. The haemodynamic effects can be reduced by a low I:E ratio so that the heart has time to fill on the expiratory phase. Patients with stiff

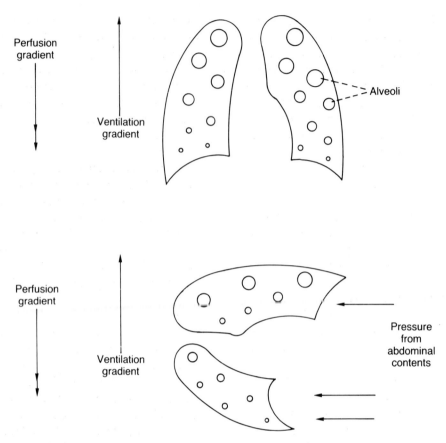

Figure 9.2 Effect of IPPV on ventilation and perfusion gradients. In contrast to spontaneous respiration, the ventilation gradient is reversed and perfusion gradient increased. Compare with Fig. 1.5.

lungs suffer less haemodynamic compromise because less of the alveolar pressure is transmitted to the pleural space.

9. Fluid retention can occur due to stress-mediated ADH secretion and redistribution of blood flow within the kidneys, leading to an average 40% decrease in urine output (Pilbeam 1992, p. 223).

10. Barotrauma is extra-alveolar air which occurs in 0.5–20% of patients (Schnapp, 1994). In the past this was thought to be due to excess pressure, which came from the reasoning that 'patients with barotrauma tend to have high peak pressures, therefore high peak pressures cause barotrauma'. But because the two occur together does not mean that the one causes the other. Alveolar overdistension and high F_IO_2 levels are usually present when pressures are high, and it is now thought that excess oxygen and excess volume cause the damage rather than excess pressure (Heulitt 1995). Most attention has been given to the excess volume because high F_IO_2 levels are often unavoidable. The excess volume versus excess pressure argument is explained by the fact that coughing (in which pressure increases

greatly but volume is unchanged) rarely causes barotrauma, and that high-volume negative pressure ventilation can cause lung injury (Chatburn 1991). The term 'volutrauma' rather than 'barotrauma' is sometimes more correctly used. Prolonged exposure and pre-existing lung damage are extra risk factors (Heulitt 1995).

Excess inflation can be monitored by inductive plethysmography (Dall 1992), which measures FRC (raised with hyperinflation) and V_T (not raised with hyperinflation). But physiotherapists may have to rely on their knowledge of conditions that are associated with hyperinflation.

Barotrauma leads to alveolar rupture, then interstitial emphysema (escape of air into interstitial lung spaces), pneumomediastinum, subcutaneous emphysema, bullae and/or pneumothorax. Early signs of barotrauma are difficult to detect radiologically except in neonates.

Barotrauma is rare in normal lungs, even during prolonged mechanical ventilation (Pierson 1988), but it is a significant risk in lungs that are stiff, hyperinflated or suffer non-homogeneous damage.

11. Overdistension of alveoli and large volume changes increase vascular pressure and cause microvascular damage, inflammation and leakage of fluid (Heulitt 1995). The contribution of IPPV to pulmonary oedema is often not recognized.

12. Patients are at risk of infection.

13. IPPV can be uncomfortable and distressing. Some patients regard their ventilator with a combination of resentment and fear of the time when it has to be removed.

14. Breathlessness can be due to loss of patients' control of their own breathing, increased perception of loading imposed by airflow resistance in the trachealtube, and lack of stimulation of lung stretch receptors.

15. Positive pressure reduces splanchnic perfusion, increases permeability of the gut mucosal barrier and leads to increased incidence of paralytic ileus, bleeding and ulceration (Pilbeam 1992, p. 225).

16. Absorption atelectasis (p. 90) may occur with high oxygen concentrations and a low V_T. Oxygen toxicity can occur with prolonged oxygen therapy.

17. Intrinsic PEEP (p. 55), unlike extrinsic PEEP (p. 227), occurs unintentionally. It is caused by obstructed airways, poor ventilator management, or plumbing problems such as a narrow tracheal tube or water clogging the ventilator tubing. This exacerbates the difference between alveolar pressure and pressure at the airway opening at end-expiration.

Intrinsic PEEP ($PEEP_i$) can lead to overdistension, decreased lung compliance, risk of barotrauma, increased work to trigger a breath, reduced V_T, impaired trigger sensitivity, misleading haemodynamic and pressure monitoring, reduced venous return, and direct cardiac compression (Sim 1994).

$PEEP_i$ is suspected in patients with COPD, asthma or ARDS. Signs of hyperinflation such as reduced breath sounds and a hyper-resonant percussion note, further increase suspicions. Confirmation is by a high plateau pressure, a flow tracing with persistent flow at end-expiration (Fig. 9.3) or sundry ventilator manoeuvres (Slutsky 1993). $PEEP_i$ has been identified in nearly half of a typical ICU population of ventilated patients (Wright 1990).

The effects of this unwanted PEEP can be mitigated by maximizing spontaneous breathing, minimizing airflow resistance, and by ventilator manipulations such as reducing

(a)

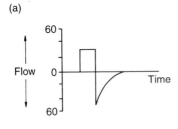

(b)

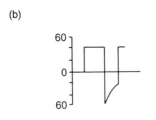

(c)

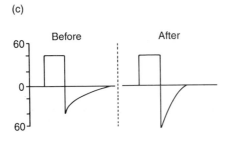

Figure 9.3 Flow curves representing different conditions: (a) normal, (b) intrinsic PEEP, showing positive flow at end-exhalation, (c) before and after bronchodilator, showing prolonged and normal expiratory flow.

minute ventilation, decreasing I:E ratio or maintaining patent airways with a pressure support mode of ventilation (Tokioga 1992) or low levels of extrinsic PEEP. It may seem paradoxical to apply extrinsic PEEP, which conventionally increases lung volume, to a condition characterized by hyperinflation, but extrinsic PEEP counterbalances intrinsic PEEP provided it is comfortable and below the level of intrinsic PEEP (Slutsky 1993).

9.3.5   Waveforms

Figure 9.4(a) shows a normal pressure curve.

Peak airway pressure is the maximum pressure recorded at the end of inspiration.

Mean airway pressure is equivalent to the average system pressure; it is associated positively with oxygenation and negatively with haemodynamic side-effects.

Plateau pressure is the nearest approximation to peak alveolar pressure. The decelerating inspiration means that rapid early-inspiration delivers gas to the small airways quickly and slow late-inspiration encourages optimum distribution once it reaches the small airways.

A negative pressure deflection (Fig. 9.4(b)) represents a patient-triggered breath, the depth of deflection indicating patient effort. Small fluctuations in pressure indicate spontaneous breathing efforts (Fig. 9.4(b)).

9.3.6   Modes

IPPV can do all the work of breathing (WOB) by controlled mandatory ventilation, or the work can be shared between ventilator and patient using a wide variety of ventilatory modes. These modes allow ventilatory support to be adjusted to the needs of individuals, leaving them more comfortable, less sedated and with fewer complications.

Ventilatory modes have to be matched skilfully to the patient because all are less efficient than spontaneous breathing (Shelledy 1995), and while too much support leads to muscle atrophy, too little overworks the patient. Most modes allow or require patients to trigger breaths. Activating the demand valve to trigger a breath requires effort because valves must have some inbuilt insensitivity to prevent artifacts triggering inspiration.

Controlled mandatory ventilation (CMV)

Fully controlled ventilation is usually only needed for patients who are unable to

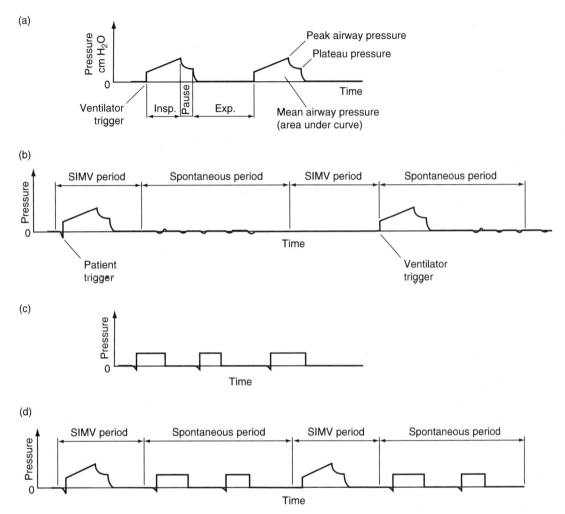

Figure 9.4 Pressure curves delivered by the ventilator:
(a) controlled mandatory ventilation, (b) SIMV, (c) pressure
support, (d) SIMV with pressure support. A negative deflection
indicates a patient-triggered breath. If PEEP is used, the baseline
would be raised above zero.

breathe at all or for whom complete control is necessary, e.g. to allow a patient to be paralysed. It is an unforgiving mode which dictates the depth and frequency of each breath and time-cycles into expiration. If patients try to breathe, they only receive gas from a relief valve, and sedation is required. Risk of intrinsic PEEP and other complica-tions is significant. Minute volume is set high enough to maintain a mild respiratory alkalosis so that spontaneous breathing is inhibited.

Intermittent mandatory ventilation (IMV)

The IMV mode allows patients to breathe spontaneously between a preset number of mechanical breaths, but without regard for the patient's breathing pattern. This can lead to the stacking of machine breaths on top of spontaneous breaths, intrinsic PEEP and up to double the WOB of a spontaneous breath (Tobin 1991).

Synchronized intermittent mandatory ventilation (SIMV)

In SIMV mode, the ventilator delivers either a patient-triggered spontaneous breath or a time-triggered mandatory breath. If the patient has not taken a spontaneous breath after a set interval, the mandatory breath is delivered (Fig. 9.4(b)). Synchrony with inspiratory effort is more comfortable than IMV and avoids breath stacking.

Pressure support or assist mode

Pressure support (PS) is a pressure-controlled, flow-cycled mode which delivers a preset pressure while allowing patients to determine their own flow, V_T, RR and I:E ratio (Fig. 9.4(c)). The preset variables are the trigger sensitivity and pressure support level.

PS reduces WOB in proportion to the pressure delivered, the patient doing up to 50% of the work (Pilbeam 1992, p. 171), which is less than with CPAP (Shelledy 1995). Newer machines increase the pressure if the patient makes more effort. PS is relatively comfortable and ensures synchrony because patients have control of ventilatory timing. It acts like IPPB, but inspiration stops according to flow rather than pressure, thus discouraging the unhelpful expiratory effort that can mar IPPB.

PS is used for patients who can reliably trigger the ventilator. It is especially useful for weaning, when 10 cmH$_2$O pressure support counteracts the work imposed by the ventilator circuit.

SIMV with pressure support or assist-control

This mode provides some minimum mandatory breaths, topped up with extra breaths triggered by the patient (Fig.9.4(d)). This is less synchronous and less comfortable than pressure support, and if not carefully set can cause excess WOB (Shelledy 1995) and may overventilate patients who get a full preset breath every time they breathe or even hiccup.

Mandatory minute ventilation (MMV)

MMV is a little-used mode in which the ventilator provides a guaranteed preset minute ventilation if the patient's spontaneous breathing drops below a preset level. Unlike SIMV, assistance is not provided until the patient's minute ventilation falls below a preset level. Pressure support is sometimes added to ensure adequate tidal volume for patients with rapid shallow breathing.

Inverse ratio ventilation

For patients with refractory hypoxaemia but for whom high peak airway pressures are to be avoided, inspiratory time can be prolonged to the point of reversing the I:E ratio up to 4:1 (Pilbeam 1992, p. 413). Long inspiration recruits collapsed alveoli, and short expiration aims to prevent recollapse. Disadvantages are risk of intrinsic PEEP and the discomfort of an unnatural breathing pattern, for which extra sedation is required. Inverse ratio ventilation is usually used with pressure control to reduce the risk of barotrauma for people with ARDS (Armstrong 1995).

Airway pressure release ventilation

In this modified form of BiPAP, spontaneous breaths are passively supported by a continuous flow, with intermittent one to two second releases on expiration so that CO$_2$ is eliminated (Pilbeam 1992, p. 124). The aim is to improve oxygenation with lower peak airway pressures, especially for people with ARDS.

9.3.7 Settings

Ventilation and oxygenation are matched to the patient according to $PaCO_2$ and PaO_2 respectively. A healthy spontaneously breathing adult maintains adequate ventilation with an approximate **tidal volume** (V_T) of 450–600 ml and **respiratory rate** (RR) of 10–20/min to give a minute volume of 5–7 l. Ventilated patients are given a relatively high V_T (500–800 ml) to minimize atelectasis and keep patients comfortable by stimulating the stretch receptors and reducing breathlessness. RR is kept relatively low (10–18/min) for optimum gas distribution.

The **minute volume**, made up of V_T and RR, is adjusted according to $PaCO_2$. V_T is adjusted for a small change in $PaCO_2$, and RR is adjusted for a larger change. Normal range for minute volume on IPPV is 8–12 l, but this varies widely, a COPD patient with chronic hypercapnia requiring a few litres while a septic patient with a high metabolic rate might need > 30 l.

Inspired oxygen concentration is adjusted according to PaO_2, although the relationship between F_IO_2 and PaO_2 is less direct than that between minute volume and $PaCO_2$ (Chatburn 1991). A higher than normal concentration is required to offset the $\dot{V}_A/\dot{Q}$ mismatch caused by the altered mechanics of breathing.

The **I:E ratio** is related to V_T, RR and flow rate. It is normally set at 1:2 to allow time for adequate venous return on expiration, but can be as low as 1:4 to prevent hyperinflation, e.g. in acute asthma, or as high as 2:1 to improve oxygenation in hypoxaemic patients.

Inspiratory **flow rate** is related to the I:E ratio. Low levels reduce peak airway pressure and improve gas distribution, but at the expense of a high I:E ratio with its associated haemodynamic side-effects (particularly decreased cardiac output). It is set high enough to meet the patient's inspiratory demand.

Inspiratory pause (plateau) is an end-inspiratory hold which enhances gas distribution by recruiting poorly ventilated alveoli. Advantages are maximum gas exchange with minimum peak airway pressure. Disadvantages are increased mean airway pressure with the risk of haemodynamic side-effects.

The maximum number of independent controls is three, the others following automatically. Examples of adapting these variables are:

- for a patient with emphysema and prolonged expiration who typically has a spontaneous I:E ratio of 1:5 or 1:6, the inspiratory flow is set for rapid inspiration and long exhalation,
- for a patient with fibrotic lungs who works hard to inhale and whose high recoil pressure speeds exhalation, the flow rate allows prolonged inspiratory time and short expiratory time.

A continuous flow system can be superimposed on the patient-demand system to allow greater responsiveness to inspiratory effort. The **flow-by** or **flow-trigger** option delivers a predetermined base flow of gas to the patient circuit so that fresh gas is available as soon as inspiration is initiated. This minimizes the delay between effort and gas supply and reduces the work load, virtually eliminating patient effort to trigger a breath. Flow-by is similar to BiPAP but based on flow rather than pressure. It should not be used during nebulizer treatment.

A **sigh mechanism** is incorporated into certain ventilators because it was once thought, mistakenly, to prevent atelectasis. The risk of atelectasis is now reduced by PEEP or high tidal volumes (Chatburn 1991).

9.3.8 Positive end-expiratory pressure (PEEP)

There are several ways to boost SaO_2. Inspired oxygen, I:E ratio or the plateau can be increased, or PEEP can be applied. PEEP maintains a constant pressure in the lungs during the expiratory phase and expiratory pause so that airway pressure does not fall to atmospheric pressure at end-expiration. Like CPAP, it aims to recruit collapsed alveoli.

PEEP can be used with any mode of ventilation, pressures varying from 3 to over 20 cmH$_2$O. The pressure gauge on the ventilator shows the pressure returning to the PEEP value instead of zero at end-expiration. For triggered breaths, the machine is set to cycle into inspiration a few cmH$_2$O below the PEEP level so that the patient does not have to make an inspiratory effort all the way to zero.

PEEP is termed 'extrinsic PEEP' when it needs to be distinguished from intrinsic PEEP.

Effects and complications

Extra positive pressure raises the resting lung volume out of the range of airway closure, thus increasing the area available for gas exchange and improving $\dot{V}_A/\dot{Q}$ match. At optimum pressures, surfactant is conserved, $PA\text{-}aO_2$ reduced and oxygen saturation improved for the same F_IO_2. Pressures of 10 cmH$_2$O can reduce lung densities, but these will reappear within one minute of removing PEEP (Brooks-Brunn 1995).

PEEP does not reverse the underlying pathology, and high levels of PEEP are associated with complications that are exaggerations of the complications of mechanical ventilation, especially the following:

1. PEEP impairs venous return to the heart and reduces cardiac output. This can offset the beneficial effects of PEEP by causing a net decrease in oxygen delivery, even with improved SaO_2. Haemodynamic compromise occurs at > 15 cmH$_2$O in normovolaemic patients, at lower pressures in hypovolaemic patients and at higher pressures in patients with stiff lungs (Pilbeam 1992, p. 392). Stability of cardiac output depends partly on intra

vascular volume, and fluid administration can therefore compensate, although this may incur pulmonary oedema when PEEP is discontinued. Haemodynamic monitoring is required and PEEP should be applied in small increments, titrated against the improved oxygenation.

2. PEEP increases the risk of barotrauma in patients who have lung disease, e.g.:
    (a) hyperinflation conditions such as emphysema (unless carefully controlled PEEP is being used to reduce intrinsic PEEP),
    (b) unilateral pathology, in which PEEP would cause hyperinflation of the normal more compliant lung, unless selective ventilation using a double lumen ETT is used.

3. Increased pressure within the chest may increase CVP and PAWP readings (p. 234) at the same time as the ventricular filling pressure that they are supposed to represent is declining because of decreased venous return.

4. High level PEEP may disrupt the alveolar-capillary barrier and redistribute alveolar fluid, leading to pulmonary oedema. Any apparent X-ray improvement may be due to recruitment of alveoli even though lung water may be rising. However, levels of PEEP at or below 10 cmH$_2$O are thought safe and, by preventing alveolar collapse, may even protect against ventilator-induced damage due to shear stresses generated by the reopening of collapsed alveoli (Parker and Hernandez 1993).

5. When disconnecting the ventilator circuit for suction, pressure from PEEP increases blow-back, with risks to staff and other patients of cross-contamination from the spray.

Best PEEP

Optimum levels of PEEP normalize oxygen delivery to the tissues, not just increase

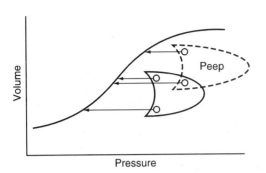

Figure 9.5 Effect of PEEP on the relationship between regional pressure and volume. Compliance is greater in the upper part of the lung without PEEP. It is greater in the base of the lung with PEEP. (Source: Nunn (1987), with permission.)

oxygen in the blood: normal cardiac output with a hypoxaemic patient may be better than half the normal cardiac output without hypoxaemia. Best PEEP is achieved with the highest value for oxygen delivery or, if tissue oxygenation monitoring (p. 236) is not available, a combination of optimum SaO_2 and cardiac output. A high lung compliance, as indicated by the least pressure swing on the ventilator pressure gauge, is also an indicator because while effective PEEP increases lung compliance, excessive PEEP decreases it by overdistending alveoli. The effect on oxygen delivery is measurable within 15 minutes of initiating PEEP (Patel 1993). Figure 9.5 shows how best PEEP can improve ventilation to the lung bases.

Precautions

High levels of PEEP should be avoided in patients with an undrained pneumothorax, avoided if possible with subcutaneous emphysema, bulla, bronchopleural fistula or recent pneumonectomy, and used with caution in patients with damaged or diseased lungs.

Hypovolaemia is a relative contraindication, but if PEEP is necessary, measures can be taken to support cardiac output with fluids and inotropes.

Indications

PEEP promotes oxygenation without toxic levels of inspired oxygen, and is often used if more than 50% oxygen is required. Its main use is for hypoxaemia caused by alveolar instability. It may also be used to overcome intrinsic PEEP. Occasionally, differential ventilation with selective PEEP is used for atelectasis (Klingstedt *et al* 1991) and to reduce haemodynamic side-effects (Veddeng 1992).

9.3.9   High-frequency ventilation

How does the Himalayan mountain shrew maintain oxygenation during copulation? With a respiratory rate up to 600/min, its V_T is less than its dead space, but it manages to achieve the feat of gas exchange by a mechanism similar to the intriguing phenomenon of high-frequency ventilation (HFV).

There are three basic methods of this form of mechanical ventilation:

1. High-frequency positive pressure ventilation uses conventional ventilation at respiratory rates of 50–100/min.
2. High-frequency jet ventilation directs short rapid jets of gas from a high-pressure nozzle down an ETT or minitracheostomy tube, pulsating gas into the airways and entraining air by the venturi principle. Expiration is by passive recoil and rates of 100–600/min are achieved.
3. High-frequency oscillation (HFO) forces minibursts of gas in and out of the airway so that both inspiration and expiration are active, thus avoiding the gas trapping that often occurs with passive exhalation (Hardinge 1995). This can be superimposed on spontaneous breathing (p. 127) or can be the sole method of ventilation. Rates up to 4000/min are achieved.

Mechanism

With such a meagre V_T, gas exchange cannot rely on the bulk flow of gas. The classic concept of 'dead' space is no longer applicable, and this space is in fact thought to play an active part in gas exchange by the following mechanisms (Bower 1995):

- high-velocity flow creates turbulent mixing in the central airways, which is propagated peripherally by convective inspiratory flow,
- gas mixing may occur by asynchronous filling and emptying of alveoli independent of each other, an effect known merrily as 'disco lung',
- diffusion is augmented, especially by the vibrating gas of HFO.

Advantages

1. HFV provides a more even distribution of ventilation than conventional IPPV because diffusion is independent of regional compliance, and gas flow does not take the path of least resistance.
2. Spontaneous respiration is inhibited and little sedation is needed, most patients finding the sensation comfortable, as if being massaged from the inside.
3. Structural lung rest can occur because alveoli are subjected to minimal volume or pressure changes, leading to less damage and less risk of oxygen toxicity (Durbin 1993).
4. Jet ventilation via minitracheostomy allows spontaneous respiration through the normal airway, which enables patients to talk, cough, sigh, eat and drink.
5. HFO is thought to aid mucociliary clearance (Natale *et al* 1994).

There is no evidence that haemodynamic compromise or barotrauma are reduced.

Disadvantages

1. Progressive atelectasis is almost inevitable because of the tiny V_T, although this can be minimized by intermittent sustained inflations at 30 cmH$_2$O pressure (Bond 1994).
2. Intrinsic PEEP can be caused by the brief passive exhalation of jet ventilators (East 1993), thus putting them out of bounds for asthma and COPD. This problem can be reduced by creating an air leak around the ETT or combining jet with conventional ventilation (Raphael 1993).
3. Secretion clearance may be adversely affected (McEvoy *et al* 1982), except with HFO.
4. Humidification is inefficient, particularly with jet ventilation. Humidifying the driving gas is more successful than humidifying the entrained gas, and special devices such as high-temperature vaporizers can be used (Rouby 1990).
5. HFV is noisy.

Indications

HFV is sometimes considered a technique in search of an application, but enthusiasts consider the following to be suited to its ministrations:

1. Patients with a flail chest, bronchopleural fistula, large air leak, acute head injury or unstable cardiovascular status, so long as low airway pressure is assured.
2. Patients with an inordinate respiratory drive, or a need for minimum sedation.
3. Patients with unilateral lung stiffness, by receiving differential ventilation to each lung.

Physiotherapy

Jet ventilation through a minitracheostomy allows patients to deep breathe and cough, and suction can be performed without interruption of ventilation. Suction has fewer adverse effects on oxygenetion or heart rhythm than with IPPV, but as bag-squeezing is not possible, it is advisable to increase the F_1O_2 for three minutes before and after suction.

9.3.10   Weaning

I was sure I would not be able to breathe on my own. The machine was put to a setting which gave me a couple of breaths and the rest was up to me. I hated that, I never knew when to take my breaths.
Ludwig 1984

Weaning incorporates removal from the ventilator, a trial of spontaneous breathing through the tracheal tube, then extubation. This may be as simple as asking the patient to breathe, but with lung disease or after long-term ventilatory support, a protracted period of weaning may be required.

Weaning and extubation decisions are made by medical staff. The physiotherapist is involved in advising on the balance of rest and exercise, and sometimes in doing extubation. The art of weaning is to identify patients who will have difficulty weaning and start working with them early, preferably by exercise from day one, either on the bed or in sitting, standing or walking connected to a rebreathing bag.

Criteria

To prevent weaning becoming prolonged and distressing, the following are required before removal from the ventilator:

*   maximum ventilatory reserve, i.e. baseline values for vital capacity, respiratory rate and oxygenation,
*   optimum bronchodilation and clear airways,
*   optimum nutritional, fluid, metabolic and cardiovascular status, including adequate haemoglobin levels,
*   maximum strength, endurance, mobility and ability to cough,
*   prior two to three hours' uninterrupted sleep,
*   reversal of sedation.

Traditional weaning indices were based on set values for maximum inspiratory pressures (see Glossary) and minute ventilation, but these have now been challenged as no better than flipping a coin, and newer indices based on breathing pattern (absence of rapid shallow breathing and abdominal paradox) appear to be more accurate (Mador 1992).

Weaning is easier with an alert patient, but analgesia should not be withheld if needed for pain or intolerance of the endotracheal tube. Even unconscious patients can breathe spontaneously.

Removal from the ventilator

The following procedure is usually followed:

1. Explanation of the procedure is given to the patient, with assurance that it is only a trial.
2. Ventilatory support is gradually reduced, e.g. by decreasing pressure during pressure support. Weaning decisions can be computer controlled to match patient data to reduced support (Strickland, 1993).
3. The patient takes up his or her preferred posture, usually sitting upright.
4. Humidified oxygen or mechanical assistance is prepared as appropriate. If oxygen is connected by a T-piece, either a one-way valve or a 30 cm extension tubing attached to the exhalation port prevents inhalation of room air and increases dead space so that CO_2 rises and stimulates breathing.
5. The airway is suctioned.
6. The patient is disconnected from the ventilator, given oxygen and/or mechanical assistance, encouraged to breathe, and monitored for signs of laboured breathing, anxiety, desaturation, rising $PaCO_2$, fatigue or drowsiness. A breathlessness visual analogue scale allows the patient to contribute to weaning decisions (Bouley 1992).
7. Several short sessions off the ventilator are better than prolonged periods. If the diaphragm tires, it may need 24 hours to recover.

Difficulty may be due to inspiratory muscle fatigue and/or atrophy, undetected diaphragmatic paralysis or the patient's fear of suffocation, which can be imagined by anyone who has been ducked in the school swimming pool. Rest is needed for fatigue. Fears are managed by providing information and truthful reassurance that return to the ventilator is available by request at any time. Relaxation with oximetry biofeedback has been shown to reduce anxiety, respiratory rate and heart rate (Acosta 1988). Another form of biofeedback is to connect the patient briefly to a rebreathing bag with an open valve, which the patient watches for reassurance that he or she is breathing. A bedside fan may decrease breathlessness. CPAP is often used for mechanical assistance, but BiPAP or nasal ventilation may be more comfortable (Restrick 1993). Patients undergoing protracted weaning usually require full ventilatory support at night.

Continuing problems may be due to weaning strategies providing neither sufficiently intense muscle activity nor sufficient rest, leading to perpetual muscle fatigue. For this reason, a T-piece should not be used for longer than half-an-hour (Armstrong *et al* 1991). For patients who cannot perform whole-body exercise, inspiratory muscle training provides brief periods of exertion alternating with rest (Aldrich 1989). This should also be achievable by manipulation of ventilatory modes.

Extubation

After liberation from the ventilator, the ETT should be removed as soon as possible because breathing through a tracheal tube can double the workload (Goldstone and Moxham 1991). Patients can be extubated once they are alert, show a stable breathing pattern and can control their airway. The cough response can be assessed by asking the patient to cough or by gently stimulating the airway with a catheter. The ability to sustain a head lift indicates sufficient strength to protect the airway (Tobin and Yang 1990). The steps for extubation are the following:

1. Give physiotherapy if indicated, or simply suction the airway. Check for a cough reflex.
2. Ensure that reintubation equipment and personnel are available.
3. Explain to the patient how the tube will be removed and that some hoarseness is commonplace.
4. Suck out the mouth and throat to clear secretions that have pooled above the inflated cuff.
5. Cut the tape holding the tube in place, insert a fresh catheter to reach just distal to the tip of the tube, deflate the cuff, remove the tube at peak inspiration when the vocal cords are dilated, suctioning during withdrawal.
6. Encourage the patient to cough out secretions that have accumulated around the end of the tube. If this is impossible, bag-squeeze while deflating the cuff, which forces secretions into the mouth from above the cuff.
7. Give oxygen, CPAP or other support, observe the monitors, listen for stridor.
8. Enjoy the patient's delight at his or her renewed voice.
9. If sputum retention is anticipated, it may be better to request a minitracheostomy as prophylaxis rather than await respiratory distress.

Removal of tracheostomy tube

Weaning for tracheostomied patients can be more leisurely, and an intermediate step is to replace the cuffed tube with an uncuffed or fenestrated tube, which can be plugged for increasingly longer periods to test for adequate breathing and coughing. When the tube has been removed, the patient is taught to hold a sterile dressing over the stoma when coughing.

9.4 MONITORING

Frankly it feels quite awful to be connected to machines through every available orifice.

plus several new medically-made ones, in spite of feeling thankful for all the life-sustaining help and healing ministrations.

Brooks 1990

From the patient's point of view, monitors bring both anxiety and reassurance. From the staff's point of view, they are useful to record sudden or subtle changes in a patient's status. They are complementary to clinical observation and not a substitute. Monitoring differs from measuring; it implies regular observation and a systematic response if a variable falls out of a specified range.

9.4.1   Gas exchange

Arterial oxygen tension

Arterial blood samples are taken by intermittent puncture of the radial artery, using local anaesthesia (Gribbin 1993), or more comfortably by an indwelling arterial catheter. PaO_2 values are subject to spontaneous variability, and patients should be undisturbed for 30 minutes beforehand, stay in the same position for each measurement and receive the same F_IO_2. Arterialized capillary blood from the earlobe is more comfortable (Dar 1995).

Arterial oxygen saturation

Oximetry is the physiotherapist's friend. It gives instant feedback on arterial oxygen saturation without trauma to the patient. The different absorption of light by saturated and unsaturated haemoglobin is detected by the oximeter, which produces a continuous display of oxygen saturation. Sensors fit comfortably on the ear, finger, toe or nose.

Oximetry is acceptably accurate at values above 75%. Desaturation is indicated by values below 95% in black people, 92% in white people, or a drop of 4% (Durbin 1994). Being dependent on perfusion, the oximeter is fooled by vasopressor drugs, hypotension, hypovolaemia, peripheral vascular disease or anaemia. When the oxygen dissociation curve is shifted to the right, the oximeter shows a slightly low SaO_2, and when shifted to the left, a slightly high SaO_2. The accuracy of finger and toe sensors is affected by movement, and finger sensors are further compromised by nicotine stains or varnished nails.

Transcutaneous monitoring (PtcO$_2$ and PtcCO$_2$)

Oxygen and CO_2 diffuse across the skin and can be measured by a sensor. This is heated to arterialize capillary blood, but measurements vary with skin metabolism and capillary blood flow, and are thought to reflect tissue oxygen tension rather than PaO_2. In haemodynamically stable patients they therefore relate to respiratory status, but with cardiovascular problems they reflect cardiac output. Skin burns are avoided by rotating sites every few hours and incorporating a temperature alarm.

In neonates, $PtcO_2$ correlates with arterial oxygenation, but in adults it is hampered by varying skin thicknesses and invalid if there is poor perfusion, critical illness or if the sensor is not applied for 20 minutes before measurement (Durbin 1994). If ideal conditions are met, the adult $PtcO_2$ is at least 10% below PaO_2, and $PtcCO_2$ is similarly higher than $PaCO_2$.

Capnography

A capnograph provides continuous non-invasive assessment of ventilation by monitoring the percentage of CO_2 in expired air (Szaflarski *et al* 1989). It monitors end-tidal CO_2, which approximates alveolar PCO_2 if ventilation and perfusion are well matched, but for patients with lung disease it is not dependable (Tobin 1991). Capnography can be combined with oximetry to produce a continuous display of both measurements.

9.4.2   Haemodynamic monitoring

The heart and vascular systems can be thought of as a continuous loop in which constantly shifting pressure gradients keep the blood moving.

Blood pressure

Continuous monitoring of BP by an indwelling catheter gives more accurate and instant feedback than cuff pressure. The most relevant reading is mean arterial pressure, which represents the perfusion pressure over the cardiac cycle.

Right atrial pressure (RAP)

The central venous pressure (CVP) is monitored by creating an extension of the patient's vascular system and measuring the pressure within it by a transducer or manometer (Fig. 9.6). A radio-opaque catheter is passed through a large neck or arm vein into or just outside the right atrium, through which all venous blood passes. The pressure within this system is equivalent to the RAP, which is the filling pressure or preload of the right ventricle. The CVP (i.e. RAP) reflects the volume of circulating blood and the ability of the heart to handle that volume. It both determines and is affected by the interaction between blood volume, right heart function and, to a lesser extent, vascular tone.

Single values are less relevant than the trend, but a raised CVP, like a raised JVP, is caused by heart failure, COPD, pneumothorax or overtransfusion of fluid. CVP provides early warning of cardiac tamponade, which causes a sudden increase in CVP, or haemorrhage, which causes a sudden drop in CVP. Haemorrhage reduces CVP before blood pressure because BP is maintained temporarily by arterial vasoconstriction.

Central venous catheterization is now a routine procedure, and is used not just for CVP measurements, but also for drug infusions, blood sampling, feeding and cardiac

output monitoring. These multiple functions are serviced by a forest of three-way taps, or more conveniently by a triple lumen catheter.

Implications specific to physiotherapy are the following:

1. A raised CVP may indicate pulmonary oedema, and a low CVP, if due to hypovolaemia, is a sign of possibly thick secretions.
2. Cannulation of a large vein near the pleura may cause a pneumothorax or subcutaneous emphysema, and the X-ray should be checked before embarking on any positive pressure manoeuvre.
3. The supine position is normally required for measurement (although Groom *et al* (1990) have claimed that side-lying is acceptable for certain patients), which means that good teamwork is needed to ensure on-going positioning for prophylactic respiratory care.

The CVP is often an adequate guide to the filling pressures of both sides of the heart, but may take 24–48 hours to rise in response to left ventricular failure (the pressure has to back up through the pulmonary circulation) and is misleading if either ventricle is impaired, e.g. if left ventricular compliance is increased by PEEP, ischaemia or vasopressors, or decreased by vasodilators.

Left atrial pressure (LAP)

LAP relates to left ventricular function in the same way that RAP relates to right ventricular function. A pulmonary artery catheter, called a Swan–Ganz, is passed along the CVP catheter route, then floated through the right ventricle into the pulmonary artery, facilitated by an inflated balloon at its tip (Fig. 9.6). Here it measures pulmonary artery pressure (PAP), which reflects the pressure that needs to be generated by the right ventricle to contract against the pulmonary vasculature. A raised PAP indicates pulmonary hypertension, pulmonary embolism or fluid overload.

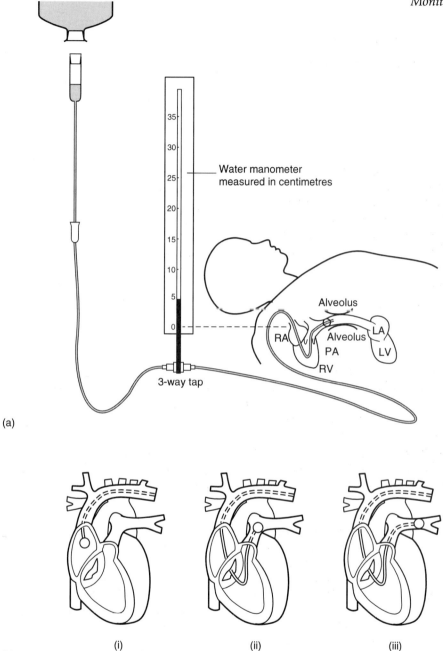

(a)

(b)

Figure 9.6 (a) Representation of haemodynamic monitoring. A multilumen catheter monitors CVP from the right atrium, PAP from the pulmonary artery, and PAWP from the pulmonary vasculature. Zero point on the manometer is at the level of the right atrium, and the CVP reading is 5 cmH$_2$O. PA = pulmonary artery. (b) Passage of pulmonary artery catheter as it measures (i) CVP, (ii) PAP, (iii) PAWP.

People with COPD show an increased PAP of up to 40 mmHg, which rises during sleep and on exercise. (Average values are given in the Glossary.)

The catheter can then be carried further by the flow of blood until it wedges in a peripheral branch of the pulmonary vascular bed. With the balloon inflated, the catheter tip is isolated from fluctuations on the right side of the heart and therefore reflects pulmonary venous pressure. So long as there is a continuous column of blood between the catheter tip and left atrium, this is assumed to reflect left atrial pressure, measured as pulmonary artery wedge pressure (PAWP). The balloon acts as a form of pulmonary embolism, so is deflated between measurements to reduce ischaemic damage.

A high PAWP implies fluid overload, 20 mmHg marking the onset of pulmonary congestion and 25 mmHg being associated with radiological evidence of pulmonary oedema. The continuous column of blood in the pulmonary vasculature is tenuous if the catheter is in the upper zone of the lungs or if the patient is severely hypovolaemic, has COPD or requires high lung inflation pressures, especially with PEEP. Therefore, the more ill the patient, the less accurate are single measurements, but the trend is still relevant.

PAWP reflects pressures in the lung vasculature, left atrium and left ventricle, and is used as a guide to left heart function and blood volume. It shows changes earlier than CVP and gives a more accurate indication of fluid status because it is affected by fewer variables. This allows fine tuning when establishing optimum PEEP, helps to rationalize fluid and drug therapy and distinguishes between hypovolaemia ($\downarrow$ PAWP) and left ventricular failure ($\uparrow$ PAWP) because hypovolaemia can coexist with peripheral oedema.

PAWP is also known as pulmonary capillary wedge pressure (PCWP) or simply wedge pressure. The glamour of this expensive monitoring system has led at times to misuse of a system whose complications include thrombosis, sepsis, arrhythmias and trauma to the delicate pulmonary vessels (resulting in blood-stained secretions). Its use is best reserved for haemodynamically unstable patients who are refractory to medical treatment after scrupulous clinical assessment.

Both CVP and PAWP measurements are limited as a guide to fluid volume because some vasoconstriction may maintain values despite hypovolaemia, and chronic lung or heart disease can also invalidate measurements. However, the trend is worth observing.

An increase in intrathoracic pressure due to IPPV, especially with PEEP, will raise both RAP and LAP values, but the common practice of discontinuing ventilation for measurement is unnecessary and can cause persistent hypoxaemia (Schwartz 1987). Readings are best taken at end-expiration.

9.4.3   Tissue oxygenation

Outcome measures for bus journeys are more relevant taken at their destination than when the bus leaves the garage. Similarly, oxygen in the tissues is more relevant than oxygen in the blood.

Mixed venous oxygenation

Oxygen delivery to the tissues is affected by many factors, such as fever, sepsis, pain and physiotherapy. Oxygen levels in the pulmonary artery measure the extent to which oxygen supply meets demand, indicating both the haemodynamic and gas exchange components of oxygenation.

Mixed venous blood in the pulmonary artery comprises venous blood from all body tissues which has been thoroughly mixed in the right heart. The oxygen and CO_2 in this pooled blood reflect events anywhere in the respiratory chain from lung to mitochondria. This measurement is especially useful in identifying problems at tissue perfusion and extraction level, beyond the reach of arterial blood gas measurements.

Mixed venous blood provides information on mixed venous oxygen saturation ($S\bar{v}O_2$), monitored continuously from the pulmonary artery catheter, or mixed venous oxygen tension ($P\bar{v}O_2$), measured intermittently in blood drawn from the catheter.

A low $S\bar{v}O_2$ reflects decreased oxygen delivery or increased demand. It drops with hypoxaemia, anaemia, low cardiac output, haemorrhage or when oxygen consumption rises with activity, pain, fever, anxiety, agitation, laboured breathing or hypermetabolic states. Values below 40% are usually associated with anaerobic metabolism. $S\bar{v}O_2$ rises with a high F_IO_2 or if the patient is paralysed or sedated. Excessively high values above 85% indicate that tissues are too damaged to extract sufficient oxygen, e.g. in severe sepsis, ARDS, acute pancreatitis or extensive burns.

An advantage of this measurement is that it indicates changes before BP, heart rate or PAWP. A disadvantage is that it does not pinpoint which of the variables is responsible for the change. It acts more as an early warning system to advise on further investigation. Cardiac output should be simultaneously monitored so that it can be distinguished from other variables.

During physiotherapy, if $S\bar{v}O_2$ varies by > 10% from the baseline for more than three minutes, or for more than 10 minutes following position change, treatment should be stopped (Hayden 1993). If it has not recovered three minutes after suctioning, increased oxygenation is required.

Gastric tonometry

Hypoxia or 20% hypovolaemia causes a 60% reduction in gastric blood flow (Ricour 1989). The gut is one of the first organs to be affected by poor perfusion and provides early warning of whole-body tissue hypoxia. Gastric tonometry entails passing a saline-filled bal-loon into the stomach to measure the mucosal pH. Acidosis indicates hypoperfusion and ischaemia, which if not corrected may lead to multisystem failure (Chang 1994).

9.4.4 Cardiac output (CO)

Accurate CO measurements require the patient to be in a steady state. If a pulmonary artery catheter is *in situ*, CO is measured by the thermodilution technique, in which a bolus of cold liquid is injected into the pulmonary artery catheter and escapes through a hole into the right atrium. The speed of its dispersal is then measured and CO calculated by computer. CO can also be assessed non-invasively through measuring aortic blood flow by Doppler and a host of other techniques (Harrington 1993).

Cardiac output usually reflects BP, but they do not always change in the same direction. If the myocardium is poorly contractile, peripheral vasoconstriction may ↑ BP and ↓ CO, and vasodilation may ↓ BP and ↑ CO.

9.4.5 Overview of electrocardiography (ECG)

Disturbances such as hypoxia, physiotherapy treatment, electrolyte imbalance, myocardial ischaemia or anxiety can cause disorders of heart rate or rhythm; some are transient but others are significant because of their effect on cardiac output. These are picked up on the ECG, which is a recording of electrical activity in the heart (Fig. 9.7).

Sinus tachycardia is a heart rate (HR) over 100 bpm with normal rhythm. **Sinus bradycardia** is an HR under 60 bpm with normal rhythm.

Supraventricular arrhythmias originate from above or in the atrioventricular (AV) node, and are known as atrial and nodal arrhythmias respectively. Ventricular arrhythmias originate from the ventricle.

Supraventricular tachycardia is recognized by a rapid rate, regular rhythm and normal

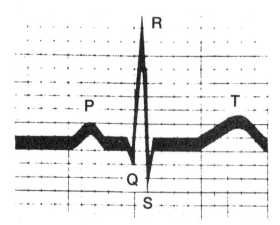

Figure 9.7 Normal ECG trace of one heart beat. P = atrial depolarization, PR = atrioventricular conduction time, Q = ventricular depolarization, R = first positive deflection during ventricular depolarization, S = first negative deflection during ventricular depolarization, QRS interval = total ventricular depolarization, T = ventricular repolarization (recovery period).

QRS complex. It is caused by excess drugs or sympathetic activity and can reduce cardiac output. **Ventricular tachycardia** is distinguished from supraventricular tachycardia by its irregularity, lost P wave, and broad and bizarre QRS complex. It can reduce cardiac output, BP and tissue perfusion, and lead to ventricular fibrillation.

Sinus rhythm is normal rhythm, activity being controlled by the sinus node. **Nodal rhythm** is abnormal and occurs when the AV node takes over from a non-functioning sinus node, resulting in lost P waves and a variable or absent PR interval. Cardiac output remains stable unless HR is severely affected.

Ectopic beats are premature beats followed by a compensatory pause, sometimes felt as missed heart beats by the patient. They are common and do not contraindicate physiotherapy unless they increase in number or cause haemodynamic disturbance, but they may signal the onset of serious arrhythmias. **Atrial ectopics** manifest as occasional abnormal P waves or an early normal beat, and are of little significance unless frequent. **Nodal ectopics** are similar to those of atrial origin and are the main cause of nodal rhythm. **Ventricular ectopics** are caused by an irritable focus in the ventricle, producing an absent P wave, a wide and wayward QRS complex and inverted T wave. They occur following heart surgery or myocardial infarction, and in smokers, and are associated with hypoxia or low potassium. **Bigeminy** means that every other beat is ectopic and **trigeminy** means that every third beat is ectopic.

Atrial fibrillation (AF) is the commonest arrhythmia, affecting 5% of people over 60 years (Rowland 1994). It occurs when ectopic foci throughout the atria discharge too fast for the atrial muscle to respond other than by disorganized twitching. It appears as a rapid rate of up to 200 bpm, irregular rhythm and the replacing of P waves with a fibrillatory baseline. It has a variety of causes including increased sympathetic tone, hypoxaemia, hypokalaemia, over- or underhydration, myocardial ischaemia, heart failure or heart surgery. It causes fatigue, predisposes to thrombosis and may reduce cardiac output. **Atrial flutter** is similar to AF but is less common, and fires at a lower rate of discharge, causing regular saw-tooth undulations on the ECG.

Ventricular fibrillation (VF) is total breakdown of ordered electrical activity, causing an ineffectual quivering of the ventricles and appearing as a chaotic line. There is no cardiac output and cardiac arrest ensues. A similar disorganized trace may also appear, but harmlessly, during percussion and vibrations to the chest or if the electrodes fall off the patient. **Asystole** is ventricular standstill and also leads to cardiac arrest. It shows as a straight line with occasional minor fluctuations.

Heart block is caused by delayed or blocked conduction between P wave atria and ventricles, shown as a disrupted relationship between P wave and QRS complex

Causes are hypoxia, myocardial infarction, digoxin therapy, heart disease or complications after heart surgery. First or 2nd degree heart block is suspected if there is a long PR interval or several P waves prior to each QRS complex. Third degree heart block is indicated by an absent PR interval and abnormal QRS complex. This may reduce cardiac output and lead to asystole.

9.5 SUPPORT

9.5.1 Pacing

An artificial pacemaker is used to deliver an electrical stimulus to the myocardium when the conducting pathways are damaged. For temporary use, pacing wires connect the patient's myocardium to an external pacing box. For permanent support, the energy source is implanted under the skin. Indications are 3rd degree heart block, arrhythmias refractory to medication and prophylactic support in the first days after heart surgery. External wires on a patient's chest postoperatively are common and not a contraindication to mobilization, so long as the cardiovascular system is stable.

An implantable cardioverter defibrillator may be implanted into patients at risk of VF that cannot be suppressed with drugs (Collins 1994).

9.5.2 Nutrition

The oft-quoted comparison between the nutritional status of prisoners of war and ICU patients is a myth that comes perilously close to the truth at times. Physiotherapists commonly watch their patients waste away on the empty calories of a dextrose infusion while they are struggling uphill to maintain the physical condition of lungs and limbs.

Critical illness can double or treble the metabolic rate, while at the same time reducing the body's adaptive response, leading to some patients being malnourished for 85% of

their stay (Lowell 1990). The causes of malnutrition are:

- increased catabolism, as shown by a study on starvation in which septic, traumatized or burned patients lost up to 200% more protein daily than healthy people (Schlichtig and Sargent 1990),
- pre-existing nutritional deficit,
- inadequate feeding in an attempt to limit weight gain following fluid overload during surgery (Lowell 1990),
- lack of recognition of a process as undramatic as starvation,
- lack of hunger, ability to express hunger or capacity to eat normally.

The effects of malnutrition are muscle wasting, difficult weaning, impaired healing, atelectasis, pulmonary oedema (Pilbeam, 1992, p. 261), increased risk of oxygen toxicity (Durbin 1993) and the effects described on p. 98.

The key is to provide early nutritional support in order to prevent rather than correct tissue breakdown. If patients are able, they should sit out of bed and eat at normal times. If patients cannot swallow, they should have nasogastric or enterostomy feeds, and those with gut dysfunction should be fed intravenously. Intravenous (IV) feeds are hypertonic in order to provide sufficient calories, and central venous access is required to allow for its rapid dilution with blood to avoid vessel damage.

Disadvantages of IV feeding are infection risk (Koretz 1995) and loss of integrity of the gut lining. The gut has long been considered dormant in critical illness, but is now known to be metabolically active and a protective barrier against gut pathogens. IV feeding or starvation can worsen the damage caused by gut ischaemia, leading to breakdown of the mucosal barrier and liberation of microorganisms into the portal circulation to wreak havoc in the rest of the body. The gut is now thought to be the 'motor' of multisystem failure (Johnston 1993). It is recommended that some postoperative patients start enteral feeding in the recovery room, using small bowel access if there is paralytic ileus (Babineau 1994).

The ability to meet the nutritional requirements of critically ill patients may be hindered by fluid restriction, impaired renal function, gut problems or glucose intolerance. Remedial measures include diuresis or haemofiltration to prevent fluid overload and early dialysis for kidney problems.

Rapid administration of high calorie (especially high carbohydrate) feeds can increase CO_2 production by 40% due to oxidation of glucose (Schlichtig and Sargent 1990). For patients with marginal respiratory reserve, this can precipitate respiratory failure (Liposky 1994). Slow administration of high-fat, low-glucose feeds is necessary for patients with hypercapnic COPD, especially during weaning, and the omnipresent dextrose infusion must be taken into account.

9.5.3 Fluids

Preload is the filling pressure in the ventricle at end-diastole, which stretches the myocardium and assists contraction. It is determined by venous return and blood volume. It is increased in heart failure or fluid overload, and decreased in hypovolaemic shock or dehydration. Left preload is monitored by PAWP and right preload by CVP.

Afterload is the amount of pressure against which the ventricle must work during systole, as if opening the door against a wind. It is increased with systemic/pulmonary hypertension, peripheral vasoconstriction or aortic/pulmonary valve disease, and decreased in septic or neurogenic shock. Left afterload is monitored by systolic BP and right afterload by pulmonary artery pressure.

Fluids are closely associated with cardiovascular function. An adequate circulating volume should be ensured before other forms of support are considered (Armstrong *et al* 1991). The detrimental effects of physiotherapy, especially suctioning, are less marked in a well-filled patient (Schwartz 1987).

Intravascular fluids are relevant to circulatory function whereas interstitial and intracellular fluids are not. **Colloids** are thick fluids such as plasma and albumin. Transfused colloid stays in the intravascular compartment and affects osmotic pressure and circulatory function (Golster 1995). **Crystalloids** are thin fluids, such as dextrose and saline. Seventy-five percent of transfused crystalloid is rapidly lost from the plasma (Armstrong *et al* 1991), so that **crystalloid transfusion** has less effect on intravascular volume or circulation and **excess transfusion** may lead to pulmonary oedema from the escaping fluid.

9.5.4 Drugs

Critically ill people often respond abnormally to drugs because of liver hypoxia, stress and circulatory or renal impairment (Park 1994). They are also subject to complex interactions of multiple medication. Many intensive care drugs have a narrow window between effective and toxic doses, and infusion pumps help the titration of dosage to patient response.

Cardiovascular drugs

The intimate relationship between heart function, vascular tone and fluid volume can be manipulated by medication to achieve optimum tissue oxygenation. Many patients need a combination of increased CO, reduced myocardial oxygen demand and redistribution of flow to vital organs.

Diuretics reduce blood volume and preload, and are used to treat hypertension, heart failure and pulmonary oedema. When mobilizing a patient who is taking diuretics, a wary eye should be kept for signs of hypotension.

Vasodilators, such as the nitrates, reduce systemic vascular resistance and are prescribed for hypertension, heart failure and angina. Side-effects include postural hypotension.

Inotropes assist a failing heart by augmenting the force of cardiac contraction. Natural inotropic influences include the patient's own adrenaline and noradrenaline. Before giving inotropic drugs, the fluid status of the patient should be sufficient to ensure that the drugs do not stimulate an empty heart. Dopamine is an inotropic drug which at low doses increases renal perfusion (possibly due to ↑ CO), at medium doses increases CO directly, and at high doses causes unwanted vasoconstriction. Dobutamine has a greater effect on oxygen delivery and does not cause vasoconstriction. Dopexamine combines the renal effects of dopamine with the haemodynamic effects of dobutamine.

These inotropic agents are used for circulatory failure and to offset the depressant effects of PEEP on cardiac and renal function. They do so at the expense of increasing myocardial oxygen requirements, and in patients with tachycardia, may actually decrease oxygen delivery and cause myocardial ischaemia. They are therefore only used after regulation of fluid, diuretic and vasodilator therapy.

Digoxin is a cardiac glycoside with mild inotropic effects that has been in and out of fashion for two centuries. It helps control arrhythmias by strengthening and slowing the HR, but tends to cause arrhythmias if there is hypoxia.

A combination of vasodilator and inotropic medication is often used. **Inolators** are combined vasodilators and inotropes which are still in the experimental stage.

Beta-blockers are 'negative inotropes' which inhibit sympathetic action, block the action of adrenaline and related hormones and slow the HR, reduce cardiac work and relieve hypertension, angina and arrhythmias. Non-selective beta-blockers such as pro-pranolol may induce bronchospasm, but this risk is reduced with the more cardioselective drugs, such as atenolol. Other side-effects are fatigue and the blunting of cardiac exercise responses. Beta-blockers should never be given to patients on beta$_2$-stimulants because of their mutual antagonism.

Sedation

Sedation is required for most patients on IPPV, but should not be used as the first line treatment of anxiety. Drugs that cloud consciousness cause delusions if anxiety stems from patients' realistic perceptions of their situation, and they are no substitute for the primary task of explanations and relief of discomfort. Commonly prescribed anxiolytics are midazolam and propofol, which reduce oxygen consumption but cause the side-effects of respiratory depression, loss of time sense and misinterpretation of voices and noises, which can paradoxically increase anxiety.

Analgesia

Treatment for pain, anxiety and insomnia is often interwoven. The pain component should be easily managed in mechanically ventilated people because respiratory depression is not a problem. Prior to physiotherapy treatment, a bolus of intravenous analgesia is often indicated, using a short-acting drug, such as fentanyl or alfentanyl. Entonox can be administered by a doctor or respiratory technician through the ventilator before and during treatment, but the initiative for this must come from the physiotherapist.

Paralysis

I couldn't turn or change position. And even though it may have been only an hour, it seemed like a week to me . . . someone would come near me and would just be working and not saying anything to me. That would be frightening because I didn't know what they were going to do next.

Parker *et al* 1984

Muscle relaxants such as pancuronium, atracurium or vecuronium are given to patients on IPPV in order to induce paralysis and prevent resistance to ventilation. These neuromuscular blocking agents are used when it is detrimental to allow patients to move, e.g. after acute head injury, or to reduce oxygen consumption in severely-hypoxic patients. Paralysing agents should not be used to keep a patient quiet. They act as a form of chemical restraint, and this can feel frightening for patients if they are not told that they are being given a drug that will make them feel weak.

The induction of weakness, not paralysis, is sufficient to prevent patient–ventilator asynchrony (Marino 1995). The drugs must be accompanied by sedation and, if appropriate, analgesia, because they obliterate the only means by which patients can indicate discomfort. Patients feel, hear and think normally, but it is easy to forget that they are conscious and need regular explanations and orientation. Extra care must also be taken to prevent ventilator disconnection. Prolonged administration sometimes leads to persistant myopathy after cessation of the drug (Bellomo 1994), especially in patients taking steroids or in renal failure.

Drugs for airflow obstruction

Airflow obstruction raises airway pressure and increases the risk of barotrauma and haemodynamic disturbance. Bronchodilators or steroids may be required, especially during weaning, and can be delivered to ventilated patients by metered dose inhaler or small-volume nebulizer. Half the drug is lost in the endotracheal tube (Kacmarek and Hess, 1991), but a spacer compensates for this, whether using an inhaler or nebulizer (Harvey 1995). The spacer is removed from the circuit when not in use. The effect of aerosolized drugs is variable and should be monitored, e.g. by ↓ wheeze on auscultation, ↓ peak airway pressure, a normalized flow curve (Fig. 9.3) or ↓ intrinsic PEEP (Wollam 1994).

An MDI with spacer delivers a greater dose than a nebulizer and is quicker and cheaper (Hess 1994). Nebulizers interfere with patient-triggered breaths and ventilator settings, so the ventilator should be put on a non-assisted mode (Pilbeam 1992, p. 311), with reduced flow and respiratory rates to maximize inspiratory time for aerosol deposition (Manthous 1994). It is placed at the Y-connector (Hess 1994).

The MDI is also placed at the Y-connector and either fired immediately after the beginning of a mechanical breath or manually ventilated through the spacer just before inspiration using slow deep breaths, a breath hold and a one minute gap between actuations if this is not contraindicated (Hess 1994). Dry powder inhalers cannot be used in ventilator circuits.

A humidifier increases particle size of either MDI or nebulizer, and decreases aerosol delivery by 40–50% (Hess 1994), so it should be removed during administration.

9.5.5   Advanced cardiac support

For patients in profound heart failure, mechanical assistance can be provided temporarily by an **intra-aortic balloon pump** (Underwood 1993). The pump, housed in a console, is connected to a catheter with a deflated balloon at its tip. This is threaded through the patient's femoral artery and into the aorta (Fig. 9.8), where it is triggered by the patient's ECG into the following cycle:

1. Diastole causes balloon inflation, which assists aortic valve closure and displaces blood to augment perfusion of the myocardium, brain and kidneys.
2. Systole deflates the balloon, which decreases afterload and allows the ventricle to empty more completely

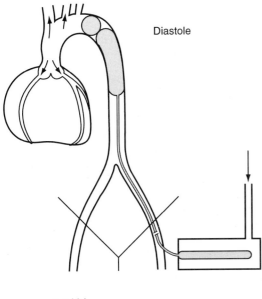

Diastole

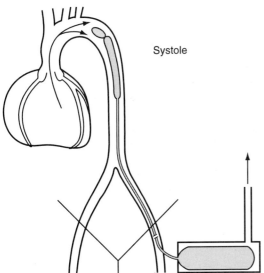

Systole

Figure 9.8 Intra-aortic balloon pump. An external balloon indicates the inflation or deflation of the intra-aortic balloon. (From Collier, P.S. and Dohoo, P.J. (1980) The intra-aortic balloon pump. *Physiotherapy*, **66**, 156–7, with permission.)

The effect is like a mechanical form of combined inotropic and vasodilator therapy, increasing myocardial perfusion and reducing the workload of the heart. Complications include vascular damage, embolism and lower limb ischaemia. The patient is heparinized to lessen the risk of thrombosis.

Indications are cardiogenic shock, low CO and difficulty in weaning from cardiopulmonary bypass. The display unit on the console shows the augmented BP, a calculated non-augmented BP, and an average of the two. When patients are ready for less support, assistance is reduced gradually from every beat (1:1) to every 4th beat (1:4). Implications for physiotherapy are the following:

1. The augmented BP should be watched because this is what the patient receives.
2. Hip flexion should be avoided at the insertion site.
3. Patients are often too unstable to turn, but if turning is indicated, care is required to avoid disconnection of the catheter.
4. If bag-squeezing is necessary, it should be performed with caution because pressure may compromise the function of the balloon and destabilize cardiac output.
5. Percussion is unwise because of interference with the ECG, and mechanical percussors and vibrators are contraindicated. If vibrations are needed, one supporting hand under the patient minimizes unnecessary movement.
6. To reduce the risk of bleeding, coughing should be avoided for some hours after the device has been removed.

The **ventricular assist device** is a supplementary pump that assists a failing heart, and is mainly used as a bridge while awaiting heart transplantation (Seche 1992).

9.5.6 Advanced pulmonary support

IPPV rests the respiratory muscles but does not rest the lung itself, which is still being intermittently stretched and released. Ventilator pressures can be reduced by augmenting gas exchange using **intravascular oxygenation**

(IVOX), by which gas exchange occurs within the body through a 2 ft-long bundle of hollow tubes sited in the vena cava (East 1993). The device can be employed for up to a month and provides half the patient's oxygen requirements.

Structural lung rest can also be achieved by **liquid ventilation**, using perfluorocarbon which has high solubility for respiratory gases (Leach 1993). This gentle non-invasive innovation is still experimental but has potential for neonates.

9.5.7 Advanced cardiopulmonary support

As a last resort for people with severe but potentially reversible cardiopulmonary failure, total rest can be provided by extracorporeal gas exchange, which is a modified form of cardiopulmonary bypass and buys time for an injured lung to recover (East 1993). ECMO is **extracorporeal membrane oxygenation** using a membrane oxygenator outside the body, CO_2 transfer occurring as a secondary effect. ECCO$_2$R is **extracorporeal CO$_2$ removal**, which separates the process of oxygenation (via the lung) from CO_2 removal (via the extracorporeal circuit), taking advantage of the rapid diffusion of CO_2 by using a low flow venovenous circuit, with less damage to the blood. Both reduce the need for IPPV and the potential for pulmonary damage. These techniques are established in neonatal practice, but logistic difficulties for adults remain daunting.

Many adults are too unstable for physiotherapy, but treatment may be indicated for neonates, in which case it is advisable to ask a technician to stand by in case the machinery needs attention during treatment. Much care is needed to avoid bleeding during suction, due to anticoagulation, but because oxygenation is maintained outside the lungs, physiotherapy is less likely to cause hypoxaemia then with conventional IPPV.

RECOMMENDED READING

Bolton, P.J. and Kline, K.A. (1994) Understanding modes of mechanical ventilation. *Am. J. Nurs.*, **94**, 36–42.

Ciccone, C.D. (1992) Cardiovascualr pharmacology. *Phys. Ther. Pract.*, **1**(4), 1–11.

Cowie, M.R. (1994) Understanding electrocardiograms. *Student Br. Med. J.*, **2**, 229–32.

Dennison, R.D. (1994) Making sense of hemodynamic monitoring. *Am. J. Nurs.*, **94**, 24–31.

Durbin, C.G. (1994) Monitoring gas exchange. *Respir. Care*, **39**, 123–37.

Gerold, K.B. and Nussbaum, E.M. (1994) Understanding mechanical ventilation. *Phys. Ther. Pract.*, **3**, 81–91.

Grant, I.S. and Nimmo, G.R. (1995) Oxygen transport. *Care Crit.* III, **11**(2) 67–9.

Graver, J. (1992) Inotropes – an overview. *Int. Crit. Care Nurs.*, **8**, 169–79.

Hansen, J., Cowen, J. and Raps, E.C. (1993) Neuromuscular blockade in the ICU: more than we bargained for. *Am. Rev. Respir. Dis.*, **147**, 234–6.

Hess, D. and Kacmarek, R.M. (1993) Techniques and devices for monitoring oxygenation. *Respir. Care*, **38**, 646–169.

Koretz, R.L. (1995) Nutritional supplementation in the ICU. *Am. J. Respir. Crit. Care Med.*, **151**, 570–3.

MacKenzie, S.J. (1993) Clinical use of PEEP. *ACPRC J.*, **23**, 29–32.

Manning, H.L. (1994) Peak airway pressure: why the fuss? *Chest*, **105,** 242–7.

Marini, J.J. (1995) Weaning techniques and protocols. *Respir. Care*, **40**, 233–8.

Meyer, T.J., Enveloff, S.E., Bauer, M.S. *et al.*, (1994) Adverse environmental conditions in the respiratory and medical ICU settings. *Chest*, **105**, 1211–16.

Parker, J.C. and Hernandez, L.A. (1993) Mechanisms of ventilator-induced lung injury. *Crit. Care Med.*, **21**, 131–42

Sassoon, C.S. (1995) Noninvasive positive-pressure ventilation in acute respiratory failure. *Respir. Care*, **40**, 282–8.

Slutsky, A.S. (1993) Mechanical ventilation. *Respir. Care*, **38**, 1389–19.

Westcott, C. (1995) The sedation of patients in ICUs. *Int. Crit. Care Nurs.*, **11**, 26–31.

10. *Physiotherapy in intensive care*

10.1 PRELIMINARIES

No-one explained . . . all they said was not to worry about it.

Thomson 1973

To reduce the risk of patients becoming disoriented by their stay in the ICU, it is advisable for them to:

- be kept informed throughout,
- visit the unit before surgery if postoperative admission is planned,
- be given advice on means of communication if they are to be intubated,
- have treatment with the same physiotherapist before, during and after admission to the unit.

Patients should not, if possible, be woken when asleep, especially if flickering eyelids indicate that they are in the REM phase of the sleep cycle, when tissue regeneration is at its maximum (Shelly 1992). We should enter the patient's space gently, introduce ourselves and explain our purpose.

If visitors are present, they can either be invited to stay or asked to leave during treatment, depending on the patient's wish. The presence of relatives means that they can become involved in patient care and be reassured that physiotherapy is not distressing, but if the patient's wish cannot be ascertained, it is best that they are asked to leave.

Before treatment, patients need adequate fluids and appropriate drug therapy to ensure optimal cardiac output and minimum pain. Although physiotherapy should not be distressing, the traditional protocol of turning, percussion, vibration and suction has been shown to release catecholamines, destabilize

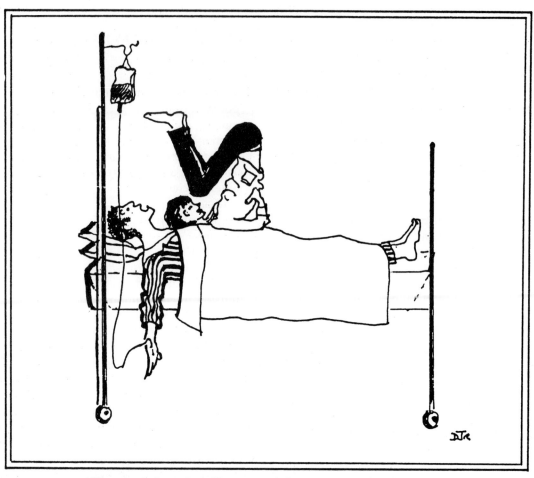

'The physiotherapist will come and do exercises on his chest'.
(Reproduced with permission from ACPRC Newsletter no. 11,
1987.)

cardiac output, ↑ oxygen consumption by
over 50%, ↑ BP and heart rate, ↑ $PA\text{--}aO_2$
and ↓ PaO_2 (Weissman 1993).

Vulnerable patients can be pretreated with
↑ F_IO_2, a sedative such as propofol (Horiuchi
1995), or 15 cmH_2O pressure support (Kemper
1993) as appropriate. Continuous tube feed-
ings are best turned off during treatment.

10.2 ASSESSMENT

Assessment is required before, during and
after treatment, especially if patients are

unable to complain of new symptoms. The
sequence of assessment described in Chapter
2 can be used, with additions described
below.

10.2.1 Notes and charts

Increased core temperature raises oxygen
consumption, the extra demand being partly
met by increased HR and respiratory rate. A
probe on the toe monitors peripheral temperature. A value < 5° lower than the core
temperature implies that patients are not well

perfused, for example they have low cardiac output or are in shock.

Fluid status may be measured by the daily weight, any change of more than 250 g/day representating fluid gain or loss (Parker and Middleton 1993). The fluid balance chart can be affected by a multitude of factors such as drug therapy, IPPV, PEEP or postoperative fluid changes. Electrolyte and haematocrit values are decreased with fluid excess and increased with fluid loss. The signs of hypovolaemia are:

- pallor
- ↑ HR
- ↑ respiratory rate
- ↓ vascular pressures (CVP, PAWP)
- ↓ systolic BP
- ↓ pulse pressure
- ↓ urine output

Urine output is also depressed by low cardiac output because of the kidneys' sensitivity to hypoperfusion. Hypovolaemia reduces pulse pressure (see Glossary) because the body compensates by vasoconstriction, which assists venous return and helps maintain diastolic pressure, so that in the early stages, systolic pressure drops faster than diastolic pressure.

Blood test results may indicate a low platelet count or long prothrombin time (see Glossary), which act as a warning to use suction with care because of the risk of bleeding. Low serum albumen is associated with reduced surfactant and a drop in osmotic pressure, leading sometimes to peripheral and pulmonary oedema. Potassium levels below 4 mmol/l predispose patients to arrhythmias, so most forms of treatment are contraindicated.

The overall trend in BP should be checked for any response to previous sessions of bag-squeezing.

10.2.2 Chest X-ray

Portable radiographs in the ICU are taken with the patient supine or slumped. In this position a pleural effusion loses its clear boundary and the fluid line is replaced by a faint smooth density throughout the lung. The boundary between air and lung may be lost when there is a pneumothorax, which shows up more clearly on a CT scan.

The tracheal tube should reach to just above the carina. If it is too long, the right main bronchus will be intubated, leaving the left lung unventilated. If it is too short, the patient's head should be moved as little as possible so that the tube is not dislodged.

10.2.3 Monitors

Monitoring of oxygenation is particularly important because physiotherapy can increase oxygen consumption by over 50% (Weissman and Kemper 1991). SaO_2 has extra significance in patients with cardiac instability because hypoxaemia can precipitate arrhythmias. If the SaO_2 falls during treatment, e.g. below 90%, the F_IO_2 should be increased and/or treatment halted. $S\bar{v}O_2$ can be used to monitor the effect of procedures such as suction, which reduces oxygen supply, or position change, which increases oxygen demand.

Changes in BP and HR can reflect factors as diverse as septicaemia, pain, drugs or fluid status. Monitors should be observed during treatment in order to identify responses relating to physiotherapy. BP usually relates to cardiac output, which is a major determinant of oxygen delivery. Systolic pressures as low as 80 mmHg are adequate so long as the patient is warm and passing sufficient urine. However, overvigorous physiotherapy can reduce cardiac output by 50% in critically ill patients (Laws and McIntyre 1969).

Although 78% of patients exhibit arrhythmias spontaneously (Artucio and Pereira 1990), the ECG should be watched during physiotherapy to check for changes related to treatment.

10.2.4   Ventilator

The ventilator will indicate which mode of ventilation is in use and whether PEEP is applied. The airway pressure dial reflects the ease or difficulty with which the lungs are inflated. It provides the following information:

- peak pressure above the norm of 20 cmH$_2$O could be due to bronchospasm, stiff lungs, pulmonary oedema, pneumothorax or obstruction by sputum, a kinked tube or clenched teeth,
- peak pressure below normal is caused by a leak in the circuit which can usually be located by a hiss,
- oscillation of the airway pressure signifies a patient breathing spontaneously between ventilator breaths,
- erratic readings signify a patient fighting the ventilator, as confirmed by observation,
- readings that dip substantially below the end-expiratory baseline indicate excess work of breathing, i.e. flow delivery is below the patient's need.
- the complete cycle is raised in proportion to added PEEP.

A high level of PEEP means that patients are at risk of severe hypoxaemia if they are disconnected from IPPV, and that cardiac output might be impaired.

A saw-tooth pattern on the flow-volume curve suggests that secretions are present (Fig. 10.1).

10.2.5   Patient

Is the patient unconscious, confused, agitated, sedated, paralysed? Paralysis, whether therapeutic or pathological, indicates the importance of clarity of communication because patients may be trying to make sense of strange sounds and sensations but be unable to give feedback. Agitation can be due to the endotracheal tube, fear, incorrect ventilator settings, gut distension, restraints,

awkward positioning or pain. What channels of communication are available? Is perception or interpretation of information altered by drugs or cerebral damage?

The location of lines and tubes should be noted and kept in view throughout treatment, especially femoral lines or unobtrusive pacing wires. The breathing pattern gives few clues for a ventilated patient, but accessory muscle activity suggests excess work of breathing, and laboured breathing may indicate an obstructed airway. Hydration is difficult to assess clinically because oedema or overhydration can coexist with intravascular depletion in critically ill people (Dobb and Coombs 1987). Warm hands usually mean warm kidneys and a healthy cardiac output.

The breath sounds of ventilated patients are slightly harsher than normal. When side-lying, the dependent compressed lung generates augmented breath sounds and more dullness to percussion than the upper lung (Gilbert 1989). Breath sounds can be heard more clearly during bag-squeezing, sometimes crackles being elicited with a sharp release on expiration. The stethoscope may pick up the wheeze-like sound of air leaking around the cuff of the tracheal tube, or the bubbling of condensed humidifier water in the tubing.

10.3   MOTIVATION AND STRESS REDUCTION

Who am I?
Where am I?
Why do I hurt so much?

Anon 1981

Treatment is most effective in a motivated patient. Motivation is reduced by stress. Stress is better prevented than treated. Examples are the following:

1.   The first priority is to establish communication. One patient commented on 'the extraordinary fact that so many believe that because you are unable to talk, you

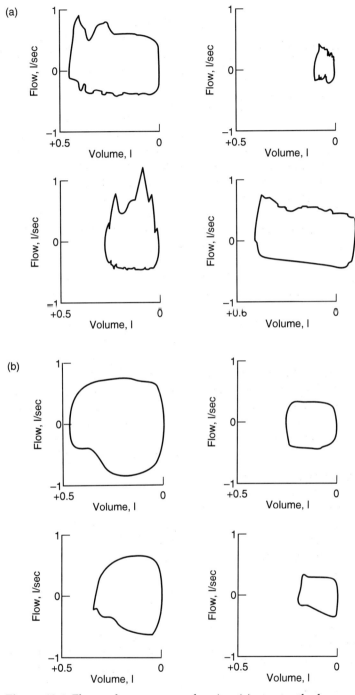

Figure 10.1 Flow-volume curves, showing (a) saw-toothed curves for patients with secretions, and (b) smooth curves for patients with clear chests. (Reproduced with permission from A. Jubran, *Am. J. Respir. Crit. Care Med.*, **150**; published by Williams & Wilkins, 1994.)

either can't or don't want to listen' (Holden 1980). Understanding and memory may be affected by anxiety or drugs, but patients who are unable to speak are neither deaf nor mentally impaired. They need:

(a) clear and explicit explanations, repeated as necessary,

(b) hearing aid or glasses if used,

(c) information on why physiotherapy is necessary, what it will feel like, how long it will last and instructions on how to ask for it to stop,

(d) if unable to speak, and lip-reading proves inadequate, communication aids, such as word or picture cards, pencil and paper or, for greater privacy, a magic slate,

(e) if unable to write, yes-or-no questions asked one at a time:

> 'Are you hot? cold? itchy? worried? tired? sleepy? nauseous? in pain? Is your ear twisted against the pillow? your mouth dry? the tube bothering you? Do you want to turn? raise/lower your head? Do you need more air? less light? less noise? more information? bottle or bedpan?'

Vigilance ensures that communication is aimed at patients, not over them. Chatting over patients has been shown to increase stress more than suction (Lynch 1978). One patient said, 'it didn't matter what they talked about, so long as they talked to me' (Villaire 1995). If a patient wishes not to communicate, this should also be respected.

2. The more helpless patients are, the more important it is that they be given a measure of control. They can choose which side to finish on, whether they would like treatment now or later (if possible), whether the bed head is the right height, and whether they would like to regain their day/night rhythm by being woken in the day or having a sleeping pill at night. Autonomy is particularly important in a situation of unequal power and knowledge.

3. ICU patients are extra sensitive to human physical contact as a contrast to the cold clinical procedures to which they are frequently subjected. One patient said, 'the most important thing for me was the human contact, the communication' (Villaire 1995). Another said, 'it surprised me how much I valued human touch' (Redfern 1985). Foot massage is accessible for the ICU patient and has been shown to reduce tension and lower the respiratory rate (Stevensen 1994). The benefits of even brief massage can be confirmed by watching the monitors. As always, it should be remembered that individuals vary and some dislike touch.

4. Measures to alleviate physical discomfort include regular turning (before the allotted time if the patient requests), minimal use of restraints, cream for dry lips, double taping all tape to protect the skin, and smoothing out all creases from the sheet after treatment. For immobile patients, creases feel like a knife after a brief period.

5. Orientation is helped by the presence of personal belongings in an area that the patient can control, a visible clock and calendar, family photographs, information on progress, interpretation of noises and voices, attendance to alarms promptly, avoidance of disagreements over the patient, patient-controlled radio and TV, and trips outside the unit when possible.

6. Expression of emotion is best accepted, even encouraged, and reduces the depression that is common in ICU patients.

7. Praise is a potent motivator and enhances a patient's self-esteem

8. Patients should not be expected to be or coerced into being popular at a time when they least need such a burden.

10.4 HANDLING PATIENTS WHO ARE CRITICALLY ILL

To be talked frankly through a complete procedure, particularly its estimated length, would help curb the deadly effects of uninformed anticipation.

Brooks 1990

10.4.1 Turning

Three people are needed to turn a helpless patient. The following steps are suggested:

1. Ensure sufficient slack in lines and tubes.
2. Clear ventilator tubing of any accumulated water that could spill into the patient's airway.
3. Inform the patient.
4. Slide the hands under the patient, digging the fingers into the bed to avoid scraping the skin (having ensured that no team members have watches or rings).
5. Disconnect the patient from the ventilator if this is safe (and advise the patient), or support the tracheal tube manually. Some trusted patients can hold an endotracheal tube briefly with their teeth during the turn.
6. Say clearly, '1, 2, 3, turn', then turn the patient smoothly and clear of the bed.
7. Check lines, check patient comfort, observe monitors.

An alternative is to cross the patient's arms over the chest and use a draw sheet for turning.

10.4.2 Handling unconscious or paralysed people

Discomfort . . . was definitely helped by being turned . . . I gained greater comfort when the positions of my legs were varied . . . Hearing was acute: every sound seemed magnified.

Gandy 1968

We need to act as the consciousness of the unconscious. It is easy to depersonalize patients who cannot respond to us, especially if we have not had the opportunity to get to know them when they were alert. It is thought that even unconscious people can hear and understand all that is said (Sisson 1990).

If a paralysing drug has been used, it is reassuring for it to be allowed to wear off once a day as a reminder that the effect is temporary. Patients also appreciate having their eyelids opened occasionally (after being informed).

When turning paralysed or unconscious patients, attention should be given to:

- protecting the eyes,
- supporting the head,
- aligning the limbs in a neutral position, with special care of the shoulder,
- checking that no objects are under the patient,
- reassuring the patient and turning firmly, to reduce fears of falling off the bed,

The use of the word 'paralysis' can be alarming to patients, and drug-induced paralysis should be explained.

10.4.3 Pressure area care

Anything can be put on a pressure sore except the patient. Hospitals are full of concoctions for putting on pressure sores, but better still is prevention, by means of:

- most importantly, frequent turning and judicious positioning (Davies 1994),
- keeping pressure areas dry,
- turning without friction,
- avoidance of excessive washing or rubbing with talc or cream,
- prevention of hypotension or hypovolaemia,

- adequate vitamin C and protein intake (Barratt 1989).

Pressure sores can be prevented by a fluidized (Clinitron) bed. This looks like boiling milk, and consists of a miriad of beads floating in a current of warm air which supports the patient happily like a semi-submerged iceberg. Turning is done with a sheet. The air compressor is switched off when the patient is side-lying so that the beads mould to the body like sand. Points to note are that:

- good teamwork is needed to ensure regular turning for preventive respiratory care, because turning is no longer required for pressure area care,
- the dry air current may contribute to dehydration,
- the bed should be switched off and un-plugged for cardiopulmonary resuscitation.

A sacral pressure sore that has developed in supine does not preclude sitting out in a chair, so long as an upright position is maintained to prevent pressure on the sacrum.

10.5 TECHNIQUES TO INCREASE LUNG VOLUME

In spontaneously breathing patients, lung volume can be increased by the techniques discussed in Chapter 5. For ventilated patients, the following can be used.

10.5.1 Exercise

Bed exercises, even when strenuous, are unable to prevent deconditioning (Sandler 1988). An attempt should be made to stand and walk all patients for whom there is no contraindication such as cardiovascular instability, fracture or paralysis. Attachment to a ventilator does not preclude getting out of bed, but solicitous attention to lines and tubes is required. A rebreathing bag provides ventilator support if the patient walks more than a few steps from the ventilator. Walking should be brief because fatigue drains motivation.

The patient needs to spend some time sitting with the legs dangling over the edge of the bed before standing. Patient and monitors should be scrutinized when he or she is upright. For patients unable to stand, sitting out two or three times a day helps prevent hypovolaemia (Wenger 1982). A tilt table is useful.

Long-term patients are excited at the prospect of their much-awaited first expedition out of bed, and some are then disillusioned by the extent of their weakness and fatigue. This is when they most need encouragement. A visit outside is rewarding, especially if the ICU has no windows, lack of outside windows has been shown to double the incidence of delirium (MacKellaig 1990).

Patients confined to bed need active or passive exercises to maintain sensory input, comfort, joint mobility and muscle strength. Special attention should be given to the Achilles tendon, hip joint, joints around the shoulder, two-joint muscles and, for long-term patients, the jaw and spine. The longer a patient is immobilized, the more time is needed for exercise. An overhead bar provides some independence.

Passive movements should be performed with caution for paralysed people, whose joints are unprotected by muscle tone. Vigorous active exercise should be avoided for patients who are (1) on inotropic support because they have limited cardiovascular reserve, and (2) on CMV because they are unable to increase their minute volume. Patients with fractures, burns or altered muscle tone need input from specialist colleagues.

10.5.2 Positioning

There may be a fine irony in the observation that our advanced knowledge and technology by themselves cannot save the patient. Instead, something so simple as turning the patient from supine to lateral to prone to lateral, at least hourly, may make the difference between living and dying for the intensive care patient.

Bendixen quoted by Ray 1974

Positioning is the main treatment for patients in intensive care, and may be the only treatment for an unstable patient. By preventing the abdominal contents encroaching on lung volume (p. 110), positioning restores ventilation to dependent lung regions more effectively than PEEP or large tidal volumes (Froese and Bryan 1974).

Supine is the least helpful position for lung function. For ventilated patients, the lateral position increases FRC (Ibañez *et al* 1981) and enhances gas exchange (Lewandowski 1992) compared with supine. The prone position is useful for some severely hypoxaemic patients (see p. 284).

Studies using rotating beds show mixed outcomes, which may reflect the limited side-lying position they achieve, i.e. patients may not be positioned forwards enough to free the diaphragm from abdominal compression.

During positioning, transient changes in HR and $S\bar{v}O_2$ are acceptable, but if HR increases or decreases by over 10 bpm, or $S\bar{v}O_2$ drops more than 10% from baseline, the patient should be returned gently to supine (Winslow *et al* 1990). Factors which modify positioning are head trauma, abnormal muscle tone, pain, spinal cord injury, fractures, pressure sores and an unstable BP.

As with spontaneously-breathing patients, ventilated patients with unilateral lung pathology show optimum gas exchange when lying with the affected lung uppermost (Rivara 1984).

10.5.3 Manual hyperinflation

It was by far the most frightening thing that happened to me. I'll never forget it.

Patient quoted by Rowbotham 1990

Manual hyperinflation (or bag-squeezing or bagging) is a technique that delivers extra volume and oxygen to the patient via an anaesthetic bag. Compared with positioning, which is accepted for the prophylactic respiratory care of most ICU patients, bag-squeezing is not used routinely. Disadvantages are the following:

- prophylactic effectiveness has not been substantiated,
- it can be uncomfortable and frightening if done incorrectly,
- haemodynamic and metabolic side-effects are common.

However, bag-squeezing has been shown to open up atelectatic lung (Nunn 1987, p. 33) and reverse deterioration in gas exchange and compliance (Novak *et al* 1987). It also assists in mobilizing secretions.

Terminology

- Manual inflation or manual ventilation refers to the squeezing of gas into the lungs at tidal volume, e.g. when changing ventilator tubing,
- manual hyperventilation is when a high flow rate of gas is used in order to supply rapid breaths, e.g. if the patient is breathless or hypoxaemic,
- manual hyperinflation is when the patient is given deep breaths, usually 50% greater than a ventilator breath, in order to increase lung volume, e.g. when treating atelectasis.

Physiotherapy is usually related specifically to manual hyperinflation.

Technique

A rebreathing bag is commonly used, which is a rubber or plastic 2 l bag connected by an adjustable valve to an oxygen supply (Fig. 10.2). Its compliance allows the clinician to feel the ease of inflation. Non-rebreathing units such as the Ambu or Laerdal bag

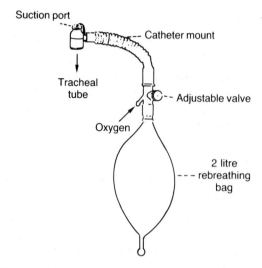

Suction port

Catheter mount

Tracheal tube

Adjustable valve

Oxygen

2 litre rebreathing bag

Figure 10.2 Rebreathing bag system.

consist of semirigid material which self-inflates from room air with added oxygen. These prevent excessive pressures being reached, but are less responsive to man-oeuvres such as the sharp release procedure.

The following technique is recommended:

1. Ensure the patient's fluid status is optimum to prevent an unnecessary drop in cardiac output.
2. Ensure appropriate analgesia and/or sedation.
3. Position the patient in side-lying. Bagging hyperinflates the more compliant upper areas and has little effect on the dependent lung. In supine, bagging would therefore treat the apical region and the lower lobes would be largely ignored. For patients who cannot turn, close attention to technique (see 8, below) will deliver some extra volume to the bases.
4. Check the monitors. Bagging should not be started until cardiovascular stability is assured in side-lying.
5. Observe chest expansion.
6. Tell patients that they will feel a deep breath with cold air. They will feel sleepy if Entonox is used. They should

be free of distractions or nursing procedures.

7. Turn off the low-pressure alarm, connect the bag to the oxygen with a flow-rate of 15 l/min, disconnect the patient from the ventilator and connect him or her to the bag.
8. Rest the tubing on the sheet to avoid tugging on the tracheal tube, tell the patient when to expect the breaths, squeeze the bag several times at tidal volume to acclimatize the patient, then give slow, smooth deep breaths, adjusting the valve to increase pressure until expansion is greater than on IPPV. Hold maximum pressure at end-inspiration for about a second to encourage filling of poorly-ventilated alveoli, especially if atelectasis is the problem. Haemodynamically unstable patients should not receive this end-inspiratory hold, and are best given one deep breath interspersed with several tidal breaths.
9. Release the bag sharply to stimulate a huff, especially if sputum retention is the problem.
10. Watch the chest for expansion, the face for distress and the abdomen for signs of unwanted active expiration. The more alert the patient, the greater is the need to co-ordinate the procedure with the patient's breathing. Continue bagging until the patient's facial expression or monitors indicate distress, or if crackles indicate that secretions have been mobilized and suction is required. Once crackles are heard, give tidal volume breaths until the patient is suctioned. If bagging causes no change, stop after six to eight breaths for a reassessment.
11. After bagging, inform the patient and reconnect him or her to the ventilator, switch on the alarm, observe chest movement and the monitors, and auscultate the chest

12. To maintain the benefits of bag-squeezing, the side-lying position should be retained as long as it is comfortable for the patient and convenient for nursing procedures.

Effects and complications

To be effective in reversing atelectasis, a sustained inflation to 40 cmH$_2$O is required (Novak *et al* 1987; Rothen 1993). But how do we know if bagging could cause lung injury? Barotrauma is an ever-present risk with diseased or damaged lungs, which should always be treated with caution. For normal lungs, pressures above 60 cmH$_2$O (Sommers 1991) should be avoided. Ensuring that inflation is slow will reduce the chance of reaching excess pressures, but it is safest to put a manometer in the bagging circuit. A manometer can often be borrowed from the neonatal unit or the respiratory technician, or bought from the manufacturers (Appendix C). All physiotherapists should test their bagging pressures with a test lung from the lung function laboratory. Pressure-relief 'pop-off' valves are available, but are not always reliable and should be checked with a test lung.

The complications of bagging are an exaggeration of the complications of IPPV, particularly barotrauma and haemodynamic compromise. BP may rise or fall, but cardiac output decreases consistently and can take 15 minutes to recover (Singer *et al* 1994). A well-filled patient is better protected from haemodynamic complications.

Complications are greatest if bagging uses large tidal volumes or is vigorous, but if bagging is too gentle it may lead to hypoxaemia. Bagging for physiotherapy is best performed by physiotherapists because nurses rarely achieve the desired effect (Singer *et al* 1994), but ICU nurses trained by physiotherapists can bag-squeeze if manual techniques are required at the same time.

Contraindications

Bagging is contraindicated if the following are present:

1. Extra-alveolar air, e.g. bulla, subcutaneous emphysema, undrained pneumothorax.
2. Bronchospasm causing a peak airway pressure above 40 cmH$_2$O.

Precautions

Bagging should be performed with caution if the following are present:

1. Pneumothorax with a chest drain, or an air leak as demonstrated by air bubbling through a chest drain bottle.
2. Low, high or unstable BP. If bagging is essential in a hypotensive patient, it should be brief, with prolonged expiration and no end-inspiratory hold.
3. Hypovolaemia, as demonstrated by low PAWP or administration of vasodilator drugs.
4. Recent lung surgery with bronchial resection, because of the risk of bronchopleural fistula at the bronchial stump. The 5th to 10th postoperative days are when the healing stump is at its most vulnerable (Pierson and Lakshminarayan 1984).
5. Acute head injury.
6. Lung disease, especially emphysema.
7. Rib fracture because a covert pneumothorax might be present. If bagging is essential, the radiograph should be scrutinized or a radiologist's opinion be sought.
8. During renal dialysis, which tends to destabilize BP.
9. Arrhythmias.
10. Intrinsic PEEP. Prolonged expiratory time should be allowed.
11. During weaning, patients with hypercapnic COPD are dependent on their hypoxic drive to breathe. If bagging is essential when the patient is off the ventilator but still intubated, the bag

should be connected to air instead of oxygen (with use of a nasal cannula if necessary), and monitors watched.

12. Severe hypoxaemia with PEEP above 5–10 mmHg. Disconnection of the patient from the ventilator will lose the PEEP. If bagging is necessary, desaturation can be minimized by:

   (a) incorporating a PEEP valve in the circuit (Schumann and Parsons 1985),
   (b) manually preventing the bag fully deflating at end-expiration, although it is difficult to maintain PEEP above 8 or 10 manually,
   (c) increasing the flow rate and/or tightening the valve, then bagging faster and/or harder to augment oxygenation, but only briefly, and only if this is safe for the patient,
   (d) using the 'manual sigh' button which is available on certain ventilators and delivers a twice normal tidal volume without disconnection from the ventilator or loss of PEEP; this can substitute for bagging even at high levels of PEEP, but does not allow subtle modifications of technique in response to the feel of lung compliance, nor is a sharp release of pressure possible,
   (e) if no 'manual sigh' button is available, the inspiratory hold facility can be used, which does not give a deep breath but encourages collateral ventilation.

10.6 TECHNIQUES TO CLEAR SECRETIONS

The secretions of patients on IPPV can usually be cleared by regular position change, suction as required and bagging if necessary. Sputum retention is seldom a problem in patients whose humidification is adequate and whose position is changed regularly (Laws and McIntyre 1969).

10.6.1 Postural drainage

The head-down tilt is rarely suitable for patients on IPPV. First, abdominal contents weight heavily against an inactive diaphragm, markedly reducing lung volume. Secondly, haemodynamics are compromised, cardiac output sometimes rising initially and then dropping precipitously. Side-to-side positioning, which is used for maintenance of lung volume, is usually adequate as modified postural drainage.

10.6.2 Manual techniques

Manual techniques are not needed routinely, but excessive or thick secretions occasionally need the extra assistance of percussion or vibrations, so long as there is not a risk of arrhythmias (Hammon *et al* 1992), and appropriate safeguards are taken to avoid further reduction in an already low FRC. Vibrations beyond FRC may cause atelectasis (Laws and McIntyre 1969), and percussion can induce atelectasis by rapid emptying of air spaces (Zidulka *et al* 1989), but these problems can usually be avoided by bagging during and after the manoeuvres. Vibrations are unlikely to add greater benefit than bagging alone because they cause less airflow (Fig. 10.3), but fine vibrations may create beneficial oscillations. Maximum benefit is obtained if they are started at peak inflation, just before the bag is released.

Monitors should be observed closely because many patients cannot meet extra metabolic demand by increasing their cardiac output. Increases in oxygen consumption of 20% and 40% have been documented during chest physiotherapy (Swinamer 1987; Kemper 1992), although technique was not clearly defined in these studies.

10.6.3 Suction

Suction reduces lung volume by an average 27% (Brochard *et al* 1991), increases oxygen demand also by an average 27% (White

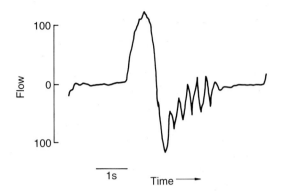

Figure 10.3 Airflow during manual hyperinflation and vibrations. (Source: MacLean, D., Drummond, G., Macpherson, C. *et al.* (1989) Maximum expiratory airflow during chest physiotherapy on ventilated patients before and after the application of an abdominal binder. *Int. Care Med.*, **15**, 396–9, with permission from the copyright holder, Springer-Verlag.)

et al 1990), decreases oxygen supply, causes haemodynamic disturbance and may repeatedly flood the lungs with bacteria which adhere to the inside of the ETT (Sottile 1986). Suction should be carried out when indicated, not routinely (Judson 1994).

Indications, contraindications and technique for nasopharyngeal suction are described in Chapter 5. Modifications for tracheal tube suction are described below.

Preliminaries

For patients with cardiovascular instability, administration of a narcotic analgesic before suction can attenuate haemodynamic disturbance (Klein *et al* 1988). Patients are advised that they will feel more in control if they let the catheter go down and avoid coughing until it is irresistible. Self-ventilating intubated patients find it helpful to hyperventilate voluntarily beforehand.

When suctioning beyond the end of the tracheal tube, the catheter normally enters the right main bronchus. If access to the left main bronchus is required, Judson (1994) recommends turning the head to the left, but this is less successful than using an angled (coudé-tipped) catheter with the tip directed to the left. Some angled catheters have a guideline to indicate the direction of the tip. For physiotherapy purposes, a straight catheter is usually sufficient because secretions have already been brought proximally.

Technique

Catheter size should be no more than half the internal diameter of the tracheal tube. A size 12 catheter is normally used, but size 14 is acceptable with large tubes. Aseptic technique should be pristine. Violations such as touching the edge of the tracheal tube opening with an ungloved hand or catheter are taboo.

Vibrations are unnecessary during suction because enforced coughing overrides outside influences, unless the patient is paralysed. Bagging should be stopped before opening the system for suction in order to prevent blow-back of possibly infected aerosol from the patient.

If more than one suction pass is necessary, this should wait until SaO_2 returns to baseline levels. Returning the patient to the ventilator at normal settings between suction passes is not adequate to prevent desaturation (Baun 1984), and other measures should be used to prevent hypoxaemia (see below). The same catheter should not be used for repeated suction because of the bacteria-ridden inner surface of the ETT (Sottile 1986) The patient's mouth often needs suction afterwards with the rinsed catheter or a yankauer sucker. Patients who are able to will prefer to do this themselves.

To minimize hypoxaemia

Suction causes hypoxaemia, and the discontinuation of ventilation that accompanies suction can cause sustained hypoxaemia for up to an hour (Schwartz 1987). The following measures reduce suction-induced hypoxaemia:

1. Manual hyperinflation and hyperventilation can be performed before and after suction. This is one of the most effective techniques (Goodnough 1985) and has the advantage of helping reverse post-suction atelectasis. If bagging is contraindicated, and especially if high PEEP is used, a manual sigh or end-inspiratory pause can be administered via the ventilator (Gronkiewicz 1983).

2. Oxygen levels through the ventilator can be raised to 100% for several minutes prior to suction, then returned to normal after suction once SaO_2 has stabilized. Goodnough (1985) claims that it takes one to two minutes for 100% oxygen to be delivered from the ventilator and an unknown additional time for alveolar gas to equilibrate, and oximetry is necessary for accurate timing. It is worth creating some personal system to remember to return the inspired oxygen back to normal.

3. A maximum of 10 seconds should be allowed for each suction pass. The physiotherapist can also breath-hold during the procedure to identify with the patient's tolerance. If longer than 10 seconds is needed, this can be accommodated by removing the thumb from the catheter port to release the vacuum, occluding the catheter mount opening (with the catheter still *in situ*), then giving the patient 100% oxygen by bagging. Suction is resumed when ready.

4. A closed circuit catheter can be used without disconnecting the patient from the ventilator. The catheter system becomes an integral part of the ventilator circuit and the same catheter is used over 24 hours. The advantages are reduced cross-infection and, for people who need high F_iO_2 and PEEP, less physiological disturbance (Johnson 1994). Disadvantages are that:

(a) atelectasis may be caused if suction flow exceeds gas flow from the ventilator,

(b) high suction pressures may occur inadvertently, so the pressure gauge must be watched,

(c) there is loss of manual sensitivity to the degree of suction pressure,

(d) there is less fine tuning of suction pressures because a control valve can be used for intermittent suction but the more gentle rocking thumb technique cannot be used,

(e) there is a tendency to suction when not necessary because of the ease of use.

Closed-circuit catheters can be more or less expensive than regular catheters, depending on the frequency of suction. There is no evidence that they influence nosocomial infection in the patient using them.

5. Double- or single-lumen catheters can insufflate oxygen either simultaneously or alternately with suction. These are expensive and difficult to use, but have the advantage of helping maintain lung volume (Brochard *et al* 1991). Between 5 and 15 l/min are used, with adequate venting of insufflated gas to ensure patient comfort and prevent pressure building up distal to the catheter.

Monitors should be observed, and suction finished rapidly if HR slows by 20 or increases by 40 bpm, if BP drops or arrhythmias develop. $S\bar{v}O_2$ is a more sensitive indicator of oxygenation than SaO_2 because suction can be accompanied by a significant rise in oxygen consumption without a corresponding rise in cardiac output (Walsh *et al* 1989).

Problems

Difficulty in passing the catheter may be due to kinking of the tracheal tube, lodging of the tube against the carina, obstruction by thick secretions or the patient biting the tube. Biting requires reassurance and sometimes insertion of a bite block. If secretions are mixed with blood, this may be due to recent tracheostomy change, trauma from a Swan–Ganz catheter, clotting disorder, heparinization or suction that is rough, frequent or used with dry airways.

Saline instillation

Normal saline is sometimes instilled into lungs with the intention of liquefying and mobilizing thick secretions. Disadvantages are the risk of infection, bronchospasm and interference with gas exchange. There are also doubts about its efficacy because one of the functions of mucus is to prevent the lungs drying out, and therefore mucus does not incorporate water easily (Dulfano 1973). The need for saline also suggests that humidification has been inadequate.

However, saline may help dislodge encrusted secretions or encourage coughing (Gray *et al* 1990); limited data suggest that it is beneficial (Judson 1994) and continuous-irrigation catheters show improved clearance (Isea 1993). If saline is used, the following points are suggested:

* warm the ampoule of saline first to minimize the risk of bronchospasm,
* administer the liquid slowly to prevent patients feeling as if they are drowning,
* not a drop must touch the tracheostomy dressing,
* 5 ml has been advised (Bostick and Wendelgass 1987), but more can be used if trickled in slowly and interspersed with bagging (or large tidal volumes on the ventilator if bagging is contraindicated) to prevent desaturation,

If this does not clear secretions, the saline can be delivered more distally by injecting it through the suction catheter or the patient can be turned to the opposite side after instillation, so that the instilled side is uppermost for treatment.

When using a closed-circuit catheter with an HME, caution is required to prevent influx of saline into the device (Martinez 1994).

10.7 END OF TREATMENT SESSION

After suction, patients should not be turned or moved immediately, so that they can stabilize (Riegel 1985). After treatment, it is advisable to check that all alarms are on, to tell patients the time, and ensure that their bell and other requirements are within reach. Patients need reassurance that they are not being left alone, and that their lines are safe so that they do not feel inhibited from moving. Some patients may be frightened for a variety of reasons, e.g. being left facing a wall, so it is worth eliciting a nod before leaving to check that they feel secure.

10.8 RECOGNITION AND MANAGEMENT OF EMERGENCIES

The key to the successful management of emergencies is informed anticipation and recognition. Physiotherapists are not immersed in life-threatening events every day, so it is advisable to review protocols regularly in order to maintain confidence and avoid the indecision that is often evident at the scene of an emergency.

10.8.1 Cardiac arrest

Cardiac arrest is the sudden cessation of heart function. It is the commonest mechanism of the old-fashioned process of death, but is potentially reversible. It is followed within seconds by loss of consciousness and within a minute by loss of respiration and dilatation of pupils.

Anticipation

Before starting work in any new unit, the first task is to locate the crash trolley. It is also advisable to have prior knowledge of patients' past medical and drug history.

Patients with pre-existing ischaemic heart disease, severe respiratory disorder or drug overdose are most at risk of cardiac arrest, especially if compounded by metabolic disturbance, arrhythmias or shock. Warning signs are a change in the patient's breathing, colour, facial expression, mental function or ECG. Hypoventilation with altered consciousness is an ominous combination.

Recognition

Loss of consciousness is the first obvious sign. The patient's colour may be pale, ashen or blue, depending on the cause. No carotid pulse can be felt in the groove between the larynx and sternomastoid muscle. Respiration becomes gasping and then stops (unless respiratory arrest has been the primary event). Monitored patients show ventricular fibrillation (VF) or asystole on ECG.

Management

The time between collapse and initiation of resuscitation is critical, and a false alarm is better than a dead patient. Irreversible brain damage will occur unless circulation is restored within three to four minutes, less if the patient is severely hypoxaemic before the arrest. If suspicions are raised by a change in consciousness and colour, do not waste time fumbling for the pulse unless skilled in this. Call out to the patient, and if he or she is unresponsive, follow the basic life support stage of cardiopulmonary resuscitation (CPR):

1. For patients whose ECG shows VF, thump the midsternum once. This may reverse VF in the early stages. At the same time, summon help by bellowing, 'cardiac arrest!'.
2. Position the patient supine and remove the pillows.
3. Establish a patent airway. Use one hand to tilt the head back (unless cervical injury is suspected) and the other to lift the chin forwards. Insert an airway from the crash trolley. Suction the mouth and throat if required. Ventilate with 100% oxygen using the face mask, resuscitation bag and oxygen at 15 l/min. For an airtight seal, pull the mask edges apart before positioning over the face. Ventilation is easier with two people. The first two breaths should be slow to minimize the risk of aspiration.
4. Kneel on the bed and apply external chest compression with short thrusts, using a degree of body weight through straight arms. With the heels of both hands two finger-breadths above the xiphoid process, depress the lower part of the sternum by 4–5 cms at 60 compressions a minute. Apply pressure smoothly and evenly to minimize fracture risk, but if rib fracture occurs, adjust hand position and continue. Most hospital beds are firm enough to support effective CPR, but if not a footboard or meal tray can be pushed under the chest. Pulling the patient to the floor to achieve a firm surface takes time, sometimes loses precious intravenous lines, and creates an awkward position for intubation. Effectiveness of chest compression is evaluated by return of a healthy colour and, when a spare person is available, palpation for a spontaneous pulse.

For in-hospital CPR, the above two stages are performed concurrently, with chest compressions and ventilation at a ratio of 5:1. For one-person CPR, the compression-to-ventilation ratio is 15:2. For physiotherapists working in the community or out of reach of a crash trolley, a pocket mask is advisable for mouth-to-mouth resuscitation, and a finger sweep across the back of the tongue may be needed to remove any obstruction.

Do not leave the patient. Check the pulse after the first minute and every few minutes thereafter. If the patient regurgitates, turn the head to the side, suction or wipe out the mouth, and continue with CPR. If recovery occurs, turn him or her into the semiprone recovery position so that the tongue falls safely to the side of the mouth and any unwanted material can drain out. Common errors are:

- not maintaining a patent airway throughout, e.g. inadequate neck extension,
- not allowing chest deflation between breaths,
- not compressing the chest with sufficient force,
- compressing one side of the sternum rather than the mid-sternum.

The addition of abdominal compressions alternately with chest compressions appears to improve outcome (O'Nunain 1993).

Spare personnel should call the crash team. When the team arrives, they will instigate advanced life support:

- intubation and continued hand-ventilation,
- medication such as atropine and adrenaline for asystole, lignocaine for VF, calcium antagonists and beta-blockers,
- ECG monitoring,
- defibrillation, which delivers direct current to the heart through the chest wall in an attempt to abolish arrhythmias and allow the sinus node to regain control of the heart beat. Staff should stand clear while the shock is being delivered.

When no longer needed, the physiotherapist can give attention to other patients who may be distressed at witnessing the event.

10.8.2 Respiratory arrest

As cardiac arrest leads to respiratory arrest, so too does respiratory arrest, if untreated, lead to cardiac arrest.

Anticipation

Predisposing factors include exacerbation of COPD (which can lead to depression of respiratory drive by inspiratory loading and hypoxaemia), airway obstruction (e.g. foreign body, swelling or bleeding from trauma, regurgitation from the stomach or smoke inhalation) or aspiration (especially following drug overdose). Warning signs are inability to speak, and violent respiratory efforts, laboured breathing or drowsiness.

Recognition

Respiratory arrest is indicated by absence of movement of the chest, loss of airflow from the mouth and nose and sometimes cyanosis. This progresses to loss of consciousness.

Management

Guidelines for dealing with a respiratory arrest are the following:

1. Call for help.
2. Establish a patent airway as described for CPR. If there is no airflow, continue as below.
3. If a foreign body is the likely culprit, attempt to dislodge it from the throat by suction or finger sweep manoeuvre. If unsuccessful, attempt to dislodge any foreign body from the airway by administering up to five piston-like Heimlich manoeuvres, i.e. inward and upward thrusts to the abdomen, below the rib cage and above the navel. This can be from behind a standing victim or kneeling astride a supine victim. If unsuccessful, turn the victim and deliver several sharp blows between the shoulder blades. If the patient is still not breathing, continue as below.
4. Hand ventilate or perform mouth-to-mouth resuscitation once every five seconds. Check the carotid pulse once a minute.

If cardiac arrest ensues, instigate full CPR. If the patient starts breathing, turn him or her into the recovery position. Vomiting is common as consciousness lightens.

If a patient with a tracheostomy suffers a respiratory arrest due to obstruction, follow these steps:

1. Suction the airway.
2. Move the head, which may relieve the obstruction.
3. Summon help.
4. Insert the suction catheter (not attached to suction), deflate the cuff, cut the securing tape, slide out the tracheostomy tube over the catheter while keeping the catheter in position in order to maintain the airway. Then follow one of two choices, depending on availability of equipment and experience:
   (a) insert a new tracheostomy tube over the catheter, using the catheter as a guide,
   (b) maintain ventilation through the catheter or via tracheal dilators, either encouraging the patient to breathe spontaneously, or blowing down the catheter or the stoma.

10.8.3 Seizure

Anticipation

The medical notes indicate whether a patient has a history of epilepsy. Other causes of fitting are fever in children, head injury or alcohol intoxication. Some patients sense an aura that warns them of an imminent seizure.

Recognition

Seizures vary from minor loss of consciousness to major muscle activity, followed by drowsiness.

Management

1. Patients subject to seizures should have the bed kept low, side rails up and padded, and oxygen and suction available.
2. If there is advance warning, insert airway. Do not attempt this once the fit is underway.

3. Protect the patient's head and body from injury. Do not use restraints or hold the victim down, but keep in side-lying if possible. Loosen tight clothing, especially around the neck.
4. Afterwards, ensure the patient is in the recovery position. Reassure as consciousness returns.

10.8.4 Haemorrhage

Anticipation

Uncontrolled bleeding can follow surgery or other trauma.

Recognition

External bleeding is not easily missed. Internal bleeding is suspected if there are signs of severe hypovolaemia (p. 247). The BP and heart rate are the least reliable of these signs because BP may be maintained by vasoconstriction and high cardiac output until 20–40% of blood volume is lost, and heart rate is responsive to many other variables.

Management

1. Position the patient flat.
2. Apply pressure to the bleeding point if accessible.
3. Elevate the affected part if possible.
4. Request assistance.
5. Explain to the patient what is being done throughout.

Fluid resuscitation is required with acute blood loss < 30% of total blood volume in order to maintain perfusion to vital organs. Haemorrhage from a tracheostomy is described on p. 196.

10.8.5 Massive haemoptysis

Expectoration of > 200–600 ml blood over 24–48 hr implies massive haemoptysis, which is rare but carries 30–50% mortality, usually from asphyxiation more than blood loss (Reid 1994).

Anticipation

Lung cancer, bronchiectasis, abscess or TB can cause massive haemoptysis.

Management

The patient should be laid head down, and if the side of the haemorrhage is known, laid on the affected side to prevent aspiration into the healthy lung. Cough suppressants and sedatives should not be given. Patients with depressed consciousness or at risk of asphyxiation require intubation and suction. Measures to identify the cause and arrest the bleeding will be taken by medical staff.

10.8.6 Cardiac tamponade

Cardiac tamponade is accumulation of fluid in the pericardium. The pericardium is not distensible and the fluid causes acute compression of the heart and a damming back of blood in systemic veins. If increasing pressure is not relieved, cardiac arrest is inevitable.

Anticipation

Tamponade can occur in the first 24 hours after heart surgery. Other predisposing factors are trauma, dissecting aneurysm, infection or malignancy.

Recognition

Progressive compression of the heart leads to precipitate loss of cardiac output and rise in filling pressure, as shown by:

- ↓ BP, $S\bar{v}O_2$, urine output,
- ↑ RAP, LAP, heart rate,
- RAP and LAP approximately equal,
- sudden change in pericardial drain output,
- distended neck veins,
- pulsus paradoxicus,
- narrowed pulse pressure,
- enlarged heart on X-ray.

Hypovolaemia masks some of these signs, but they become apparent after fluid administration.

Management

When medical staff have been notified, they will relieve pressure by aspirating fluid with a needle inserted into the pericardium.

10.8.7 Tension pneumothorax

Pneumothoraces are more likely to be under tension in ventilated patients than in spontaneously breathing patients, which means that gas enters the pleural space on inspiration but cannot escape on expiration. If not relieved, cardiac arrest follows.

Anticipation

Patients are vulnerable to tension pneumothorax at the following times:

- immediately after intubation, when inadvertent tube placement into the right main bronchus leads to hyperinflation of the intubated lung,
- in the hours following instigation of mechanical ventilation, when air is forced through a previously unknown leak in the pleura.

Predisposing factors are mechanical ventilation in patients with COPD, and surgery or other trauma to the chest. The presence of a chest drain on the affected side does not preclude a tension pneumothorax because the drain may be malpositioned. Subcutaneous emphysema in the neck can be a warning sign.

Recognition

Tension pneumothorax is sufficiently rare to be sometimes mistaken for bronchospasm. Both of these conditions cause respiratory distress, wheeze, increased airway pressure and laboured breathing. The added features of tension pneumothorax are:

- ↓ amplitude in ECG (often the first sign),
- unequal chest movement,
- hyperresonant percussion note on the affected side,
- ↓ breath sounds on the affected side, or both sides if severe,
- ↓ PaO_2 or SaO_2,
- distended neck veins, ↑ CVP,
- displaced apex beat,
- for self-ventilating patients, dyspnoea and tracheal deviation away from the affected side,
- for ventilated patients, high airway pressure, and expired minute volume less than preset minute volume,
- ↓ BP, ↑ heart rate, progressing to cardio-vascular collapse,
- if there is time for a radiograph, this shows the mediastinum pushed away from the affected side and an inverted diaphragm.

Management

Immediate insertion of a needle into the pleura is required to let the air out. While waiting for this assistance, reduce positive pressure by disconnecting the patient from IPPV and bagging with high flow rate and low valve pressure.

10.8.8   Pulmonary embolism

Sudden patient distress and the signs described on p. 86 raise suspicions of pulmonary embolism. Disconnection from the ventilator and bagging do not help. Monitors will show ↑ HR, BP and respiratory rate, and ↓ SaO_2. See p. 86 for management.

10.8.9   Fat embolism

Anticipation

Fat may be released from bone marrow into the circulation after orthopaedic surgery or other injury. Fat emboli can become lodged in the pulmonary circulation, which may prove fatal.

Recognition

Warning signs are breathlessness, agitation, tachycardia, pyrexia and cyanosis within 72 hours of trauma.

Management

Inform the doctor. Treatment is aimed at maintenance of gas exchange, vital functions and hope.

10.8.10   Air embolism

Anticipation

Air may enter the circulation after cardiac or neurosurgery, or occasionally from a pneumothorax or during insertion or removal of a central venous catheter.

Recognition

A large air embolus causes respiratory distress, palpitations, dizziness, weakness, pallor or cyanosis.

Management

Summon help. Place the patient head down in left-side-lying, which diverts air away from the pulmonary artery and the pulmonary circulation. Apply pressure over the original dressing. Give high-percentage oxygen. An embolus > 100 ml may cause cardiac arrest, which requires cardiac compression with heavy and deep pressure to disperse air bubbles to peripheral segments of the pulmonary artery.

10.8.11   Equipment malfunction or disconnection

Astute eyes and ears need to be cultivated in the ICU in order to pick up the slight hiss of an air leak, identify from an orchestra of alarms which is the offending malfunction, or notice the subtle change in a drowsy patient's demeanour which signifies that something is amiss. This can distinguish equipment malfunction from physiological change.

Prevention includes reading the manufacturer's manual in order to understand the workings of the ventilator, and familiarity with the alarms to help distinguish what each signifies.

Alarms

The most relevant alarms for the physiotherapist are the high-pressure alarm, low-pressure alarm, F_IO_2 alarm and humidifier overheating alarm.

The high-pressure alarm is set at 5–10 cmH$_2$O higher than peak airway pressure and is activated if:

- suction is needed,
- water condenses in the tubing,
- the patient coughs or fights the ventilator,
- bronchospasm or pneumothorax develops,
- the ETT slips into the right bronchus,
- the cuff herniates over the end of the tube,
- tubing is obstructed by kinking or the patient biting.

If the patient bites the ETT, this requires discouragement, sedation or change to a nasal tube. For a displaced ETT, the doctor will deflate the cuff, reposition it, inflate the cuff and listen for equal breath sounds.

The low-pressure alarm indicates that pressure has fallen more than 5–10 cmH$_2$O below the desired limit and goes off if there is a leak or disconnection in the system. A disconnected circuit should be reconnected, the patient's condition checked, the cause determined and appropriate adjustments made or the nurse informed.

It should be remembered that alarms are fallible, and observation of the patient comes first.

Patient distress

If a patient becomes agitated or fights the ventilator (Fig. 10.4), patient-related problems include:

- pain or fear,
- pneumothorax, pulmonary oedema, abdominal distension, bronchospasm or mucus plug,
- biting the tube.

Ventilator-related problems include:

- kink or leak in the circuit,
- intrinsic PEEP,
- inappropriate settings for minute volume, F_IO_2 or trigger sensitivity.

After checking airway pressure and monitors, ask the patient, 'Do you want more air?'. If the answer is 'no', continue with questions requiring yes or no answers in order to identify the source of distress.

If the answer is a nod, or the patient is unable to respond, disconnect the patient from the ventilator and attach him or her to the bag with oxygen. Either hand-ventilate or allow the patient to self-ventilate through the bag, with the valve open for minimal resistance and a high flow rate for comfort. If distress continues, it is a patient-based problem, but if it resolves, there is some mechanical mischief. Bagging may itself settle the patient.

If the problem is not solved, suction the airway, which will indicate whether there is a blocked tube or excess secretions.

If still unsolved, deal with problems as follows:

- leaking tracheal tube cuff: inflate the cuff with air from the syringe, just enough to eliminate the leak,
- tube disconnection: reconnect if the tubing is sterile, otherwise continue bagging until a replacement is available,
- inability to locate disconnection: inform the nurse or technician,
- air entry present on one side of chest only: inform the doctor of suspicions of a malpositioned tracheal tube,
- other tracheal tube malfunction or bronchospasm: inform the doctor.

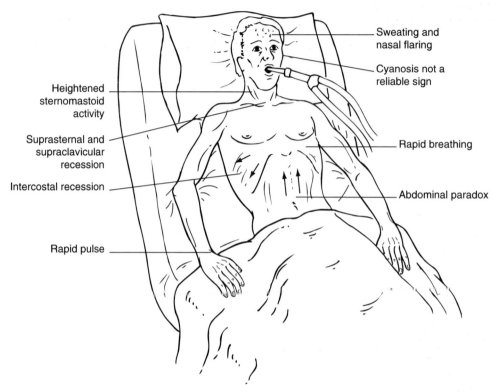

Figure 10.4 Physical signs of patient distress. (Source: Tobin, M.J. (1991) What should the clinician do when the patient 'fights the ventilator'? *Respir. Care*, **36**, 395–406, with permission.)

Arterial line disconnection

If an arterial line becomes disconnected, apply firm pressure immediately to the site and request assistance. Reassure the patient, who may be frightened at the amount of blood, and observe both the patient and monitors for signs of hypovolaemia.

Other less common emergencies are described by Tobin (1991).

10.9   ON CALLS

A well-managed on-call system can sustain many a sick patient through a difficult night. The key to success lies in education, so that all parties understand the scope and limita-

tions of physiotherapy. Education should be targeted at the following staff:

1. **Doctors**. All levels of medical staff need advice on the indications for out-of-hours physiotherapy, with particular attention to new staff. This advice can take the form of handouts, informal talks and formal induction for house officers. Discussion of individual patients is particularly useful. Medical training hardly brushes the subject of physiotherapy and this is an educational opportunity to be grasped gladly.
2. **Nurses**. Nurses and physiotherapists work closely and have an understanding of each others' work. Day-to-day exchange of information lays the foundation for co-operation, and this can be developed into

Table 10.1 Criteria for on-calls

Indications
Patients who cannot be left until the normal working day for fear of deterioration in their condition, e.g.:
  atelectasis or consolidation with worsening blood gases,
  certain patients who may need mechanical ventilation unless treated, e.g.:
    fractured ribs,
    exacerbation of COPD with drowsiness.

Non-indications
Patients for whom physiotherapy is ineffective, e.g.:
  pulmonary oedema,
  sputum retention due to dehydration (until rehydrated),
  atelectasis due to pain (until pain is controlled).

General questions to ask when called (to be asked diplomatically)
Doctor's name and how to contact him/her again.
Patient's temperature.
Cardiovascular status.
Breath sounds.
Hydration.
Result of X-ray.
Result of blood gases.
Pain, outcome of analgesia.
Productive of sputum – if not, is there sputum retention, or no sputum?

Examples of specific questions
Acute asthma:
  level of fatigue,
  bronchospasm relieved with drugs?
Pneumonia
  dehydration?
  acute or unresolving (on-call physiotherapy not indicated)?
Exacerbation of COPD: level of consciousness?
If pulmonary oedema is suspected, check Table 2.2.

If physiotherapy not indicated
Politely explain the indications for emergency physiotherapy.
Say that if the situation changes, please call again.

If physiotherapy indicated
Before coming in, ask for analgesics, antiemetics, bronchodilators, as necessary.
Ask for the patient to be positioned appropriately.

After treatment
Liaise with nursing staff re: on-going management, e.g. positioning/rest/incentive spirometry.

teaching sessions so that nursing staff are able to perform maintenance chest care and know when it is appropriate to suggest that the physiotherapist be called.

3. **Physiotherapists**. Junior and non-respiratory physiotherapists need confidence in making informed decisions. Useful time can be spent working alongside juniors, going through equipment,

and ensuring that all staff are proficient in identifying respiratory problems. It is easy to forget how frightening the first on-call experience is, and several steps can be taken to facilitate a sound night's sleep for those on duty:

(a) set aside time on the preceding afternoon for the on-call physiotherapist to see any patient whose respiratory status is borderline,

(b) talk through a handout such as that set out in Table 10.1 (also to include location of equipment), to be kept by the on-call physiotherapist's phone,

(c) clarify departmental policy on who is authorized to call out the physiotherapist, e.g. junior or senior registrar,

(d) give inexperienced on-call physiotherapists the phone number of a respiratory physiotherapist who is willing to advise them over the phone.

The interest of the patient and good relations with other disciplines can be fostered by the physiotherapist taking responsibility for prearranging call-outs when appropriate. Communication is improved by explaining in advance that the physiotherapist can act as adviser and consultant over the phone and that it is not always necessary to give hands-on treatment. Unnecessary call-outs can be followed up by diplomatic chats between the respective managers.

RECOMMENDED READING

Bergbom-Engberg, I. (1989) Assessment of patients' experiences of discomfort during respirator therapy. *Crit. Care Med.*, **17**, 1068–72.

Judson, M.A. (1994) Mobilization of secretions in ICU patients. *Respir. Care*, **39**, 213–25.

Odell, A., Allder, A., Bayne, R. *et al.* (1993) Endotracheal suction for adult non-head-injured patients. A review of the literature. *Int. Crit. Care Nurs.*, **9**, 274–78.

Selsby, D. and Jones, J.G. (1990) Some physiological and clinical aspects of chest physiotherapy. *Br. J. Anaesth.*, **64**, 621–31.

Singer, M., Vermaat, J. and Hall, G. (1994) Hemodynamic effects of manual hyperinflation in critically ill mechanically ventilated patients. *Chest*, **106**, 1182–7.

Snow, N., Bergin, K.T. and Horrigan, T.P. (1990) Thoracic CT scanning in critically ill patients. *Chest*, **97**, 1467–70.

Stone, K.S., Talaganis, S.A.T., Preusser, B. *et al.* (1990) Effect of lung hyperinflation and endotracheal suctioning on heart rate and rhythm in patients after CABG. *Heart Lung*, **20**, 443–50.

11. *Conditions in intensive care*

11.1 LUNG DISEASE

11.1.1 COPD

Mechanical ventilation is not indicated for people with COPD who are suffering an irreversible deterioration in their disease, but it may be needed to buy time during an exacerbation.

For hypercapnic patients, minute ventilation is titrated to the patient's normal $PaCO_2$ so that compensatory renal bicarbonate retention is maintained and will be adequate for buffering during weaning. Small levels of PEEP are added to counterbalance intrinsic PEEP (Rossi 1994).

A person who has acclimatized to complex acid-base compensations may find that the sudden change to IPPV has a destabilizing effect, leading to arrhythmias, hypotension and the unmasking of hypovolaemia. If physiotherapy is needed within 30 minutes of starting IPPV, close monitoring is necessary. Bagging is inadvisable unless essential because positive pressure is distributed unevenly to the damaged lungs, causing over-distension and risk of barotrauma.

Weaning is often tiring, frightening and protracted, and 48 hours of rest and sleep are required before the first attempt.

11.1.2 Asthma

IPPV for people with acute severe asthma is a perilous venture, carrying an average mortality of 10% (Grunberg 1991). The non-homogeneous state of the lungs means that patients are at risk from hyperinflation and intrinsic PEEP, which can lead to baro-trauma, reduced venous return, hypotension, arrhythmias and right heart failure due to compressed pulmonary capillaries. Dehydrated patients are particularly vulnerable.

IPPV is indicated if there is an intractably rising $PaCO_2$, exhaustion, apnoea, worsening consciousness or coma. Sixty–100% oxygen is delivered, and cautious ventilator management is required in an attempt to maintain airway pressures below 40 mmHg. Complications are minimized by deliberately using a low minute volume, even at the expense of retaining CO_2. This 'permissive hypercapnia' allows $PaCO_2$ to rise up to 12 kPa (90 mmHg), with oxygenation being monitored continuously. Hypercapnia is well tolerated, the drop in pH being counterbalanced within hours by bicarbonate retention, but it may not be safe for older people or those with a cardiac history (Bellomo 1994).

Intrinsic PEEP is controlled by a low I:E ratio and administration of extrinsic PEEP. Intractable bronchospasm may require inhalation agents (Bellomo 1994), and damaging levels of ventilation may be reduced by continuous IV anaesthesia (Grunberg 1991), or hypothemia (Browning 1992). Prolonged paralysis should be avoided unless essential because of its association with myopathy when combined with the inevitable steroids (Bellomo 1994).

Physiotherapy is contraindicated immediately after initiation of IPPV because a combination of anaesthesia, dehydration and high airway pressures may cause profound hypotension. Rapid infusion of fluids, sometimes with vasopressors, usually restores BP, but physiotherapy is still mainly limited to stress reduction. Instillation of warmed saline to help loosen thick mucus plugs, e.g. 2 ml every 15 minutes, may be indicated (Branthwaite 1985). When pressures have settled to normal, other treatment is given as necessary.

Any sudden deterioration should raise suspicions of tension pneumothorax, because the usual signs (p. 263) are obliterated in ventilated asthmatic patients.

11.2   NEUROMUSCULAR DISORDERS

11.2.1   Guillain–Barré syndrome

The physiotherapist was a most welcome person, as, despite the discomfort endured to have 'dead' limbs stretched and repositioned, this left me comfortable for several more hours.

Clark 1985

Guillain–Barré syndrome is a demyelinating neuropathy that causes a predominantly motor deficit and sometimes paralysis. Two-thirds of patients have preceding infections (Hund 1993). Presenting features vary widely and include backache (often leading to misdiagnosis), parasthesia and weakness. Weakness may progress for up to a month, but respiratory failure sometimes develops with alarming speed. The signs of respiratory muscle weakness (p. 27 and p. 49) raise suspicions, and difficulties with speech or swallowing indicate imminent ventilatory failure. Vital capacity measurements can predict ventilatory failure (Chevrolet 1991).

Treatment is mainly supportive, but plasmapheresis hastens recovery by removing or diluting the offending factors circulating in the blood (Hund 1993).

Exercise should be started early and done regularly, including spinal movements by double knee-and-hip flexion, knee rolling and neck movements. Relatives may assist with some exercises. Pain occurs in up to 72% of patients (Pentland 1994), especially aching and burning sensations arising from denervated muscles and inflamed nerves. Pain is accentuated by immobility, but initially exacerbated by exercise. Regular gentle exercise is therefore essential, and can be preceded by anti-inflammatory drugs or Entonox. Stress reduction strategies are necessary because of the combination of paralysis and consciousness. Extremities may be hypersensitive, and a cradle eases the weight of the bedclothes.

Autonomic involvement leads to unstable BP and heart rate, and sustained hypertension can alternate with sudden hypotension. The risk of hypotension is reduced by ensuring that turning is gentle, avoiding any intervention if the CVP is below 5 cmH$_2$O, and acclimatization to the upright posture with a tilt table. The risk of bradycardia is reduced by oxygenation before and after suction. Rehabilitation is improved by hydrotherapy, trips outside and information on self-help groups (Appendix C). Recovery takes weeks or months, but 80% of patients recover fully (Hund 1993).

11.2.2 Acute quadriplegia

You can't appreciate what it is to be paralysed unless you are. The big things you get used to easier, like not getting up and walking around. The trivial things – like not being able to scratch your nose or feed yourself – they hurt.
Patient quoted by
Stewart and Rossier 1978

People whose lives have been devastated by trauma or disease to the cervical spine are overwhelmed at first and find it difficult to comprehend how savagely their life has been reduced.

Physiotherapists who care for people with acute quadriplegia need to allow them to work through their grieving at their own pace, while endeavouring to prevent the respiratory complications that are the leading cause of death.

Pathophysiology and clinical features

Lesions above T6 to L1 paralyse the abdominal muscles and impair coughing. Higher thoracic lesions paralyse the intercostals and destabilize the rib cage, causing paradoxical inward motion on inspiration. The commonest picture is maintenance of accessory muscle and diaphragmatic action but loss of intercostal and abdominal action, leading to a vital capacity (VC) between 1250–2500 cc. If VC is below this with a high thoracic lesion, further pathology such as unilateral diaphragmatic paralysis is suspected. Lesions above C4 denervate the diaphragm, leaving only the sternomastoid and trapezius muscles to shift a trace of air into the lungs.

Paralysed abdominal muscles lead to reduced venous return and an exaggerated response to hypovolaemia. Sympathetic outflow is impaired in traumatic lesions above T6, leaving parasympathetic tone unopposed

and causing hypotension and bradycardia, especially during suction or exertion. Cardiac monitoring is required for the first two weeks, and oximetry is advisable to detect nocturnal desaturation and monitor treatment. DVT is a high risk, especially if there is multiple trauma.

Physiotherapy

If hypoxia is allowed to develop, the spinal cord may be further damaged. The 3rd to 5th crucial days after injury are when lung complications are commonest. McMichan et al (1980) have shown how the need for IPPV can be reduced by two-thirds with regular preventive measures in the form of frequent position change and hourly incentive spirometry to maintain lung volume, and percussion and assisted coughing to clear secretions.

The head-down position is unwise, but if it is essential for postural drainage, care is needed to ensure that tipping is done slowly, not fully, that traction is maintained, that patients are not left unsupervised in case of sudden sputum mobilization, and that arterial and venous pressures are monitored because of the loss of compensatory cardiovascular reflexes.

Coughing is assisted with manual pressure upwards and inwards using the heel of the hand from below the xyphoid process, in synchrony with any expiratory force that the patient can muster. Some patients require two helpers for this. Care should be taken to avoid disturbing neck traction, jarring the fracture site, exacerbating associated injuries, or pushing towards the spine instead of the diaphragm. This form of assisted coughing should not be attempted if there is a paralytic ileus.

Early minitracheostomy is advisable if there is a hint of sputum retention, especially as the neck cannot be extended for effective nasopharyngeal suction. If suction is required, whether for an intubated or spontaneously breathing patient, it should be accompanied by monitoring and measures to minimize hypoxia.

Treatment of the limbs involves meticulous attention to positioning and range of movement (Bromley 1985). Between a half and three-quarters of patients develop shoulder pain (MacKay–Lyons 1994), which is particularly disabling in this group of patients. The key is prevention in the form of education to all team members on the need for continual attention to positioning, especially if there is cervical traction or a rotating bed. Early range of movement and judicious use of the 'crucifixion' position have also been advocated (MacKay–Lyons 1994).

Mobilization takes the form of head elevation very gradually, preferably with a tilt table to minimize hypotension. Standing is less comfortable than supine because the floppy abdominal muscles allow bulging of the abdomen. The application of a stabilizing abdominal binder is helpful for standing or sitting (Goldman 1986). Physiotherapy in the acute stage should be little and often to prevent fatigue.

Respiratory rehabilitation is lengthy for people with high lesions and may be hindered by depression. This is eased by facilitation of communication, sometimes with the help of a speech therapist, and ensuring that patients have as much control over their environment and treatment as is feasible.

Ventilator-dependent patients can be assisted to gain some degree of independence using biofeedback (Morrison 1988b), glossopharyngeal breathing (p. 127), phrenic nerve stimulation to coax the diaphragm to life (Moxham 1993), short periods on a portable ventilator with a mouthpiece, or possible use of β_2-stimulants to improve muscle strength (Signorile 1995). Exercise training in the form of arm ergometry and incentive spirometry has shown a 24% increase in FVC (Crane, 1994). Inspiratory muscle training, using abdominal weights or a threshold resistor, can improve talking, eating and confidence (Schweitzer 1994), and training the surviving

expiratory muscles may improve coughing (Gounden 1993).

After the first two years, mortality parallels that of the normal population. With support and encouragement in the early stages, patients find the determination to rebuild their lives, and it is a tribute to the human spirit that many go on to find fulfilment.

11.3 FRACTURED RIBS AND LUNG CONTUSION

A third of patients with traumatic rib fractures develop pulmonary complications (Ziegler 1994), especially if ribs are fractured in more than one place, creating a flail chest and paradoxical breathing (Fig.11.1). The accompanying pain and derangement of the chest wall cause a restrictive defect. Palpation over fractured ribs elicits exquisite pain, but this test is not necessary because X-ray signs are usually apparent. Fractures are commonly seen at the lateral border of the rib cage.

Blunt trauma, with or without fracture, can cause lung contusion, i.e. bruising with inflammation and oedema which fills alveoli with blood and further reduces lung compliance. Signs of contusion are rapid breathing, progressive hypoxaemia, which may be refractory to oxygen therapy, bloody secretions and, after about 12 hours, mottling on X-ray.

Early pain control for rib fractures is essential, usually by epidural analgesia. If drainage is initiated for a pneumothorax or haemothorax, local anaesthetic can be administered through the chest drain. TNS may be applied locally (Sloan *et al* 1986) or on acupuncture points (4 cm bilateral to T1/2 space and T2/3 space). Entonox can be administered if there is no pneumothorax, and a cough belt or towel supports coughing. Early mobility is encouraged.

IPPV may be needed for contusion, but CPAP is preferable for fractured ribs because it provides pneumatic stabilization without

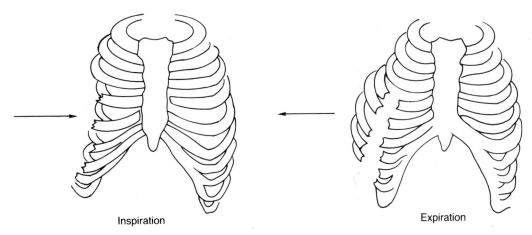

Inspiration   Expiration

Figure 11.1 Flail chest caused by fractured ribs, leading to an unstable segment being sucked in on inspiration and pushed out on expiration.

the risks of IPPV (Bolliger and Van Eeden 1990). Contused lungs do not take kindly to percussion and vibrations, and postural drainage can spread bloody secretions to other parts of the lung. Mechanical vibrators may help to mobilize secretions, and an oscillating bed has been found to reduce chest infections (Fink *et al* 1990). If frank bleeding is present, suction is contra-indicated.

11.4 ACUTE HEAD INJURY

Nowhere is accurate assessment and finely-tuned clinical judgement more vital than in the management of a person with acute head trauma. Methods to control intracranial pressure and prevent lung complications are often in conflict, and this is further complic-ated if other trauma is present.

The effect of most injuries is maximal at onset, but head injury may precipitate a process that converts a mild injury to a life-threatening condition. Primary damage sus-tained at the time of impact is irreversible, but secondary damage can double mortality by reducing oxygen delivery to the brain (Wald 1993). Secondary damage includes

hypoxaemia, hypotension, anaemia (due to bleeding), infection and intracranial hyper-tension. These can be made worse or better by the quality of management.

11.4.1 Effect of head injury on gas exchange (Fig. 11.2)

Chest infection is second only to intracranial hypertension as the main cause of death following head injury (Rudy *et al* 1991). Reasons for this and other respiratory com-plications are legion:

1. Damage to the respiratory centre may cause abnormal breathing, leading to either hypercapnia, which causes vaso-dilation and raised intracranial pressure, or hypocapnia, which causes tissue hypoxia (Fig 11.3). Cheyne–Stokes or ataxic breath-ing are signs of severe damage.
2. Regurgitation and loss of protective pharyngeal reflexes in an unconscious patient may cause acute aspiration.
3. Associated injuries such as facial injury, fractured ribs, haemopneumothorax or lung contusion compromise the airway or impair gas exchange.

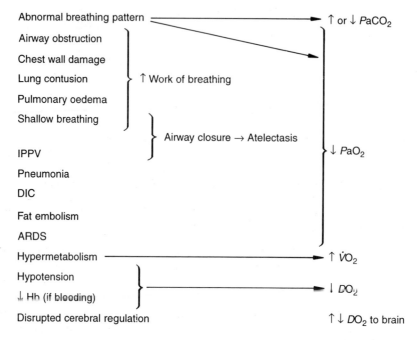

Figure 11.2 Effect of acute head injury on oxygenation.
$\dot{V}O_2$ = oxygen consumption; DO_2 = oxygen delivery.

4. Immobility, recumbency and depressed consciousness cause shallow tidal volumes and impaired cough.
5. Over-enthusiastic fluid restriction, in an attempt to reduce cerebral oedema, can lead to hypotension and reduced oxygen delivery.
6. Pulmonary oedema may occur for two reasons. In severe cases, a massive sympathetic discharge creates vasoconstriction and a surge of fluid into the pulmonary circulation (Dettbarn and Davidson 1989). Iatrogenically, over-enthusiastic fluid administration, in an attempt to maintain cerebral perfusion, can create or exacerbate pulmonary oedema.
7. Pneumonia is common in the early stages if acute aspiration has occurred at the time of injury or emergency intubation. It is less common in the later stages because many patients are young and few have underlying medical illness (Hsieh *et al* 1992).
8. Later problems may arise, e.g. DIC (p. 281) because the brain is a rich source of thromboplastin, or fat embolism from fractured long bones, which causes lung damage from fatty acids.

11.4.2　Effect of head injury on the brain

CSF Cerebrospinal fluid.
ICP Intracranial pressure (normal < 15 mmHg).
CPP Cerebral perfusion pressure (normal > 70 mmHg).
MAP Mean arterial pressure.

Like other tissue, the brain will swell when damaged, reaching a maximum 24–48 hours after injury. Initially, swelling can be accommodated by displacement of CSF and venous blood into the spinal subarachnoid space and jugular veins. When these compensating

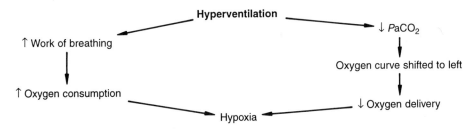

Figure 11.3 Effect of hyperventilation in acute head injury.

mechanisms have been exhausted, a small increase in cerebral oedema within the rigid container of the skull causes a disproportionate upsurge in ICP, as shown by Fig. 11.4.

Raised ICP is implicated as the major cause of secondary brain injury because it impairs CPP. CPP must be kept above 60 mmHg in order to perfuse the brain. CPP needs an adequate blood pressure but is compromised by a high ICP. MAP (related to BP) and ICP are in effect competing for space in the contused brain, i.e.:

$$CPP = MAP - ICP$$

The picture can be further complicated if pressure autoregulation is affected. Normally cerebral blood flow remains constant over a CPP range of 50–150 mmHg due to compensatory vasodilation as a response to hypoxia or hypotension. If this mechanism is damaged by brain injury, ICP follows MAP passively rather than maintaining independence. Medical intervention may be needed to regulate cerebral vascular resistance (Zhuang *et al* 1992).

Intracranial dynamics are reflected in a vicious cycle that exacerbates the secondary effects of head trauma (Fig. 11.5). Lung complications cause hypoxia to which brain tissue is particularly sensitive because of its high oxygen requirements and dependence on aerobic glucose metabolism. Hypoxia causes cerebral oedema, and disturbances in $PaCO_2$ add to this woeful picture. It is no wonder that head injuries have a reputation for being treacherous.

11.4.3 Factors which increase ICP

ICP is keenly sensitive to a multitude of factors:

1. Head-down postural drainage increases arterial, venous and intracranial pressures, impairs compensatory venous outflow, and is contraindicated in the acute stage (Lee 1989). Beware of literature that gives unreferenced reassurance about this position or suggests that advice be sought from doctors, who cannot be expected to know about the effect of physiotherapy procedures.

2. Turning the patient increases ICP (Chudley 1994), much of this being due to head

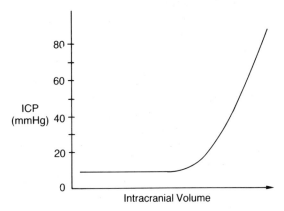

Figure 11.4 Intracranial pressure–volume curve, showing the steep rise in ICP once compensation for increased volume has reached its limit. Reproduced with permission from J.M. Cloeheny *et al.*, *Critical Care Nursing*; published by W.B. Saunders Company, 1993.

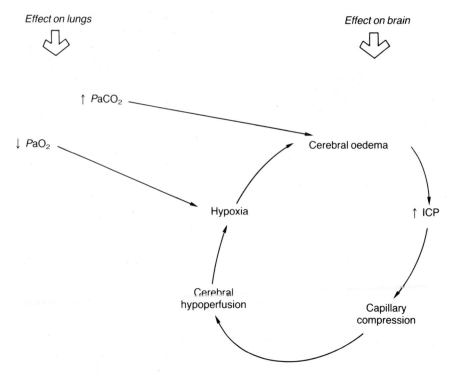

Effect on lungs

Effect on brain

↑ $PaCO_2$

↓ PaO_2

Cerebral oedema

Hypoxia

↑ ICP

Cerebral
hypoperfusion

Capillary
compression

Figure 11.5 Vicious cycle set up by acute head injury.

movement obstructing drainage from the brain.

3. Coughing, suction, bagging, vibrations and percussion impede compensatory outflow from the brain and raise ICP (Paratz 1993; Garradd and Bullock 1986). Outflow is also obstructed by extreme hip flexion (Mitchell and Mauss 1978), PEEP, tight tracheostomy tape and a cervical collar that may be applied for some days after trauma until cervical injury has been ruled out (Raphael 1994).

4. Hypertension increases ICP and hypotension reduces CPP. If pressure autoregulation is lost and cerebral perfusion is related linearly to blood pressure, BP can be monitored as a surrogate for cerebral blood flow.

5. Even deeply comatosed patients show a surprising sensitivity to conversation over their beds, discussion about their condition increasing ICP more than a

general discussion (Mitchell and Mauss 1978). When relatives talk to them, a reduction in ICP may be seen (Chudley 1994).

6. ICP is increased by stress such as noise, pain, restraints, movement of the tracheal tube, arousal from sleep or emotional upset (Mitchell *et al* 1981).

Most of these factors warn physiotherapists to keep their distance, but the importance of maintaining adequate gas exchange is a cogent reminder not to stray too far.

11.4.4   General management

Monitoring

ICP monitoring (Fig. 11.6) is needed because assessing neurological function by clinical examination means that secondary damage has already occurred (Harrington 1993). The intraventricular catheter has the capacity to withdraw CSF for diagnosis or therapy.

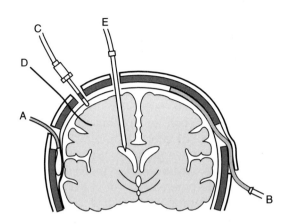

Figure 11.6 ICP monitoring: A = epidural sensor, which leaves the dura intact. B = subdural bolt, inserted into the subdural space. C — subarachnoid bolt, inserted into the subarachnoid space. D = parenchymal catheter, implanted in brain substance. E = intraventricular catheter, implanted into the nondominant lateral ventricle. (From Vos (1993), with permission.)

Head elevation

It is common practice to elevate the head to 15–35° in order to reduce ICP and encourage CSF outflow, although there is some argument about whether this compromises CPP (Rosner and Coley 1986; Feldman 1992). In either case, the head should always be kept aligned with the body to allow outflow.

Fluid management

Fluid balancing is a crucial but delicate task. Free fluid rushes into injured brain cells and increases cerebral oedema, but hypotension reduces brain perfusion and can double mortality (Pietropauli *et al* 1992). The danger of hypotension is not widely appreciated and occurs particularly at the following times:

- on admission, when a patient may be quietly bleeding into the abdomen and losing consciousness because of hypotension rather than brain injury,

- during surgery, when the BP may be deliberately kept low in the mistaken belief that this will keep a tenuous clot in place (Pietropauli *et al* 1992).

Fluid decisions vary from encouraging fluids (Scalea 1994), to keeping PAWP at a modest 4–6 mmHg (Vos 1993) using fluid restriction, hypertonic feeds, hypertonic saline and osmotic diuretics such as mannitol (Freshman 1993), all of which may also thicken secretions. Rapid maintenance of cerebral perfusion without fluid overload is sometimes achieved using vasopressors or inotropes.

Nutrition, temperature control and drug therapy

Nutritional support is needed because energy expenditure may be doubled for up to four weeks (Borzotta 1994), a carbohydrate-free diet being recommended to prevent hyperglycemia exacerbating cerebral ischaemia (Robertson 1995). If gastric feeding is contraindicated, other enteral routes are preferable (Borzotta 1994).

Temperature is tightly regulated. A pyrexia of 1° can increase cerebral metabolism by up to 10% (Vos 1993), but hypothermia causes arrhythmias and shifts the oxygen dissociation curve to the left.

Sedative drugs may be used in an attempt to reduce brain metabolism and control ICP, but they can reduce CPP without reducing ICP (Papazian 1993), especially in hypovolaemic patients. Steroids such as dexamethasone reduce cerebral oedema if taken before the injury, which is possible before neurosurgery but not generally feasible before an RTA!

Mechanical ventilation

Intubation may be needed to maintain a clear airway. IPPV may be needed to regulate an unstable breathing pattern, ensure oxygenation, control ICP or manage chest complications. Paralysis also reduces oxygen consumption, but its routine use has been questioned because Hsiang (1993) found that it increased complications. Hyperventilation is sometimes used to lower $PaCO_2$ and induce cerebral vasoconstriction, but this can itself cause cerebral ischaemia (Ruta 1993), as signalled by slowing of the EEG. PEEP may be needed for severe hypoxaemia, its effects balanced against the disadvantages of hypotension and further impairment of venous outflow from the brain. High frequency ventilation may be beneficial in eliminating BP fluctuations and maintaining venous return. DVT is a significant risk (Gersin 1994).

11.4.5 Physiotherapy

The hallmark of physiotherapy is maximum involvement but minimum intervention. Involvement is twofold:

- frequent assessment to assist the balancing act of deciding whether to intervene and the method of intervention,
- supervision of handling to minimize ICP disturbance.

The first priority is to establish a means of communication for patients who are not comatosed. For unconscious patients, explanations should be maintained, but noise and unnecessary conversation avoided.

Assessment should avoid moving the patient. SaO_2 is the main guideline. Observation of BP and ICP monitors is required prior to and throughout any treatment. In the absence of an ICP monitor, signs of ↑ ICP are:

- ↓ conscious level,
- change in vital signs, breathing pattern or muscle tone,
- vomiting.

CSF leak through the nose or ear is a sign to avoid nasal suction because it indicates a possible route for infection. If a non-intubated patient with CSF leak requires suction, a minitracheostomy or oral airway should be used.

Pain relief for associated injuries reduces oxygen consumption. TNS is useful for fractured ribs, but Entonox should be avoided in acute head injury (Moss and McDowall 1979) and opioids can raise ICP (Sperry 1992). Gentle input such as stroking the skin has shown beneficial effects (Chudley 1994).

Further intervention is unwise in the presence of cardiovascular instability, particularly hypotension, or ICP above 15 mmHg (Paratz 1993). If it is essential, a drug such as thiopental should be given beforehand to moderate ICP (Borel *et al* 1990). Treatment can also be timed to follow withdrawal of CSF.

Positioning is safe with ICP < 15 and CPP > 50 mmHg (Chudley 1994). Patients should be log-rolled slowly using a turning sheet, with one person solely responsible for maintaining head alignment, or a kinetic bed can be used (Tillett 1993). Accurate positioning in side-lying with a neutral head position assists prophylactic chest care. However, minimum movement is the priority, and it may be best to not turn the patient at all in the early stages if there is a suitable mattress for preventing pressure sores and if gas exchange is adequate. When the patient is supine, one small pillow or no pillow should be used to avoid neck flexion (Mitchell *et al* 1981).

If bagging is essential, it should be brief, and for the first few days rapid enough to maintain hypocapnia, preferably checked with an end-tidal CO_2 monitor. If manual techniques are essential, percussion is less detrimental than vibrations (Garradd and Bullock 1986). Percussion should be rhythmic, smooth and gentle, while vibrations should be fine and with minimal effect on intrathoracic pressure. A mechanical vibrator is preferable.

Suction can precipitate a dramatic increase in ICP, either immediately or on the rebound after approximately 10 minutes (Rudy *et al* 1991). This is caused by hypoxia, impairment of venous outflow due to coughing, and increased heart rate and BP. If suction is indicated, the patient should be rested from previous activity, hyperventilated with 100% oxygen before and after, monitored and have the head strictly in alignment. Multiple suction passes without a rest in between are dangerous (Rudy *et al* 1991).

Extreme hip flexion should be avoided in the acute stage to prevent a rise in intra-abdominal pressure. If flaccidity is present with no pattern of activity, then it may be best to avoid any movements in the first few days. If postural tone indicates that spastic patterning is developing, extra attention should be given to avoiding factors which exacerbate abnormal activity, e.g. poor positioning, infection, pain, anxiety, pressure under the feet and the weight of bedclothes. Staff and carers should be taught positioning and handling to encourage inhibitory control over spasticity. If increased tone is identified, serial splinting to maintain dorsiflexion is indicated immediately (Moseley 1993).

Preplanning is needed to avoid a cumulative rise in ICP. Most teams work to space physiotherapy, nursing and other interventions as far apart as possible, although some find it best to do everything at once and then let the patient settle. Co-ordinated teamwork is a priority, especially in the first vulnerable week. It is worth remembering that many patients are better with no hands-on physiotherapy at all in the very acute stage.

It is also worth remembering that rehabilitation is now expected to start in the ICU. MacKay (1992) showed that length of coma can be cut to a third by an early multidisciplinary programme of orientation, sensory stimulation, exercise and family involvement.

11.5 SMOKE INHALATION

Thermal damage by inhalation of hot gas is inflicted on the airways, which filter heat at the expense of bronchospasm, mucosal swelling, pulmonary oedema, paralysis of cilia and ulceration. These 'heat sink' filtering properties are overwhelmed by inhalation of steam or crack cocaine, which penetrates to alveoli, burns lung and destroys surfactant (Haponik 1992).

Respiratory complications are the major cause of death following fire entrapment, although X-ray changes may not appear for days. Upper airway obstruction is the most treatable of respiratory complications, but deaths still occur from delayed intubation. Oxygen delivery is impaired by shock and inhaled carbon monoxide, which displaces oxygen from haemoglobin and shifts the dissociation curve to the left. Infection can be transmitted to the lung from the hospital environment or infected burns. Epithelial damage may lead to long-term small airway injury and hyperreactivity (Kinsella *et al* 1991). Lung expansion may be restricted by a tight armour of scarring around the chest.

General treatment follows a fourfold approach:

- pain management, e.g. by PCA (Choiniere 1992),
- judicious fluid administration with crystalloids and colloids to replace lost water and protein without incurring pulmonary oedema,
- supplementary feeding to compensate for hypermetabolism that can last for months (Milner 1994),
- oxygen, CPAP (if the face is not burned) or IPPV as required to maintain gas exchange.

Inhaled nitric oxide may also be given to assist gas exchange by vasodilating pulmonary vessels (Ogura 1994).

Respiratory physiotherapy is aimed at maintaining lung volume and clearing the thick and prolific secretions caused by airway damage. Lavish humidification is needed. Precautions include the following:

1. Treatment should be little and often because of the importance of prophylaxis and the inevitable fatigue.

2. Percussion and vibrations should be avoided over chest burns, whether dressed or not. If manual techniques are essential, a vibrator is reasonably comfortable.
3. If suction is necessary, it should be gentle, minimal and scrupulously aseptic to prevent further damage to the mucosa.
4. Patients need extra attention to communication if facial oedema affects vision or speech. Many are deeply distressed at what has happened to them.
5. If there is oedema around the head or neck, postural drainage is contra-indicated and patients are often nursed upright.
6. If stridor develops in non-intubated patients, this should be reported because of the risk of obstruction.

Two-hourly exercises are required for burned limbs, especially the hands (Keilty 1993), using Entonox or other analgesia.

11.6 POISONING, PULMONARY ASPIRATION AND NEAR-DROWNING

Poisoning is often associated with pulmonary aspiration, in which case vigorous and early measures to clear and re-inflate the lung are required, including CPAP or IPPB as appropriate. The X-ray will identify the opacity to be targeted. Associated trauma should be checked because any person found on the floor has to get there first.

Most poisoning is self-inflicted and there is sometimes a tendency for the patient to be dismissed as attention-seeking or time-wasting, but these patients are often at the extremes of depression or desperation, and the professional approach is to withhold personal judgement and care for the patient in such a way that he or she believes that life might be worth living after all.

Near-drowning is defined as submersion followed by survival for 24 hours, but death from pulmonary complications can still occur. Patients suffer a form of aspiration, leading to pulmonary oedema, cerebral oedema, inactivation of surfactant and bronchospasm. If water is swallowed, there is often further vomiting and aspiration. Frequent physiotherapy may be needed for at least 48 hours in order to prevent atelectasis.

11.7 SHOCK

In contrast to the layperson's shock-horror understanding of the term, the sober clinical definition of shock is 'failure of oxygen supply to meet oxygen demand', and the signs on p. 247, leading to inadequate tissue perfusion, anaerobic metabolism and lactic acidosis. It commonly falls into into three main categories.

Hypovolaemic shock is caused by loss of fluid, e.g. haemorrhage or burns. It is accompanied by a low CVP. **Cardiogenic** shock is caused by sudden heart failure, as in severe myocardial infarct. It is characterized by high CVP and pulmonary oedema. The central feature of these two forms of shock is low cardiac output, represented by tachycardia, profound hypotension, poor urine output, rapid shallow breathing, confusion and cold clammy skin.

Septic shock occurs when endotoxins cause uncontrolled vasodilation, which in effect reduces circulating blood volume. Oxygen delivery (DO_2) is therefore depressed while oxygen consumption ($\dot{V}O_2$) is excessive, so the aim of treatment is to achieve supranormal levels of DO_2 to prevent tissue hypoxia. A high cardiac output may double oxygen supply but cannot sustain an adequate BP. Damaged tissues cannot extract sufficient oxygen, as shown by $S\bar{v}O_2$ rising to 85% or more. Just one hour of gut ischaemia can liberate gut bacteria into the circulation (Brown 1994), and within two to three weeks multisystem failure may develop. Patients are pyrexial, flushed, tachypnoeic, hypotensive, confused and have a bounding pulse.

Treatment is by fluids, inotropes, infection control, oxygen and IPPV. Vasopressors are given in septic shock but may compromise regional blood flow. This formidable array of options may improve oxygen delivery, but does not touch oxygen extraction and has not notably reduced the high mortality from this condition.

Other examples of shock are **obstructive** shock as occurs with severe pulmonary embolism, and **anaphalactic** shock, which occurs as a reaction to certain drugs, allergans and poisons, causing widespread vasodilation and hypotension.

11.8 DISSEMINATED INTRAVASCULAR COAGULATION (DIC)

Most people with septic shock go on to develop a massive activation of the coagulation process known as DIC. Other precipitating factors are fat embolism, lung contusion or burns. Traumatized cells release thromboplastin, leading to vessel blockage by clumps of platelets and fibrin. When clotting factors and platelets are depleted, bleeding can occur from the slightest trauma, including suction. DIC is a strong predictor of multisystem failure and death (Fourrier 1992).

The syndrome is suspected if a patient with predisposing factors shows signs of spontaneous bleeding, produces blood-stained secretions on suction, or has abnormal clotting studies. Nasopharyngeal suction is contraindicated in such patients, and tracheal suction should be done with extra care.

11.9 ACUTE RESPIRATORY DISTRESS SYNDROME (ARDS)

The commonest cause of death in a non-coronary ICU is not the original disorder, but progressive damage to other organ systems, known as multisystem failure. This is a response to both the initial disorder and to medical interventions.

11.9.1 Causes

Multisystem failure is best recognized in people who suffer a catastrophe leading to excessive oxygen demands. Causes include the following:

- shock/prolonged hypotension,
- major sepsis,
- aspiration,
- overtransfusion,
- smoke inhalation,
- head injury,
- near-drowning,
- fat embolism,
- lung contusion,
- DIC,
- poisoning/drug abuse,
- acute pancreatitis,
- cardiopulmonary bypass,
- trauma including major surgery,
- multisystem disease.

11.9.2 Pathophysiology

If an amputated limb is reimplanted after a period of ischaemia, the body is subjected to hypoperfusion, reperfusion and release of endotoxins, a domino effect which sets off generalized inflammation. Reamputation is required to prevent the rest of the body becoming poisoned. This scenario provides an analogy for multisystem failure. Hypoperfusion and reperfusion activate a deadly cascade of mediators from damaged cells, leading to 'rogue inflammation', which escapes the usual control mechanisms and exacerbates rather than repairs injury, leading to increased permeability of body membranes. Gut ischaemia–reperfusion is thought to be either the engine of this process or an early victim, leading to leakage of toxins into the circulation. The main victim is the lung because it is exposed to the entire venous effluent.

There follows progressive failure of other systems, the highest mortality occurring with kidney and liver failure. Of particular relevance to the physiotherapist is haematological insufficiency, which leads to clotting abnormalities, and the most common and dramatic manifestation, acute respiratory distress syndrome (ARDS).

Both alveolar and vascular functions of the lung are ravaged by the inflammatory response. Non-cardiogenic pulmonary oedema floods the alveoli and makes the lungs four or five times their normal weight, almost drowning the patient from the inside. Invading plasma proteins deplete surfactant, which exacerbates atelectasis, increases $PA\text{-}aO_2$ to 250 mmHg or more, and leads to refractory hypoxaemia.

Hypoxaemia is exacerbated by bronchospasm, and hypoxia is exacerbated by (1) reduced gas diffusion at tissue level because of interstitial oedema, (2) impaired oxygen extraction due to damaged cells and (3) excess oxygen consumption due to a twice-normal metabolic rate.

The water-logged lungs suffer a restrictive defect, which worsens as fibrosis sets in. The lungs become progressively and irregularly damaged, showing areas of hyperinflation, compression atelectasis and a small area of undamaged compliant lung. The capacity of this so-called 'baby lung' may be one-third of normal (Slutsky 1993).

As demand exceeds supply, oxygen consumption ($\dot{V}O_2$) becomes dependent on oxygen delivery (DO_2), even if delivery is well above normal. If anaerobic metabolism occurs, blood lactate levels rise, further impairing the normal mechanisms of oxygen extraction.

Vascular injury leads to pulmonary hypertension, which exacerbates oedema formation and inhibits right ventricular function. Circulating catecholamines may increase cardiac output and total body blood flow, but deranged autoregulation means loss of control of capillary blood flow, increasing perfusion to nonvulnerable systems such as skin and muscle, and further depriving needy systems such as the gut and liver.

ARDS is also called leaky lung syndrome because of the seive-like characteristic of the alveolar-capillary membrane. It is also called shock lung because it first came to light in soldiers resuscitated from shock in the Vietnam war.

11.9.3 Clinical features

Following the provoking insult, there is a latent period of 24–72 hours before the syndrome develops. In the next 24 hours there is rapid shallow breathing and respiratory distress. The following one to two days show reduced PaO_2 and $PaCO_2$ and minor X-ray changes. Diagnosis is not usually made until the third phase, when virulent hypoxaemia develops, $PaCO_2$ rises as the patient tires, and the X-ray shows diffuse ground-glass shadowing which characteristically spares the costophrenic angles. CT scanning shows opacities in dependent regions, representing lung areas compressed by the weight of oedematous lung above, and will show up any barotrauma (Fig.11.7).

The incidence of pneumothorax varies according to ventilator management and is demonstrated in 8–77% of patients (Heullit 1995). Breath sounds are surprisingly normal, with just a harsh edge to them. Fibrosis sets

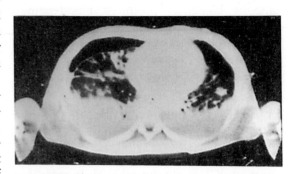

Figure 11.7 CT scan of a patient with ARDS, showing dense areas of atelectasis in dependent regions, and pneumothorax in right non-dependent region.

in after the first week. Pulmonary artery catheterization shows a high PAP, reflecting increased pulmonary vascular resistance. PAWP is < 18 mmHg because ARDS is not a condition of generalized overhydration, in contrast to cardiogenic pulmonary oedema, which causes a high PAWP.

11.9.4 Medical treatment

Gastric tonometry can detect gut ischaemia before mucosal injury occurs. Then vigorous efforts are made to find and eradicate septic foci. Management is then aimed at restoration of normal homeostasis rather than attempts to reverse individual components of the syndrome, because support of a single system may place an intolerable burden on another. The principle is to sustain tissue perfusion by supranormal DO_2, using ventilatory and haemodynamic support. The balance between beneficial and damaging interventions is a fine one.

Skilled fluid management is required because transfused fluid tends to escape into the lung, while inadequate circulating volume hinders DO_2, Renal impairment may complicate the picture. PAWP is kept as low as is consistent with optimum DO_2 and haemodynamic stability, and overload may require slow continuous ultrafiltration (Anderson 1994).

DO_2 is promoted by inotropic support, packed red blood cell transfusion and vasodilators. VO_2 is reduced by sedation, paralysis and avoidance of stress and pyrexia. Added oxygen is limited to 60% if possible to prevent oxygen toxicity, which resembles the effects of ARDS itself. Haemodynamic support is by manipulation of preload, heart rate, myocardial contractility and afterload.

Paralysis and IPPV can reduce VO_2 by 20% (Manthous 1995). However, IPPV squeezes the bulk of the ventilation into the 'baby lung', creating stretching forces that can cause secondary lung injury (Parker and Hernandez 1993).

Complications include the following:

1. Barotrauma, which becomes more likely as lung damage progresses.
2. Intrinsic PEEP, because non-homogeneous loss of elasticity causes uneven distribution of expiratory time, leading to increased expiratory resistance (Pesenti and Pelosi 1992, p. 328).
3. Impaired cardiac output because of high-pressure IPPV.

Various ventilatory manoeuvres help to maintain DO_2 with minimal damage:

1. To recruit alveoli and maintain DO_2, levels of PEEP up to 30 cmH$_2$O are imposed, even though this may overdistend some areas of lung.
2. To discourage barotrauma, low tidal volumes may be used, sometimes to the point of permissive hypercapnia (Hickling 1994). High $PaCO_2$ is well tolerated if established over several days, but $\dot{V}_A/\dot{Q}$ mismatch may be exacerbated.
3. Pressure control ventilation limits peak pressure and minimizes overdistension of the more compliant areas of lung. The decelerating inspiratory flow also allows a more equal distribution of gas to lung units with varied filling speeds.
4. Techniques can be tried such as airway pressure release ventilation, inverse-ratio ventilation (p. 226) or high-frequency oscillation (Imai, 1994), which minimizes overdistension by using small tidal volumes.
5. Extracorporeal gas exchange allows reduced ventilation pressures and lower F_IO_2, but causes bleeding in 75% of patients (Anderson 1994).

Medical management is mainly supportive, but curative measures include haemofiltration to wash out circulating mediators (Lingnau 1995), inhaled surfactant (Spragg 1994) or inhaled nitric oxide. Despite nitric oxide's reputation as the car exhaust killer of rain forests, its ability to cause selective pulmonary vasodilation and bronchodilation in ARDS led it to be elected the 'molecule of the year' in 1992 (Anggård 1994).

11.9.5   Physiotherapy

Like medical management, physiotherapy aims to maximize DO_2 while causing the least harm. Gratuitous increase in stress and energy expenditure must be avoided.

In spontaneously breathing patients, CPAP or BiPAP may delay or prevent IPPV (Martin 1995). For ventilated patients, the main problem is loss of lung volume, secretions usually being of little note. Positioning is the first approach. Occasionally, patients who are well hydrated can sit up in bed. Side-lying may or may not be beneficial, as guided by the monitors, but regular position change in a kinetic bed has been shown to reduce atelectasis and improve gas exchange (Hormann 1994). Barotrauma is less likely to occur in the dependent lung (Stewart 1993).

A more dramatic improvement in SaO_2 may be found by gently turning the patient into prone. This can reverse atelectasis in the non-dependent lower lobes, which improves overall gas exchange because there is more space in the lungs posteriorly due to the chest's triangular cross-section and the space taken up by the heart anteriorly. Lung expansion is also more uniform in prone than supine because the heart is supported by the sternum and there is less parenchymal distortion (Yang 1991). By opening previously deflated lung, oxygenation may improve to such an extent that PEEP and F_IO_2 can be reduced (Lamm 1994). The benefits are reversed on returning to supine and many patients are best left in prone for extended periods, most comfortably on a fluidized bed. Not all patients benefit. Problems of the prone position are:

- it can be a frightening experience for the patient,

- care is needed to protect the eyes, secure the tracheal tube and guard against shoulder joint damage,
- potential cardiac arrest must be planned for and a procedure prepared in case rapid return to supine is necessary, although CPR can be achieved in prone with a fist under the sternum and compression of the mid-thoracic spine (Sun 1992).

Bagging is undertaken only if necessary. However, the literature on barotrauma during extended periods of IPPV should not be extrapolated to the brief bagging used for physiotherapy. Enright (1992) has shown how patients with atelectasis or sputum retention show sustained improvement in DO_2 after positioning, bagging, vibrations as necessary and suction. This caused no barotrauma (Enright, personal communication). If bagging is anticipated, the X-ray should be examined for any precursors to a pneumothorax such as thin-walled air cysts beneath the visceral pleura or linear streaking towards the hilum (Albelda 1983; Haake *et al* 1987). Pneumomediastinum is suspected if there is air outlining the mediastinum or aorta. Patients fare better if well filled before treatment. Disconnection for suction should be avoided when possible (Schwartz 1987) by using a closed circuit catheter.

The observant physiotherapist is a useful team member because treatment is more effective if the syndrome is recognized early. Suspicions are raised if a patient with the relevant predisposing factors develops tachypnoea and hypoxaemia more severely than would be expected from the clinical picture, or if a ventilated patient develops high airway pressures.

A concerted approach of regular position change, permissive hypercapnia and inhaled nitric oxide has shown that mortality can be brought down to 16% (Lewandowski 1992). However, the past 20 years have shown no general reduction in mortality from ARDS, and 50–75% of patients still perish overall (Heulitt 1995), mostly because of superinfection and multiple organ failure, and rarely because of lung injury (Pearl 1993). High-risk factors include infection as a cause, and lack of response to treatment in the first 24 hours. Low-risk factors include trauma as a cause, and younger age groups (Beale *et al* 1993). Survivors show a remarkable capacity to regenerate lung tissue; most show abnormal gas transfer and many a mild restrictive defect, but rarely is there functional impairment.

RECOMMENDED READING

Bellomo, R. (1994) Asthma requiring mechanical ventilation – a low morbidity approach. *Chest*, **105**, 891–6.

Bone, R.C., Balk, R., Slotman, G. *et al.* (1992) Adult respiratory distress syndrome. *Chest*, **101**, 320–6.

Bullock, R. and Teasdale, G. (1990) Head injuries. *Br. Med. J.*, **300**, 1515–18, 1576–9.

Johnson, J. and Silverberg, R. (1995) Serial casting of the lower extremity to correct contractures during the acute phase of burn care. *Phys. Ther.*, **75**, 262–6.

Jones, B. (1994) The effects of patient repositioning on intracranial pressure. *Austr. J. Adv. Nurs.*, **12**, 32–9.

Keilty, S.E.J. (1993) Inhalation burn injured patients and physiotherapy management. *Physiotherapy*, **79**, 87–90.

Pinsky, M.R. (1994) Through the past darkly: ventilatory management of patients with COPD. *Crit. Care Med.*, **22**, 1714–17.

Senekal, M. and Eales, C. (1994) The optimal physiotherapeutic approach to penetrating stab wounds of the chest. *S. Afr. J. Physiother.*, **50**, 29–36.

Wake, D. (1995) Near drowning. *Int. Crit. Care Nurs.*, **1**, 40–3.

12. Physiotherapy for children and infants

12.1 PHYSIOTHERAPY FOR CHILDREN

12.1.1 Introduction

Adult patients can say to themselves: 'I understand that I am not in hospital for the rest of my life, that my family will visit, that the nasty things they are doing to me are for my own good.' Young children do not have these resources of reasoning and may be overwhelmed by bewilderment, feelings of abandonment, uncertainty about the behaviour expected of them and sometimes the impression that they are being punished. Despite progress over the last decades in humanizing children's experience in hospital, long-term emotional disturbance can still be caused. Children need to be listened to, believed and given some control over what is done to them. Teenagers in particular need autonomy because they are already resenting their illness and feel extra sensitive to the paternalistic environment that is inherent in many paediatric units.

Children appreciate having the same physiotherapist throughout their stay. Those over three years old should not have their treatment discussed in their presence without being included. Children need their own toys and belongings, and all but the sickest are best dressed in their normal clothes. Their siblings benefit from involvement because they may feel a variety of responses including anxiety, grief, jealousy, isolation, resentment and guilt. Parents need confidence in their own competence, and acknowledgement that they are the experts on their own children. Their anxiety is otherwise contagious.

It is normal for adults to adopt the sick role when hospitalized, and children may also act as if younger than their years when finding themselves in a dependent position, often showing an exaggeration of the behaviour patterns that they normally use to cope with stress.

Young children tend to react more severely to acute respiratory infection than older people because of their narrow airways. The incidence of infant infections is reduced by breast feeding (Wright 1989), and increased by factors such as damp homes (Brunekreef 1989) and parental smoking (Couriel 1994a) Childhood respiratory infection tends to leave a legacy of sensitized airways and a higher incidence of COPD in adult life (Shaheen *et al* 1994).

12.1.2 Aspects of assessment

Parents should be welcomed during assessment and treatment. If this causes the child to express anxiety more noisily than when unaccompanied, this is healthier than withdrawal. The younger the child, the greater the need for a parent.

The presence of an intravenous needle can inhibit children from moving, and they should be reassured that it will be watched and supported during assessment and treatment. The presence of a nil-by-mouth sign may indicate considerable distress if the child cannot understand why he or she is so thirsty, and parents can be enlisted to help with explanations and mouth care. Children should be allowed oral fluids up to two hours before surgery to reduce the risks of dehydration, hypoglycaemia and misery (Phillips *et al* 1994).

Before auscultation, children can be given the opportunity to see and feel the stethoscope, and use it to listen to themselves

Table 12.1 Vital signs in children (source: Prasad and Hussey 1995)

	Newborn	1–3 years	3–7 years	Over 7 years
RR	40–60	20–30	20–30	15–20
PaO_2	60–90	80–100	80–100	80–100
HR	100–200	100–180	70–150	80–100
BP	60–90 / 30 60	75–130 / 45 90	90–140 / 50 80	90–140 / 50 80

or a doll. The diaphragm or bell should be warmed before use.

Normal respiratory rate, blood gas and cardiovascular measurements during childhood are shown in Table 12.1.

Laboured inspiration is represented by intercostal recession because of a compliant chest wall. Laboured expiration is represented by grunting, which acts as a form of PEP to splint open the narrow airways. Other signs of respiratory distress are:

- tachypnoea,
- asynchronous or paradoxical breathing, shown by a see-saw motion between chest wall and abdomen, with the over-compliant rib cage being sucked inwards during inspiration,
- nasal flaring,
- apnoea associated with bradycardia or cyanosis.

Breathlessness may hamper communication, interfere with the child's sleep or that of the parents, and affect eating or drinking.

Deterioration in gas exchange may be indicated by pallor, sweating, restlessness agitation, glazed eyes and, in ventilated young children, fighting the ventilator. Hypoxaemia must be excluded before sedating an unsettled child.

12.1.3 Physiotherapy management

Before treatment, clear and honest explanations should be given to the child, including descriptions of what the treatment will feel like, how long it will last and reassurance that it can be stopped by request at any time. Resistance to treatment can often be overcome by giving the child a choice, such as either incentive spirometry or a walk outside. Requests to stop treatment must be respected, and if further treatment is refused despite cajoling, distraction, joking and enlisting the parent's help, serious thought should be given to whether the benefits of continuing treatment outweigh the effects of enforced intervention. In the UK, a child's consent to treatment is required if he or she is of 'sufficient understanding to make an informed decision' (Children Act 1989).

The parent is encouraged to take part in, as well as learn from, the treatment. Two-year-olds can do breathing exercises if taught imaginatively, and all but the youngest appreciate explanation about their disease and the purpose of physiotherapy.

Methods to increase lung volume

The use of paper mobiles, bubble-blowing, blowing through a straw or simply blowing a tissue utilizes the deep breath that is taken before blowing out. Paediatric incentive spirometers are enjoyable and encourage deep breathing without a subsequent forced expiration. Abdominal breathing can be taught by placing a favourite toy on the abdomen.

Young children need particular attention to maintenance of lung volume, because lack of elastic tissue in immature lungs means that they share with elderly people a tendency towards airway closure at low lung volumes.

Any suggestions that children should be made to cry to encourage deep breathing should be rejected.

When positioning for gas exchange, the distribution of ventilation is opposite to the adult pattern (p. 7), which means that ventilation is directed preferentially to upper regions. In side-lying, the lower lung is poorly ventilated because airway closure occurs above FRC until age five or six (James

1991). This is due to the compliant chest wall being unable to counteract fully the elastic recoil of the lungs, and lack of connective tissue support for the small airways. This pattern predominates in the first 10 years (Davies *et al* 1990). In the presence of unilateral lung pathology, gas exchange is optimal with the diseased lung dependent, which is opposite to the adult pattern.

Many young children have gastro-oesophageal reflux (GOR). Most improve spontaneously by 18 months, but up to 30% remain symptomatic until aged four (Phillips *et al* 1994). Persistent wheezing and vomiting are the main manifestations, and GOR is often underdiagnosed. Management is by feeding little and often, and maintainance of 30° head elevation, although this should match the needs of the child because occasionally children aspirate in this position only.

CPAP is particularly suited to children to compensate for the floppy chest wall. Administration can be via the closed system of an endotracheal tube, or by an open system using face mask, nasal prongs or nasopharyngeal tube. The open system allows the infant to generate more distending pressure in moments of need by grunting. CPAP is usually indicated for intubated children under age six and for 24 hours after extubation (James 1991) because of the loss of the ability to grunt. For spontaneously breathing children, it is used if adequate oxygenation cannot be maintained with high inspired oxygen. A starting pressure of $5 \, cmH_2O$ is used, which is gradually increased until grunting stops or oxygenation is optimum. Pressures above $10 \, cmH_2O$ bring risks of gastric distension and pneumothorax. When ready for discontinuation, CPAP should be reduced slowly to prevent atelectasis.

Methods to clear secretions

Postural drainage can be enjoyable over a bean bag or on the helper's lap in a rocking chair. In infants, who spend much time supine, the sitting position is included to drain the apical segments of the upper lobes. Percussion is often more soothing than vibrations. Huffing can be encouraged by blowing cotton wool or using the story of the big bad wolf who 'huffed and puffed and blew the house down'. Coughing can be motivated by laughter and rewarded by earning a star on a cough score sheet. From age four, children can do the ACBT and are able to spit out and blow their nose to prevent secretions spilling into the airways. In infants, coughing can be stimulated by gentle inward pressure against the trachea in a circular pattern during exhalation. Nasotracheal suction is usually unnecessary if the child is coughing effectively, even if secretions are swallowed. When suction is necessary, the child's saliva should be used as lubricant, unless the nose is already clogged up with mucus.

Although the level of suction pressure is related to mucosal damage, there is little original research examining at what level this occurs. Howard (1994) claims that greater negative pressure does not remove more secretions, and Hazinski (1984) recommends the following pressures:

- 60–90 cmH$_2$O for infants
- 90–110 cmH$_2$O for young children
- 110–150 cmH$_2$O for older children.

Minitracheostomy is indicated for children who need repeated suction (Allen and Hart 1988).

A specimen of nasopharyngeal aspirate may be requested in order to obtain epithelial cells for diagnostic purposes. Nasal suction is used to reach the post-nasal pathway, and the procedure followed is described on p. 143.

12.1.4 Specific measures for children with medical conditions

Asthma

Most cases of asthma appear before the age of two (Pinn 1992). The disease affects 10% of children (Deaves 1993), twice as many as any other chronic illness, and mortality is increasing (Ryan-Wenger 1994). But it is widely underdiagnosed, one study showing that children consulted a general practitioner an average of 16 times before asthma was diagnosed (Levy and Bell 1984). Asthmatic children are sometimes given non-specific diagnoses such as 'wheezy bronchitis' or simply 'chestiness', possibly because it is thought that the word 'asthma' causes parents to worry. But explanation of a child's persistent symptoms relieves worry and brings relief to both parents and child. Recurrent cough or wheeze is sufficient to suspect childhood asthma. Diagnosis is aided by a six-minute exercise test, a positive result being a drop of more than 15% in peak flow within 10 minutes after exercise (Jones and Bowen 1994).

Parents, teachers and doctors may have different perceptions of the needs and potential of children with asthma. The child's view of the disease is often based on fear, reinforced by continuing anxiety about future attacks. Two-thirds of children outgrow their asthma (Sears 1994), and it is thought to be more than coincidence that this is when they outgrow their fears (Gillespie 1989). Education is therefore the foundation of physiotherapy. This is achieved most effectively through an asthma group because there is little time for education during the brief hospitalization for an acute attack. The group involves the family, whose attitude is crucial. The programme could include:

- prevention (p..62),
- practice in using inhalers, preferably in front of the group to improve confidence at school,
- for children over six years, practice in monitoring their own peak flows,
- voice work such as humming to control expiration,
- hard, enjoyable, controlled physical activity (a warm swimming pool is particularly suitable).

If bronchospasm following exercise is not prevented by the normal measures (p. 62), activity should be followed by positioning, relaxation and abdominal breathing using the concept of 'tummy balloons'. Other ideas are described in Capen *et al* (1994).

School staff, too, need educating. Inhalers must be accessible to children and not locked in cupboards. Many asthma organizations have a junior asthma club which provides diary cards for children, parents and teachers (see Appendix C).

During acute episodes, young children are best positioned on a parent's lap. An oxygen mask can be frightening for children in respiratory distress. If an acute episode causes middle lobe collapse, this is one of the few cases in which bacterial infection is likely.

Bronchiolitis

Bronchiolitis is inflammation of the small airways due to viral infection, and is seen in children under two years old, especially those born prematurely. Mucosal oedema and mucus plugging lead to airway obstruction and hyperinflation, causing excessive oral secretions, breathlessness, wheeze, chest retractions and a fivefold or more increase in the work of breathing (Milner and Murray 1989). Some infants are too breathless to manage a cough, and a respiratory rate > 50/min warrants admission to hospital (Isaacs 1995). Treatment is by humidity, oxygen, fluids and maintenance of the head-up position. The acute illness subsides into apparent sudden recovery in about a week, but damaged epithelium may lead to permanent small airways changes, often causing these children to merge into the childhood asthmatic population.

Physiotherapy tends to cause desaturation and increased wheeze in the acute stage, but if sputum retention becomes a problem, percussion in modified side-to-side positions is indicated, with suction if necessary. Close evaluation is required by assessing post-treatment wheeze, oxygen saturation and how the child settles.

Croup

Croup, or laryngotracheobronchitis, is an acute syndrome of upper airways obstruction caused by a viral infection. It usually occurs in children aged from three months to five years (Hess 1991). Signs are a barking cough, fever, sore throat and stridor. Traditional treatment includes humidification, but this is of unproven benefit and it is unclear how a mist might reduce an inflammatory obstruction. Nebulized steroids may speed recovery (Landau and Geelhoed 1994).

Epiglottitis

Epiglottitis is a less common but more vicious form of upper airways obstruction, occuring in children aged from two to seven years (Hess 1991). It is caused by fulminant bacterial infection involving the soft tissues around the entrance to the larynx, and without prompt recognition and treatment it can be fatal. Intubation may be needed to protect the airway, and antibiotics are given. In both croup and epiglottitis, physiotherapy is not indicated for non-intubated babies, and only if there are excessive secretions in intubated babies.

12.1.5 Specific measures for children undergoing surgery

Preoperative management

Appropriate management of preoperative anxiety has been shown to lead to easier postoperative management (Goresky 1994). Preoperative explanations can be augmented with pictures, books, rehearsal of procedures, visits to hospital facilities and encouragement to discuss the experience with children who have had the same operation. It should not be assumed that parents have explained the operation to the child. Care should be taken with terminology, because

Figure 12.1 Faces scale for pain assessment in children. (From Carter, B. (1994) *Child and Infant Pain*, Chapman & Hall, London, with permission.)

children have been known to mistake a bone marrow test for a 'bow-and-arrow test' or a dye injection for a 'die injection'. Young children have a protracted sense of time and will benefit from being told in advance that postoperative pain will go away after a few days. Physical sensations should be described, and the reason for the sensations explained. Without explanations, the boundary between reality and fantasy can be blurred. Truth is essential because if the child's trust is shaken co-operation is lost.

Separating a screaming child from its parent at the door of the operating room is distressing for all concerned. It is now understood that a parent should be present during induction of and emergence from anaesthesia (Goresky 1994; Hall 1995).

Pain management

If postoperative pain is poorly managed in adults, this tendency is exaggerated in children and even more so in infants. One survey found that the majority of children who had had major surgery or burns received no analgesia at all (Eland 1985). Similarly, it is unfortunately fairly common for young children to undergo intubation and chest drain insertion without analgesia; and older children have described the pain of medical procedures as the worst aspect of their condition (Yaster 1995). In animals, such treatment would bring prosecution, and the psychological impact on children can be long-term and profound (Beyer and Byers 1985).

The causes of poor pain management in children include the following:

- children's subjective complaints may not be taken seriously, health staff tending to rely on assumptions and personal beliefs when assessing children's pain (Beyer and Byers 1985),
- children's analgesia needs meticulous prescription, which is often not met and leaves children as 'therapeutic orphans' (Yaster 1995),
- children may minimize complaints because of fears of the dreaded needle,
- children may not express pain in terms that are easily understood by adults, and an absence of crying does not indicate an absence of pain,
- some health staff do not realize that children are able to feel pain from birth, and even before birth (Abu-Saad 1994).
- children are easily held down by force.

For pain assessment of young children, the parent gives a more accurate indication than health staff, but this information must be actively requested because parents tend to assume that everything is automatically done to minimize pain. For older children, it is better to ask the child, especially as this gives an indication of the associated fear (Manne *et al* 1992). Children over seven years can use a visual analogue scale, those over three years can use colour intensity scores, scales with happy-sad faces (Fig. 12.1) or comprehensive charts with body outlines (Qureshi 1994). Prelingual and non-verbal children can be observed for signs of withdrawal, face and body reactions, irritability, pallor, momentary breath-holding, prolonged sleeping and, in older babies who have been subjected to traumatic procedures over some time, an expression of frozen watchfulness similar to the abused child. Further details are in Beyer and Byers (1985) and Sparsholt (1989). Physiological measures, such as changes in respiratory rate, heart rate, BP and SaO_2 can be used as adjuncts, but are not specific as indicators of pain and are not sustained with continued pain.

Any method used for adult pain relief can be adapted for children (Rice 1989) using a painless route. An exception is the rectal route, which is not advisable because absorption is slow and variable, it can be perceived as abusive by children, and there has been one known fatality (Gourlay and Boas 1992). Children benefit from TNS (Lander 1993), and patient controlled analgesia can be adapted for children from age four years. For younger children, 'parent-controlled' analgesia provides similar benefits. Nausea is common in children and may need treatment. Infants given opioids exhibit no more respiratory depression than older children (Nichols 1993). For ventilated children, of course, respiratory depression is not a concern.

Methods to reduce pain perception include:

- according to 99% of children, the presence of a parent (Broom 1990),
- information on what will occur and what it will feel like,
- distraction with toys, stroking, stories, games or television.

Postoperative management

After heart surgery, atelectasis may be more extensive than in adults. For optimum SaO_2, the atelectatic lung is theoretically better in the dependent position, but oxygen saturation varies (Polacek *et al* 1992).

Children like to be touched as little as possible after surgery. If coughing is necessary, they prefer to splint the incision themselves by leaning forwards with their arms crossed or hugging a teddy bear. Children

must not be discouraged from crying or told to be brave. If they are difficult, it is usually because they are frightened.

12.2   THE NEONATAL UNIT

12.2.1   Introduction

The emergence of the baby into the outside world is perhaps the most cataclysmic event of its life.
West 1994

Normal babies have undergone the trauma of birth and the complex transition from respiration via the placenta to gas exchange through the lung. Premature babies, who are in effect displaced fetuses, have the added shock of being delivered into a world against which they have limited defence mechanisms, and sometimes they are without a basic capacity for respiration, feeding or temperature control. The lower the gestational age, the more keenly sensitive they are to their environment. A neonatal unit (NNU) provides the technology and skill to care for sick babies, whether full term or premature. But it is not always the ideal emotional environment, with its bright lights, chorus of noises and frequent disturbances. Recognition of this has led to an acknowledgement that as well as the importance of saving life, there is the need to prevent physical, intellectual and emotional impairment.

Central to the baby's universe is his or her mother. Bonding between child and mother is hindered by the barrier of the incubator and the mother's reticence in disturbing equipment. Since the discovery that NNU 'graduates' run an above-average risk of suffering abuse in later life (Anon 1985), attention now focuses on facilitating attachment between parents and child in this vulnerable early period. Parents need to be involved in the care and comfort of their child, and the child needs to hear and feel his or her mother. Handling by health staff can destabilize preterm infants (Murphy 1991), but handling by the mother can reduce stress and oxygen consumption (Ludington 1990). Parents need to be encouraged but not pressurized into stroking and, if possible, holding their baby. Monitoring will indicate if handling is detrimental.

Babies are known as neonates for the first month of life, and neonates born before 37 weeks' gestation are considered preterm. Most of the untoward effects of the adult intensive care environment apply to neonates, amplified by the babies' limited understanding. The majority of babies in an NNU have respiratory problems, which may be abrupt and severe because of the differences in the respiratory system, as described below:

1. The immature respiratory centre causes irregular breathing patterns and occasional periods of apnoea.
2. For the first year of life the intercostal muscles are immature, the ribs cartilagenous and horizontal, and the rib cage nearly three times as compliant as the lung (Papastamelos 1995). The diaphragm does most of the work of breathing, despite containing fewer fatigue-resistant fibres and working at a disadvantage because of its horizontal rather than oblique angle of insertion. Work of breathing is two to three times that of adults (Hoffman 1995). By age two the rib cage and lung are equally compliant (Papastamelos 1995) and by age three or four, when more time is spent upright, rib cage configuration is oblique rather than horizontal.
3. The response to heavy work loads is an increased rate rather than increased depth of breathing.
4. Hypoxaemia tends to cause bradycardia rather than tachycardia. Immature myocardium has less capacity to increase stroke volume, and bradycardia often causes a fall in cardiac output.

5. Collateral ventilation is not established until age two or three, leaving the lungs vulnerable to atelectasis.
6. The peripheral airways are narrow and contribute up to 40% of total airways resistance from birth to about age five, leaving young children prone to obstructive diseases of the small airways such as bronchiolitis (James 1991).
7. Until the age of three, the right and left main bronchi diverge at equal angles from the trachea (Bush 1963).
8. Maturity of the surfactant system occurs at about 35 weeks' gestation, so that preterm infants are at extra risk of atelectasis.
9. Blood pressure regulation is less refined than in older children or adults.

Two previous assumptions about infants have now been questioned. It had been thought that they were obliged to breathe through their nose because of their large tongues occluding the oropharynx, but this has been discounted for most babies, although they are still preferential nose breathers (Sporik 1994). It had also been thought that infants were unable to respond to bronchodilators, but these drugs have now been proved effective, although response is varied and should be monitored (Holt 1995), and mucosal oedema may create more obstruction than bronchospasm.

12.2.2 Care of the parents

I longed as I have never longed for anything so badly, to hold her . . . to put her face against mine, whisper that I was here, that it was all right . . . I stroked her hand with my finger . . . and feeling her minute pink fingers holding so hard to mine, I was hit sideways and bowled over by the purest, tenderest, most passionately committed love I have ever felt . . .

I couldn't bear to . . . not be able to help her myself at all . . . It hurt me so much, to see her weak, in distress and apparently struggling so hard . . . I wanted to drag everything away from her, every bit of machinery, to pick her up and hold her to my breast, even if it meant that she died in a few minutes. That would be better than having her suffer this, the pain, fear, noise, bewilderment, being surrounded and handled by strangers . . .

Every time I touched her, she relaxed and the monitors showed it, her heart rate settled, her limbs were calmer, her eyes searched less frantically about . . .

I had never held her to me and I ached to do so, she seemed so alone in there amongst all the wires and drips and tubes and monitors.

Hill 1989

When working in a neonatal unit, we need some understanding of the powerful feelings between parent and infant.

12.2.3   Management of pain and stress

Inadequate pain control increases morbidity and mortality in infants (*Lancet* 1992). Premature neonates feel more pain than full-term infants (McIntosh *et al* 1993), immature neurons are particularly sensitive to damage (Tyler *et al* 1991), and repeated pain causes hypersensitivity to further pain (Barker 1995). The gut is more sensitive to stress-related disorders in children than in adults, and even more sensitive in infants (Ricour 1989).

Neonates exist in a precarious metabolic milieu, and disturbances such as loud voices, knocking the incubator or even rearranging a limb, can lead to bradycardia, disorganized breathing and hypoxia. Stress leads to tachycardia, hypertension, hypoxaemia and hypercapnia (Wessel 1993).

Dimmed lights at night allow sleeping and weight gain, and reduced noise decreases episodes of desaturation, crying and intracranial hypertension. Other beneficial influences are the mother's voice, a sheepskin to lie on and a soft blanket to nest in to reduce the insecurity of feeling exposed (Sparsholt 1989).

Stressed parents mean a stressed baby, and parents benefit from help to cuddle their

child when attached to awesome equipment, advice on baby massage, and a rocking chair and other comforts for them and their child. Rocking beds have also been advocated because of the beneficial effects on ventilation, feeding, crying and length of stay (Sammon 1994). Neonatal oxygen consumption is reduced by skin contact with the mother, hearing the mother's heartbeat and voice, and being held between the breasts (Ludington 1990). Visiting should be unrestricted and include grandparents and siblings (Johnstone 1994).

A team approach to this form of stress reduction results in a more stable cardiopulmonary system, with benefits lasting for months after discharge (Mann 1986).

12.2.4   Temperature and fluid regulation

The more immature the baby, the less efficient is heat conservation because of scant subcutaneous fat, fragile skin and a large surface area in relation to body mass. Up to 50% of calorie intake may be used for maintaining body temperature, a process which consumes oxygen. Warmth by overhead radiant heat allows easier access to the baby than an incubator, but promotes water loss. Dehydration or fluid overload are risky for the immature kidney.

12.2.5   Oxygen therapy

Supplemental oxygen is given via plastic head box or, for long-term use, nasal cannula or catheter (Coffman and McManus 1984). Hyperoxia can lead to retinopathy of prematurity (Greenough 1994). This is caused by excessive oxygen pressures reaching the retinal artery, leading to constriction, proliferation and fibrosis of the delicate retinal capillaries, causing blindness. It can also be caused, paradoxically, by hypoxia (Salyer 1991). Oximetry cannot detect hyperoxia, and SaO_2 should be kept between 87% and 92% in preterm infants to ensure that there is no hypoxia or hyperoxia. For babies on trans-cutaneous monitors, $PtcO_2$ should be kept between 6.7–10.7 kPa (50–80 mmHg) and $PtcCO_2$ between 5.3–7.3 kPa (40–55 mmHg).

12.2.6 Mechanical ventilation

If neither oxygen therapy nor CPAP maintain oxygenation, IPPV may be needed. Elaborate systems for endotracheal tube fixation are required to prevent such a heavy contraption becoming disconnected from such a tiny nose. Tracheal tubes are uncuffed, allowing a slight air leak and less risk of mucosal damage, especially as the subglottic area is the narrowest part of the child's airway and babies tend to move more than adults. Pressure-controlled ventilators are used for infants up to one year old, so that flow can increase automatically to compensate for the cuff leak, and high peak airway pressures can be avoided.

A quarter of ventilated babies develop some form of barotrauma such as pneumothorax (suspected if there is rapid deterioration without apparent cause) or pulmonary interstitial emphysema (PIE), which is identifiable as black-and-white streaks radiating from the hila which do not branch or taper towards the periphery, unlike vascular markings. The high compliance of the chest wall and low collagen and elastic content of lung tissue affords little protection against lung overdistension (Parker and Hernandez 1993), and the lungs are subjected to the alternating effects of positive pressure, which repeatedly stretches the more compliant regions, and lung deflation, which induces regional atelectasis of less compliant regions. Babies with RDS (p. 300) are particularly at risk of PIE because of their lack of surfactant, whereas those with more compliant lungs are more at risk of pneumothorax (Chatburn 1991). A pneumothorax is treated by chest tube drainage, but PIE is difficult to treat and often leads to lung damage, up to a third of ventilated low-birth-weight babies develop-

ing chronic lung disease of prematurity (Coghill *et al* 1991). These complications can be reduced by low tidal volume, high-frequency ventilation, negative pressure ventilation (Samuels and Southall 1989), ECMO or liquid ventilation (Chapter 9).

PEEP is generally used in all neonates at 2–5 cmH$_2$O, but is specifically required if PaO_2 is < 6.7 kPa (50 mmHg) with oxygen > 60% (Pilbeam 1992, p. 554). Weaning from IPPV is by gradual reduction in peak pressure, PEEP, inspired oxygen and/or I:E ratio.

Secretions in the endotracheal tube can double airflow resistance (Chatburn 1991), and shallow suction is indicated as required. Physiotherapy may be indicated after extubation if airway irritation has created excess secretions.

12.2.7 Advanced life support

Prolonged extracorporeal gas exchange and other life support systems are being used with increasing success as a rescue therapy for full-term infants with severe but reversible respiratory failure (Bower 1995). Bleeding may occur during suction.

12.3 PHYSIOTHERAPY FOR INFANTS

The main role of the physiotherapist is to judge if and when intervention is appropriate. Treatment itself may be carried out by the physiotherapist, specialist nurse or in part by the parent.

The maxim that routine treatment is taboo is never more apt than in the NNU. Infants should not, for example, be treated just because they are on a ventilator. The approach is to assess, identify the problem and balance up the benefits and risks of intervention.

12.3.1 Indications

Physiotherapy may be needed if there are excess secretions that cannot be cleared by suction alone, if there is poor gas exchange, increased work of breathing or radiological evidence of atelectasis. All babies need assessment, although not necessarily hands-on assessment. Intubated babies need a check on their humidifiers. Auscultation, oxygen saturation and liaison with their nurse on the quality of secretions will indicate whether their tracheal tubes may have become encrusted with secretions. Post-extubation physiotherapy may be indicated in case of thick secretions. Babies need assessment after surgery, and all neonates who have aspirated meconium need treatment unless contraindicated.

12.3.2   Precautions

Physiotherapy is contraindicated for babies who are hypothermic, show cardiac instability (unless this is due to hypoxia), have an undrained pneumothorax or are producing fresh blood-stained secretions.

Because of the poorly developed defences of neonates, all health workers should wash their hands meticulously and avoid the NNU if they have even a minor infection.

Treatment should be scheduled before feeds or at least one hour after feeds. If physiotherapy is essential within these times, the gastric contents should be aspirated by syringe before treatment and replaced afterwards.

Both infant and monitors should be observed before, during and after treatment. Casual handling should be avoided and physiotherapy sessions structured so that the infant is rested before and after treatment. Cumulative procedures or major disturbances such as suction can drop the PaO_2 by as much as 5.3 kPa (40 mmHg) (Speidel 1978).

If the infant is receiving phototherapy for treatment of jaundice, the light can be removed temporarily for physiotherapy, but the baby's protective eye shields must be replaced afterwards.

Vigilance is needed to avoid dislodging drips, drains or the tracheal tube.

Good teamwork is required to ensure periods of undisturbed sleep. Sleep fragmentation brings risks of hypoxaemia, hypertension and apnoea (Cole *et al* 1990).

12.3.3   Assessment

Notes, charts and reports give information on birth and other history, weight gain or loss (indicating general health), response to handling and suction, results of the last suction, mode and frequency of feeds and whether the baby has rested since the last intervention. A recent history of self-limiting bradycardia or periods of apnoea suggests that suction might be needed. Much reliance is placed on this information because of the limitations of clinical and subjective examination.

Monitors should be observed for baseline levels and for changes during treatment. Physiological distress shows as bradycardia (HR < 90 bpm), tachypnoea or apnoea. Worsening oxygenation may be a sign of accumulating secretions or infection.

Auscultation seems to pick up every sound in the unit except a baby's breath sounds. Rapid shallow breathing, or ventilator noise and other referred sounds, can thwart the listener. Wheezes and crackles may be picked up, but are often easier to feel than hear.

X-ray findings may indicate atelectasis or consolidation, with the right upper lobe needing special attention because of its tendency to collapse. Babies have a large thymus that looks similar to right upper lobe consolidation. The appearance of blebs suggests pulmonary interstitial emphysema and contraindicates bag-squeezing.

12.3.4   Methods to decrease the work of breathing

Work of breathing is increased by stress (Wessel 1993). Measures to reduce stress are the following:

- limit the total treatment time to between 10 seconds and 10 minutes, depending on the infant's response,
- talk to the infant as required (but not a continuous chatter),
- keep other sounds to a minimum to avoid risk of hearing loss (Cole *et al* 1990),
- minimize bright lights by keeping the incubator partially covered,
- avoid restraints unless essential (Sparsholt 1989),
- prevent unnecessary heat loss, especially from the head,
- avoid procedures that cause crying because this leads to irregular breathing, apnoeic episodes, increased pulmonary artery pressure and hypoxaemia (Murphy 1991).

Positioning is used both to decrease the work of breathing and increase lung volume, as described below.

12.3.5 Methods to increase lung volume

Positioning

For spontaneously breathing babies, raising the head of the mattress eases the load on the diaphragm, lessens the risk of gastro-oesophageal (GOR) and is especially important in prematurity.

Compared with supine, the prone position leads to ↓ heart rate, improved synchrony of breathing, ↑ SaO₂ by an average 25% (Hussey 1992), ↓ energy consumption, ↑ sleep, ↓ GOR and ↓ aspiration (Hallsworth, 1995). The head of the mattress should remain raised in this position. Extended time in prone may lead to a flattened frog position with abducted, flexed and externally rotated hips, but postural abnormalities can be prevented by raising the pelvis on a roll (Downs *et al* 1991).

At home, the prone position puts babies at greater risk of cot death than supine (Hallsworth 1995). This is not a problem in hospital under continuous monitoring, and parents

must be reassured of this, but before discharge there should be a gradual change to spending more time in supine.

The side-lying position allows greater diaphragmatic excursion than supine. If there is a pneumothorax or unilateral interstitial emphysema, side-lying with the affected lung dependent is preferable (Swingle *et al* 1984). When babies are in side-lying, they respond best when the trunk and limbs are supported in the flexed position.

Precautions to observe when positioning a neonate are to monitor the effects of handling, avoid dragging on the tracheal tube and check for any air leak around the tracheal tube after position change.

Manual hyperinflation

The younger the child, the less advisable it is to use bag-squeezing because of the risk of pneumothorax. Contraindications are similar to adults but with two additions:

- hyperinflation conditions, such as meconium aspiration and bronchiolitis,
- prematurity, unless bagging is essential, because the risk of pneumothorax is too great.

The indication for bag-squeezing is loss of lung volume that does not respond to positioning or clearance of a mucus plug. Suggested technique is as follows:

- use a 500 ml bag with an open end to vent excess pressure,
- incorporate a manometer in the circuit to check pressures (Howard-Glenn and Koniak-Griffin 1990),
- check the monitors,
- turn the oxygen flow rate to 4–6 l/min (but the gas flow to the infant is controlled manually),
- bag-squeeze using fingers rather than the whole hand, interspersing one hyperinflation with three or four tidal breaths,

- the pressure is controlled manually through the open end of the bag, the chest rising only slightly more than when attached to the ventilator,
- the manometer should indicate a rise in pressure of no more than 10 cmH$_2$O above the peak airway pressure for term babies, 5 cmH$_2$O for preterm babies,
- maintain some positive pressure at the end of expiration to mimic PEEP and prevent airway collapse,
- between watching the manometer and monitors, do not forget to observe the patient.

12.3.6   Methods to clear secretions

Postural drainage

Unstable preterm neonates who cannot tolerate handling should not have their position changed for treatment. Other babies can be treated in alternate side-lying. If the head-down tip is necessary, it should be combined with observation and monitoring because of the baby's reliance on diaphragmatic function.

Percussion and vibrations

Manual techniques are fruitful in infants because of the compliant rib cage. They are often necessary because of the narrow airways. Percussion is usually well tolerated and indeed soothing. It can be performed with a soft-rimmed face mask, using firm pressure directly on the skin and taking care to stay within the surface markings of the little lungs. Vibrations with the finger tips can be applied on every second or third expiration.

Contraindications are similar to adults, with extra caution for preterm babies and those at risk of intraventricular haemorrhage or rickets. Some neonates respond poorly, so monitors should, as always, be observed throughout.

Suction

Suction via nose or tracheal tube should only be done if necessary because it is a stressful experience for neonates and can cause bradycardia, arrhythmias, atelectasis, abrupt peaks in blood pressure and raised intracranial pressure (Durand *et al* 1989). Figure 12.2 shows how the blood pressure of a baby increased by 20 mmHg during endotracheal suction.

For non-intubated infants, positioning and percussion may shift secretions so that they are swallowed. If not, suction may be necessary. The technique described on p. 140 and p. 289 is modified by the following:

- have the baby in side-lying and wrapped up comfortably but firmly,
- for preterm infants, preoxygenate by no more than 10% to avoid retinopathy of prematurity (Parker 1993),
- set the vacuum pressure (p. 289),
- use a size 6 FG catheter,
- lubricate the tip with water-soluble jelly or the baby's saliva,
- upper airway suction is usually sufficient to stimulate a cough, and passing the catheter further is considered unsafe (Kleiber *et al* 1988),
- ensure that the suction time does not exceed five seconds,
- suction the nostrils afterwards because of preferential nose-breathing.
- invite the parent to cuddle the baby afterwards.

Tracheal suction for ventilated infants is required if recent history suggests that suction is productive, or if monitors indicate hypoxaemia. It may not be possible to feel or auscultate for the presence of secretions.

Modifications to the above protocol are the following:

1. Lubrication is not necessary.
2. Avoid suction if the baby's temperature is below 36°C.

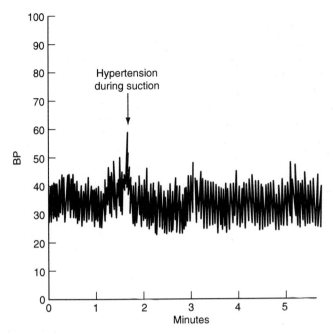

Figure 12.2 Hypertension in an infant during suction. (Source: McIntosh, N. (1989) MARY – a computerised neonatal monitoring system. *Int. Care Clin. Monit.*, **10**, 272–82, with permission.)

3. Liaise with medical staff about the advisability of predosing with a drug to blunt the stress response (Hickey *et al* 1985).

4. Observe the monitors.

5. Preoxygenate by increasing the ventilator oxygen by 10%.

6. Avoid impinging the catheter on the carina or allowing deep suction, which causes extra damage (Hodge 1991). The catheter should not advance more than 1 cm beyond the end of the tracheal tube, and its length can be checked against the length of an equivalent-sized ETT, or a calibrated catheter (Fig. 5.12(f)) can be used (Kleiber *et al* 1988).

7. Ensure the catheter diameter is less than half the diameter of the airway:

   5 FG for ETT size 2.5 mm
   6 FG for ETT size 3 mm
   8 FG for ETT size 3.5 mm (Bertone, 1988)

8. Observe the monitors and check for signs of decreased cardiac output or shock (pallor or cyanosis, sweating, decreased peripheral temperature), which mean that suction is contraindicated.

9. For postoperative infants, ensure that someone supports the wound.

10. Draw up normal saline into a 1 ml syringe, disconnect the infant from the ventilator, instil saline down the tracheal tube (0.5 ml for preterm neonates, 1–3 ml for term babies), reconnect for a few breaths, then disconnect and suction. If hypoxaemia is not a problem, an alternative technique is to inject the saline into an unconnected suction catheter until the catheter is filled with a drip visible at the other end, insert the catheter into the tracheal tube, plunge the syringe to instil saline directly to the distal end of the tracheal tube, then withdraw saline, along with some of the

mucus, using the syringe. The catheter is then disconnected from the syringe, connected to the suction circuit and suction applied in the normal way (Downs 1989). This is thought to provide more accurate saline delivery to the area of potentially encrusted secretions.

11. After reconnection to the ventilator, suction the mouth and nostrils.

12. When SaO_2 has returned to baseline, turn the ventilator F_1O_2 back to its previous value slowly. If the oximeter or other monitors do not show that values have returned to baseline, or the child does not settle, further suction may be indicated.

Caution should be observed after extubation, because suction-induced bronchospasm may add to the effects of mucosal oedema and cause obstruction.

12.4. MODIFICATIONS FOR SPECIFIC NEONATAL DISORDERS

12.4.1 Respiratory distress syndrome (RDS)

RDS, also known as hyaline membrane disease, occurs in immature lungs. It is characterized by lack of surfactant, leading to patchy atelectasis, stiff lungs and increased work of breathing. Alveoli inflate with difficulty and collapse between respiratory efforts.

Signs of respiratory distress develop over the first few hours of life, and auscultation shows reduced breath sounds and occasional fine crackles. The radiograph shows a hyperinflated chest with diffuse mottling and air bronchograms, indicating areas of atelectasis. Distress persists for 24–48 hours, then the condition either stabilizes and improves over several days as surfactant is produced, or the disease is protracted and severe. Mortality is 50%, with little morbidity in survivors (Heulitt 1995).

Prevention is by prophylactic instillation of artificial surfactant on delivery of preterm babies, administered in boluses in different positions rather than infused continuously (Ueda 1994). Management is by regulation of temperature, fluid and nutrition, inhaled nitric oxide (Abman 1994) and respiratory support using oxygen, CPAP or IPPV. Normal ventilation pressures for infants are 15–20 cmH$_2$O, but those with RDS require 20–40 cmH$_2$O.

Physiotherapy is limited to advice on positioning in the early stages, because anything more energetic is unnecessary and can be destabilizing. Intubation may irritate the airways and cause excess secretions, in which case the debris needs to be cleared in the recovery phase when the infant is stable, usually with suction but occasionally also with percussion.

12.4.2 Meconium aspiration

Full term babies who suffer asphyxia during prolonged labour may respond by passing meconium (faecal material) before birth and then making gasping movements and sucking it into their mouth. It stays safely there until delivery, but emergence of the chest causes any material that is in the mouth to be drawn deep into the lungs. This results in aspiration which causes acute obstruction of small airways and hyperinflation. The sticky meconium sets up a chemical pneumonitis and provides an ideal medium for infection.

If labour is prolonged or monitoring suggests that the baby is in distress, suction at birth before delivery of the thorax minimizes the risk. If aspiration has occurred. IPPV should be witheld until the airways have been cleared so that particulate material is not forced into distal airways. The lungs are difficult to ventilate because they behave as if full of treacle. Immediate and intensive physiotherapy is needed in the form of postural drainage, percussion, vibrations and suction, until secretions are free from the dark colour of meconium. Treatment is continued until the airways are clear so that secondary infection is prevented. Nurses should be taught this technique unless physiotherapy is available straight after birth.

12.4.3 Intraventricular haemorrhage

Bleeding into the cerebral ventricles may occur in the first week of premature life, when swings in BP or blood gases can cause the fragile capillaries in the ventricles to burst. Precipitating factors are suction, endotracheal obstruction or intubation without sedation (Wren 1989). Small haemorrhages are asymptomatic, but massive bleeding causes cerebral damage. The head-down tip is contraindicated if this condition is diagnosed.

12.4.4 Pneumonia

Pneumonia is relatively uncommon in neonates. The pathology is similar to pneumonia in adults, but the clinical course is more acute and ventilator assistance may be needed. Clinical features are a respiratory rate > 60, chest indrawing and an X-ray similar to RDS. Physiotherapy may be indicated in the later clearing-up stages.

12.4.5 Chronic lung disease of prematurity

Premature infants who receive prolonged mechanical ventilation may develop chronic lung disease of prematurity, also known as bronchopulmonary dysplasia (BPD). This is a form of barotrauma resulting from high-volume, high-oxygen ventilation, and is considered to be present if there is oxygen dependency for more than 28 days following IPPV in the first weeks of life (Hess 1991). Inflammation, opportunistic infection and exudation of fluids and protein flourish, leading to varying amounts of scarring and disordered growth. Signs are persistent respiratory distress, high oxygen requirements, pulmonary interstitial oedema, pulmonary hypertension and radiological evidence of cyst formation and ill-defined opacification.

Prevention is by strict attention to ventilator management in order to minimize inflation pressures (Greenough 1990), or the use of CPAP to reduce F_IO_2. Treatment is by diuretics, bronchodilators and, ironically, increasing levels of oxygen and higher inflation pressures as the disorder progresses. The child may need long-term hospitalization.

Physiotherapy is indicated if secretions are present because pulmonary defence is disrupted and the lungs are prone to recurrent atelectasis and infection. However, it may be contraindicated if the child is wheezy or has pulmonary hypertension. If necessary, it is best carried out after bronchodilators and stopped if wheezing is precipitated. Percussion in alternate side-lying and sometimes suction can be given, with extra attention to the upper lobes. This may be needed after discharge, either directly or through parent education. After long hospitalization, parents need comprehensive preparation for discharge so that they build up confidence and do not feel that they have just 'borrowed' their baby from hospital to take home. Domiciliary oxygen, BiPAP or nasal ventilation may be required (Teague 1995).

About 30% of infants with BPD die, but if infections are prevented, the lungs repair as they grow. Survivors may have neurological problems, are at risk of cot death and are thought to carry airways obstruction and bronchial hyperreactivity into adulthood (Hess 1991).

12.5 EMERGENCIES IN THE NEONATAL UNIT

12.5.1 Sudden hypoxaemia

If oximetry is not available, bradycardia may be the first sign of hypoxaemia, especially if the infant is fighting the ventilator. Bagging with gentle pressure should be carried out until the cause is found. A sudden disturbance in blood gases could mean a displaced or blocked tracheal tube (no change in CVP), or barotrauma (increased CVP).

12.5.2   Apnoeic attacks

Neonates who stop breathing can usually be revived by skin stimulation. If unsuccessful, intubation may be needed.

12.5.3   Pneumothorax

Any sudden deterioration in the condition of a ventilated infant raises suspicions of barotrauma. A pneumothorax is evident on X-ray, but clinical signs can be elusive. Breath sounds may still be present because sound is easily transmitted through the small chest from the unaffected lung. A tension pneumothorax causes bradycardia and a plunge in cardiac output.

12.5.4   Cardiorespiratory arrest

Most cardiorespiratory arrests in infants and children are of respiratory origin. Establishing a patent airway by head positioning may prevent progress of the event. Care should be taken to avoid pressing on the soft tissues under the chin or overextending the neck because this may occlude the trachea.

If an oral airway is required, it is not turned upside down for insertion, as in the adult. In the NNU, oxygen by bag and mask is usually available, but if mouth-to-mouth breathing is necessary, both mouth and nose should be covered with the rescuer's mouth and gentle puffs given.

If artificial ventilation does not restore the heart beat, chest compression is started by encircling the chest with both hands and squeezing the mid-sternum to a depth of 2 cm, with the thumbs one finger's breadth below an imaginary line joining the nipples, and ensuring that the chest fully re-expands between compressions. The ratio of breaths to compressions is 1:5 in infants and children, repeated 20 times per minute. The easiest pulse to locate is the brachial pulse on the inside of the upper arm (Zideman 1994).

RECOMMENDED READING

Downs, J. and Parker, A. (1991) Chest physiotherapy for preterm infants. *Paed. Nurs*, **3**(2), 14–17.

Gillespie, D. (1989) Let's listen to the children. *Respir. Dis. Pract.*, **6**(5), 23.

Howard, F. (1994) Endotracheal suctioning and the neonate. *Paediatr. Nurs.*, **6**(7), 14–17.

James, I. (1991) Respiratory management in paediatrics. *Care Crit. Ill.*, **7**, 47–50.

Hall, S.J. (1995) Paediatric pain assessment in intensive care units. *Int. Crit. Care Nurs.*, **1**, 20–5.

LaMontagne, L.L. and Pawlak, R. (1990) Stress and coping of parents of children in a pediatric ICU. *Heart Lung*, **19**, 416–21.

Parker, A. (1993) Paediatrics, in *Physiotherapy for Respiratory and Cardiac Problems* (eds B.A. Webber and J.A. Pryor), Churchill Livingstone, Edinburgh.

Ratcliffe, J.M. (1994) Sedation in the ICU. *Curr. Paeds.*, **4**, 106–9.

Rau, J.L. (1991) Delivery of aerosolized drugs to neonatal and pediatric patients. *Respir. Care*, **36**, 514–40.

Rees, J. and Price, J. (1995) Asthma in children: treatment. *Br. Med. J.*, **310**, 1522–4.

Russell, R.I.R. (1993) Complications of mechanical ventilation in children. *Paed. Resp. Med.*, **1**, 17–20.

Shield, J.P.H. and Baum, J.D. (1994) Children's consent to treatment. *Br. Med. J.*, **308**, 1182–3.

13. Evaluation of chest physiotherapy

13.1 INTRODUCTION

Respiratory therapy is one of those technical orphans that grew up eluding the cold eye of scientific enquiry.

Hughes 1980

If a patient who is receiving physiotherapy gets better, is this due to the physiotherapy, the physiotherapist or divine intervention? The credibility of physiotherapy in respiratory care is being much challenged in the pages of learned journals and on the shop-floor. This we must welcome.

Busy clinicians have resisted evaluation in the past with the comment that 'treatment of patients comes first'. This has now been replaced by 'effective treatment of patients comes first'. Practice and evaluation are not in competition. Indeed, practice without evaluation should be unthinkable; it would lead to tunnel vision and a misapplied concept of clinical experience, i.e. 'we always do it this way because we've always done it this way'. Experience is a tool to be nurtured mindfully, not used for anecdotal justification. Our finest clinicians should analyse their intuitive process so that they can pass on to others how they recognize subtle changes in a breathing pattern, modify the pressure of their hands, sense a patient's motivation or adjust their treatment in response to barely-perceptible clues.

Progress is inhibited by attitudes such as that quoted by Stiller and Munday (1992):

'Some may question the need for studies, given the generally accepted and extensive use of chest physiotherapy.' Other obstacles are:

- the ease of routine, of this routine becoming automatic, then enshrined in tablets of stone,
- difficulty in accepting that years of using a certain technique have been invalid,
- a perceived threat, e.g. one study showed that it was not detrimental to reduce the amount of respiratory care given to patients (Zibrak *et al* 1986),
- lack of a definition of respiratory physiotherapy.

But thankfully we now resist being prescribed like a drug. We evaluate the patient's need rather than what we imagine other staff expect from us, and no longer do we feel obliged to make a hearty clapping noise from behind the patient's curtain in order to convince others that we have 'done' something.

Evaluation is notoriously difficult because literature is scarce and ambiguous, and respiratory physiotherapy is replete with variables such as simultaneous medical input and the placebo effect. The placebo effect is interwoven with respiratory care because of the close connection between breathing and feelings. Indeed, the physiotherapist's attitude can provide a powerful and useful placebo.

Preliminary steps in evaluation are:

- to clarify the definition of respiratory physiotherapy to include the full spectrum of respiratory care, including education, not just passive sputum clearance,
- to build into treatment plans a system of continuous evaluation so that it does not become a luxury to be tagged on at the end if there is time,
- to ensure that goals are directed towards patients' needs.

Only about 15% of all contemporary clinical interventions are supported by objective scientific evidence that they do more good than harm.

White 1988

13.2   STANDARDS

The perception is, if chest physiotherapy doesn't help, it won't hurt.

Eid 1991

Evaluation needs standards against which outcome can be measured. Standards must be measurable, understandable, desirable and achievable. Minimum acceptable standards of practice aim to be acceptable to the patient and all grades of clinician. Quality assurance is not a specialist matter.

Standards include both the resources related to input and the process related to output, but should not get bogged down in examining just facilities and the environment, which are easy to agree and measure. It is also best that they are not imposed from above because staff are motivated by setting their own standards. Some suggestions follow.

13.2.1   Personal standards

1. All surgical patients will be seen who are having chest surgery, upper abdominal surgery, head-and-neck surgery, mastectomy or any surgery if they are high-risk.

2. Physiotherapists will introduce themselves, explain the purpose of their visit, and the expected outcome and limitations of treatment.

3. Plans and goals will be agreed between patient and physiotherapist. Any changes will be discussed as they arise.

4. Informed consent to treatment will be obtained.

5. Curtains will be used, and the patient's privacy, dignity and identity will be respected.

6. Permission will be asked before first touching the patient, or if talking to another person over the patient during treatment.

7. Patients will be assessed before, after, and, if appropriate, during each treatment.

8. Unnecessary pain will be avoided.

9. Unnecessary treatment will be avoided.

10. Preventive measures, education and self-management will be incorporated into all treatments as appropriate.

11. Hands will be washed between patients.

12. Children will be allowed to have their parents with them throughout treatment.

13. Confidentiality will be respected.

14. Discharged patients in need of further treatment or assessment will be referred as appropriate.

15. Inpatients will be assessed for treatment within 24 hours, immediately if urgent.

16. Outpatients will be seen within two weeks, within 24 hours if urgent.

17. Liaison with the multidisciplinary team will include:
    (a) attendance at relevant case conferences, ward rounds and meetings,
    (b) communication with referring doctors by phone calls, reports and visits,
    (c) regular contact with the respiratory nurse, occupational therapist, social worker and/or other team members,

(d) respiratory teaching sessions on the wards.

13.2.2 Departmental standards

1. Education for the respiratory team will comprise:
   (a) one teaching session per week,
   (b) supervision of one hour per week for each team member,
   (c) journal club once a month,
   (d) one project per rotation each,
   (e) one case presentation per month each,
   (f) suitable respiratory courses to be attended by one team member and information shared.
2. Students will be in contact with, or know how to contact, their supervisor at all times.
3. New staff will not do on-call duty until objectively and subjectively prepared.
4. Twenty-four-hour on-call cover will be provided.

13.3 AUDIT

Research determines good practice and audit determines how well this practice is carried out. Clinical audit is the systematic analysis by peers of each other's standards to determine the outcome and quality of life for the patient (DoH 1994). It educates, identifies gaps between expected and actual objectives, and dispels myths. It can be perceived as threatening by some, but suspicions are mitigated if it is voluntary, confidential, without sanctions and if all staff are involved in its development.

The following is a typical arrangement:

1. Set up the appropriate format in a department or special interest group, with arrangements to meet every six to eight weeks.
2. Define standards.
3. Choose the topic to be measured and the method of measurement.
4. Randomly select physiotherapy notes from the designated caseload.
5. Analyse the notes to compare actual practice with standards.
6. Discuss with and encourage the audited physiotherapist.
7. Recommend change if required.
8. Share information with others.
9. Rotate auditors so that all staff can audit and be audited.
10. Monitor change.

The topic chosen should be simple, e.g.:

- percentage of problems resolved,
- percentage of patients receiving discharge advice,
- percentage of call-outs that are considered appropriate,
- percentage of surgical patients discharged with full function four days post-operatively,
- percentage of objectives achieved by juniors on rotation.

Methods of measurement can be chosen from Chapter 2, or a questionnaire used to evalaute the patient's viewpoint. Other areas to be looked at include teamwork, on-calls and time management. Other methods include discussing videos of treatment sessions.

13.4 SELF-ASSESSMENT

We are the most available and abiding judges of our own work. For example:

- am I allowing myself to get swamped with acute respiratory work and unable to tackle prevention or rehabilitation?
- do I favour patients who are appreciative and co-operative, while neglecting those who are demanding or depressed?
- have I achieved the appropriate balance between patients' needs and my professional development?
- am I aware of my reactions to the intensive care environment, or blocking my feelings and becoming insensitive?

- am I continuing to learn?
- how do I handle my mistakes?

Self-assessment is enhanced by a work diary to clarify time management and work pattern, regular appraisal interviews with a trained supervisor and the setting of aims and objectives to include both opportunities and duties.

Intellect and experience should be accompanied by wisdom, and reflection should become embedded in practice in order to bridge the theory–practice gap (Driscoll 1994).

By analysing our decisions, hunches are converted into conscious deliberation of what is a complex selection of choices. How did we identify the patient's problem? Why did we choose incentive spirometry? How did we decide on the intensity of treatment, progression, or patient involvement? A decision tree (Watts 1985) or decision diagram (Horseman 1989) helps to work through a selection of choices.

Clinical judgment is both art and science. Evaluation and treatment occur almost simultaneously as we link our performance to that of the patient (Watts 1985). It is this process that needs to be harnessed. Without analysis, experience leads to imprecision and ritual. Decision analysis may well validate what we already do, but without it we run the risk of trying to solve problems before knowing what they are.

13.5 OUTCOME EVALUATION

The reference point for evaluation is the outcome of treatment. Does it work, and at what cost? What would happen if we were not here?

Subjective evaluation is by listening to the patient and using a questionnaire. Objective evaluation is by a selection of the methods used to assess patients

13.5.1 Patient questionnaire

What are patients' expectations? Are we fulfilling their needs or ours? Have we helped them towards independence? A patient questionnaire can be filled out before discharge, in which case completion is ensured, or it can be sent by post, in which case there may be less of the bias that gratitude exerts on the patient's response. Anonymity should be guaranteed. Visual analogue scales or open boxes can be used for the patient's response. Examples of questions are the following:

1. Was the greeting and information given during your first treatment: poor/fair/good/excellent?
2. Were you invited to make decisions about your treatment: never/sometimes/often?
3. If you had pain/breathlessness, did the treatment make it: worse/unchanged/better?
4. Were you granted respect and privacy: never/sometimes/always?
5. Do you feel that you yourself are now able to deal with your problem: no better/slightly better/very much better?

General questionnaires or specific questionnaires for patients with COPD (p. 151) or asthma (Hyland 1991) can be developed.

13.5.2 Outcome measures

Obstacles to measuring outcome include the following:

- SaO_2 depends on factors other than physiotherapy,
- treatment may reduce peripheral airway obstruction with little effect on SaO_2 (Menkes and Britt 1980).
- natural histories are variable,
- postoperative atelectasis may be self-limiting,
- quality of treatment cannot be assessed from the number and length of treatments,
- patients and other members of the health team may be reduced by mechanical aids that make exotic noises,

- patients with chronic respiratory disease are notoriously vulnerable to suggestion,
- mouthpieces and other methods to study breathing objectively interfere with what they are trying to measure,
- respiratory disease is often complicated by multipathology.

However, several measurements are valid if taken in the context of the full clinical picture:

- increase or maintenance of lung volume, e.g. clearer breath sounds or chest X-ray,
- ↓ work of breathing, e.g. less breathlessness or fatigue,
- clearance of secretions in greater quantity or more easily than before treatment,
- ↑ oxygenation, i.e. ↑ PaO_2, SaO_2 or $S\bar{v}O_2$,
- ↑ ventilation, i.e. ↓ $PaCO_2$,
- improved breathing pattern, e.g. greater depth of breathing or reduced paradoxical breathing,
- ↑ or maintenance of exercise tolerance, e.g. shuttle test or functional activities,
- ↓ pain,
- greater acceptance and improved management of disability,
- ↑ independence or well-being,
- lack of deterioration.

A selection of these criteria can be documented or tabulated to assess effectiveness and analyse trends.

13.6 LITERATURE CRITICISM

Why do kamikaze pilots wear helmets?

A questioning and indeed a suspicious mind is essential when reading articles because research can prove or disprove almost anything, and even the most prestigious journals publish articles based on false premises, poor design and with inaccurate conclusions. Many researchers are biased towards proving their own techniques or ideas, and it is advisable not just to evaluate the studies critically, but to relate them to the physiology.

Beware of literature that contains:

- unreferenced statements of 'fact',
- assessment of more than one modality, thereby assessing none,
- no distinction between correlation and causation,
- jargon,
- extrapolation of results from healthy young volunteers to people who are ill, e.g. oxygen toxicity, 'addiction' to analgesia, using CPAP on normals to simulate hyperinflation,
- variables not stringently controlled, thus masking the effect of an independent variable,
- physiotherapists used simply as agents to collect data, not as designers of the study,
- conclusions which state that 'chest physiotherapy was of no value', instead of the inelegant but more accurate: 'postural drainage with percussion in this way for this amount of time for these patients showed no evidence of effectiveness by these criteria'.
- assuming that studies on animals necessarily extrapolate to humans, e.g. dogs have a different chest shape and their pleural space communicates bilaterally unlike humans.

Other pitfalls are illustrated by the following examples.

1. Connors *et al* (1980) showed that postural drainage (PD) and percussion caused hypoxaemia in patients with little or no sputum. But (a) a mixture of pathologies was used including pulmonary oedema, and (b) suction was included in an unspecified number of patients. And why, we might also ponder politely, were PD and percussion used for patients with little or no sputum?

2. An oft-quoted study by Boeck and Zinman (1984) stated that chest physiotherapy offered no benefit over cough alone for cystic fibrosis patients,

but chest physiotherapy consisted of PD for two minutes in each position, which is unlikely to shift the tenacious secretions of these patients.

3. Newton and Stephenson (1978) confined their description of physiotherapy to three lines of text and failed to define 'breathing exercises'.

4. Medical journals are laden with revelations that 'physiotherapy' does not help acute pneumonia, but a passing acquaintance with the pathology of pneumonia would indicate that this form of treatment is unlikely to influence a lung that is solid with consolidation. It does not fit the physiology so why test it? Britton *et al* (1985) reached this familiar conclusion by comparing advice on deep breathing and expectoration with 'physiotherapy', which did not include these but incorporated undefined 'external help with breathing'. Poelaert *et al* (1991) reached a similar conclusion and added the intriguing but unreferenced assertion that percussion, vibration and PD can cause barotrauma.

5. Laws and McIntyre (1969) found that cardiac output and $\dot{V}O_2$ were adversely affected by treatments in which patients 'actively resisted hyperinflation and found the procedure extremely unpleasant'. Perhaps these adverse effects were caused by hurting the patients, rather than the treatment itself.

6. If techniques with different aims are compared, is it surprising that they have different outcomes? (a) Nosworthy *et al* (1992) announced that exercise performance improved with leg muscle training but not with PD or inspiratory muscle training. (b) Mulholland *et al* (1994) found that twice daily prone positioning produced less sputum than three times daily 'physiotherapy' consisting of nebulized bronchodilators, PD, ACBT, percussion and vibrations. Also not surprising is that prone produced a greater improvement

in SaO_2 than during 'physiotherapy', especially as SaO^2 should be taken after 30 minutes rest, not during the treatment being evaluated.

7. Ciesla (1994) justified percussion over rib fractures, even though there was no statistically significant improvement in outcome, commenting that it caused less pain than coughing. She concluded that 'the use of percussion over rib fractures remains controversial', although it is difficult to see what is controversial about a technique that hurts patients without benefitting them. Just don't do it.

8. MacKenzie and Shin (1985) subjected their ICU patients to over an hour of PD, percussion, vibration and suctioning, but the significance of this ordeal was questionable because the long-term clinical effect was unknown. Needless to say, the effect on their hapless patients with lung contusion was deleterious.

9. Torrington *et al* (1984) imposed four-hourly IPPB, four-hourly incentive spirometry, two-hourly deep breathing and two-hourly nebulization on obese postoperative patients, then expressed surprise that additional four-hourly PD and percussion increased discomfort, fever and cost, without reducing atelectasis.

10. Shapiro *et al* (1992) produced a classic example of a global generalization when they said that 'inspiratory muscle rest confers no benefit' when patients using negative-pressure apparatus were mostly too uncomfortable in their body suits to sleep.

11. Wollmer *et al* (1985) used supine as their PD position, defined coughing as huffing, and concluded that 'chest percussion should not be used uncritically in patients with . . . low to moderate sputum production', implying (a) that there might be logic in percussing patients with little sputum, and (b) that

it could be used uncritically in other patients.

12. Ng and Stokes (1992) attempted to evaluate respiratory muscle activity during 'unilateral' chest expansion, but did not distinguish inspiratory and expiratory muscles, used 'subjective observation' to judge this notoriously ambiguous manoeuvre, and did not explain the physiology or implications in relation to aeration of the lung.

13. King and Morrell (1992) quoted references relating to ARDS patients and extrapolated them by inference to normal patients, thus giving unrealistically low levels for safe bag-squeezing pressures.

14. Emotive language and dogmatic statements raise suspicions. Christensen *et al* (1990) concluded that 'the widely indiscriminate use of PEEP-masks is without any clinical documentation and therefore cannot be recommended in patients with irreversible COPD'. Incidentally, 'irreversible' was defined as FEV_1 of about 1 l.

15. Weissman *et al* (1984) did not define chest physical therapy in a paper associating it with major haemodynamic and metabolic stress.

16. Eales *et al* (1991) used IPPB for patients with pulmonary emboli, used it in the standing position, and expressed surprise that it was no better than deep breathing.

17. The temptation to use a plethora of treatments seems to overwhelm some researchers. Alison *et al* (1994) described an uncontrolled trial in which people with an exacerbation of CF benefitted from 'rest, intravenous antibiotics, physical therapy, high-calorie diet and regular medical review'. Maybe it was just the rest, maybe the so-called medical review, maybe none was beneficial because exacerbations usually get better.

18. Logic-defying attempts to prove that treatments that could not help do not

help continue to flood the journals. Eales *et al* (1995) announced that manual hyperinflation, vibrations and suction did not help in the 'supine position with the head and trunk elevated 20° off horizontal'. This position was chosen because it was 'routine'.

13.7   RESEARCH

All who drink of this remedy recover in a short time, except those whom it does not help, who all die. Therefore it is obvious that it fails only in incurable cases.

Galen, second century AD

Research is not mystical. It is about common sense. It enriches as well as validates our work and should be integrated into all levels of practice. To maintain credibility we must not leave it to the medical profession and we must take responsibility for putting the results into practice.

Transferring the rigours of traditional research into a bustling clinical setting is not easy, but there are methods that are responsive to the realities of the bedside:

1. **Case study presentation** involves sharing with others an example of patient management, with interpretation and discussion.

2. **Descriptive research** combines description of a certain patient population, discussion of physiotherapy management and presentation of the associated literature.

3. **Single case study research** is a quantitative approach in which treatment periods are alternated with non-treatment periods. Patients act as their own controls and a large homogeneous group of patients is not needed (Sim 1995).

4. **Pilot studies** are required for more ambitious projects in order to refine methodology and uncover potential flaws.

5. **Controlled trials** include a group of subjects who do not receive the treatment under investigation to ensure that

the outcome is attributable to what is being investigated.

6. **Randomized controlled trials** allocate subjects randomly so that certain characteristics are unlikely to be over-represented in any group.
7. **Blind trials** keep subjects in the dark about which side of the study they are participating in, so that the placebo effect is minimized.
8. **Double-blind trails** prevent investigators knowing the subjects' allocation.
9. **Meta-analysis** combines results from different studies on the same question into 'master results' (Jones 1994).

Commonly encountered obstacles are:

- lack of defined categorization in physiotherapy compared with medicine,
- statistical significance not necessarily representing clinical significance,
- unfamiliarity with the research process,
- shortage of time, money or support,
- anxiety about ethics.

The ethical question 'What right do I have to withhold treatment from some patients?' is offset by 'What right do I have to give treatment that has not been proved effective?'.

There are no known facts, only the present theory of the day.
Howell quoted by Conway 1992a

13.8   CONTINUING EDUCATION

Sometimes learning requires courage. To become a learner is to become vulnerable.
Berwick 1991

Updating knowledge requires structured planning and the fostering of a non-judgemental atmosphere in which staff feel free to discuss uncertainties about their work. Lack of this freedom leads to routine treatment. Physiotherapists are now expected to update themselves continually. As Alfred North Whitehead said in 1933, 'knowledge keeps no better than fish'.

Students and junior staff require the following:

- a balance of guidance and responsibility,
- clarification of expectations on both sides,
- feedback,
- assistance in setting feasible objectives and assessing whether these are met,
- praise when due,
- encouragement to work creatively and not become a clone of their seniors,
- correction in a way that does not undermine their confidence or belittle them in front of patients,
- space for reflection,
- enjoyment in their work.

Senior students expect to be asked how closely they want to be supervised (Onuoha 1994).

Seniors have the privilege and opportunity to inspire as well as educate, and indeed it is their human qualities that are often considered of equal or more importance than their clinical skills (Neville and French 1991). Learning through role modelling takes place through:

- enthusiasm, honesty and commitment,
- willingness to say 'I don't know',
- self-evaluation,
- respect for juniors so that they in turn respect their patients,
- setting priorities,
- toleration of a wide range of normality,
- use of language, e.g. 'this person with COPD', rather than 'this chronny bronny',
- avoidance of labelling patients as difficult or not liked,
- coaxing the nervous patient, soothing the fearful, encouraging the weary,
- constructive relationships with medical and other staff.

Communication skills and empathy are not incompatible with technical competence. Both need to be learnt, not left for uncertain assimilation. Sensitivity should be developed rather then blunted, e.g. by discussing a ward round in which a patient's needs are ignored, rather than accepting this behaviour as normal.

It is common to become inured to the distress of patients by prolonged exposure, and easy to forget the reactions of young staff or students when fresh to the intensive care unit: 'What can the patients be feeling? Why are ICU staff not upset at working closely with such ill people? Whence this light-heartedness?' Seniors need to maintain awareness of these reactions lest juniors feel obliged to conform.

Case presentations and a journal club can be enjoyable methods to update ideas and evaluate practice. New staff may need help in selecting articles from respiratory journals and analysing their contents. A file of articles written by patients can be compiled (e.g. Appendix D).

Continuing education lays the foundation for lifelong self-evaluation. It incorporates the opportunity to show that compassion is fundamental to effective respiratory care, not an old-fashioned, unscientific luxury reserved for the naïve and uninitiated.

RECOMMENDED READING

Barnard, S. (1995) Models for intervention audit. *Physiotherapy*, **81**, 202–7.
Hartigan, G. (1995) Choosing a method for clinical audit. *Physiotherapy*, **81**, 187–8.

Glossary of definitions, abbreviations, symbols and normal values

See also index for definitions in the text.
Values in [square brackets] are from the USA
(all values are approximate).

2,3-DPG Enzyme in red blood cells, ↑ in chronic hypoxaemia, shifting O_2 dissociation curve to right and allowing easier unloading of O_2 to hypoxic tissues.

A Alveolar, e.g. P_AO_2.

a Arterial, e.g. PaO_2.

ACBT Active cycle of breathing techniques.

ACE inhibitors Angiotensin-converting enzyme inhibiter drugs, for hypertension, e.g. captopril, enalapril.

ACPRC Association of Chartered Physiotherapists in Respiratory Care.

ADL Activities of daily living.

Adult respiratory distress syndrome Alternative name for acute respiratory distress syndrome.

Aerosol Suspension of particles in a gas stream. Therapeutic aerosols are for humidification and drug delivery, other aerosols spread some lung infections and allow damage from noxious agents.

AIDS Acquired immune deficiency syndrome.

Air trapping Retention of inspired gas in poorly ventilated areas of lung.

Airway closure Closure of small airways, mostly in dependent lung regions during expiration.

Airway resistance Normal: 0.5–2.0 cmH$_2$O/l/sec.

Albumin Plasma protein responsible for providing most osmotic pressure in blood.
Normal: 40–60 g/l, [4.0–6.0 g/100ml].
↓ albumin suggests malnutrition, blood loss, liver failure, nephrotic syndrome.

Anaerobic threshold Highest oxygen consumption during exercise, above which sustained lactic acidosis occurs. Normally a useful measure of aerobic capacity for monitoring endurance training, but of limited value in severe COPD because peak exercise levels are often reached below the anaerobic threshold. In normal subjects, anaerobic threshold can be increased by 25–40%.

Angioplasty Invasive but non-surgical dilatation of coronary artery stenosis, using catheter via femoral puncture, or laser.

Anoxia Synonymous with hypoxia, although implying a more complete oxygen lack.

AP Anteroposterior.

APACHE Acute Physiology And Chronic Health Evaluation (scoring system to measure severity of illness).

Apgar score Combined measurement of heart rate, respiratory effort, muscle tone, reflex irritability and colour (scoring system to measure birth asphyxiation).

Apneustic breathing Prolonged inspiration usually due to brain damage.

Apnoea Absence of breathing for > 10 seconds.

ARDS Acute respiratory distress syndrome.

Arteriovenous oxygen difference Assessment of oxygen delivered to, and returning from, tissue, related to metabolic rate and calculated from arterial and mixed venous blood samples.

Ascites Fluid in the abdominal cavity.

Aspiration (1) Inhalation of unwanted substances (e.g. gastric acid, sea water) into the lungs, or (2) therapeutic removal of fluid or gas from a cavity such as the pleural space.

Atelectasis Alveolar collapse due to poor lung expansion or complete obstruction of an airway.

Base deficit Negative base excess.

Base excess (BE) Normal: from −2 to +2 mmol/l.

BB 'Blue bloater' patient.

Bicarbonate Normal 22–26 mmol/l.

Biot's respiration Irregular cycles of deep gasps and apnoea.

BiPAP Bi-level positive airways pressure.

Bleb Collection of air under visceral pleura, outside alveoli (*see also* bulla).

Blood culture Blood taken from a pyrexial patient to identify responsible micro-organism.

bpm Beats per minute.

Bradypnoea Slow breathing.

Bronchomalacia Degeneration of elastic and connective tissue of trachea and bronchi.

Bulla Collection of air inside distended alveoli, over 1 cm in diameter, caused by alveolar destruction (*see also* bleb).

CABG Coronary artery bypass graft.

Cachectic Emaciated.

CAL Chronic airflow limitation, i.e. COPD.

Calcium Normal: 2.2–2.6 mmol/l.

CCF Congestive cardiac failure.

CaO₂ Arterial oxygen content.
Normal: 17–20 ml/100ml.

Cardiac enzymes Enzymes released from damaged heart muscle after myocardial infarction.

Cardiac index Cardiac output divided by body surface area.
Normal 2.5–3.5 l/min/m².

Cardiac output (Q̇) Heart rate × stroke volume (stroke volume depends on pre-load, afterload and contractility), i.e. amount of blood ejected by left ventricle per minute.
Normal; 4–6 l/min at rest, up to 25 l/min on exercise.

Catecholamines Collective term for compounds having a sympathomimetic action, e.g. adrenaline.

CF Cystic fibrosis.

Chest wall Rib cage, diaphragm, abdominal contents and abdominal wall, i.e. structures outside lung that participate in breathing movements.

Closing capacity Volume at which airway closure begins (as lung volume is reduced towards residual volume, dependent airways begin to close); rises with age until it equals FRC at about 66 years in standing, 44 years in supine.

Closing volume Closing capacity minus residual volume.
Normal: 10% of vital capacity in young people with normal lungs.
Age 65: 40% of VC.
Increases (i.e. becomes a greater proportion of FRC) with small airways disease, smoking and extremes of age.

Clotting studies
Platelet count
Normal: 140 000–400 000 mm⁻³.
Low enough to cause spontaneous bleeding: 20 000–30 000.
Prothrombin time (PT)
Normal: 12–30 seconds.
Expressed as internalized normalized ratio (INR)
Normal: < 1–1.3.
If on warfarin: 4–4.5 (pulmonary embolus), 2–4 (myocardial infarct), 1.8 (postoperative).
With DIC: up to 1.5–2.2.
Expressed as activated partial thromboplastin time (PTT)
Normal: 25–35 seconds.
DIC: 50 seconds.

CMV Controlled mandatory ventilation.

CNS Central nervous system.

CO Cardiac output.

COAD Chronic obstructive airways disease (= COPD).

Collateral ventilation Exchange of inspired gas between adjacent lung units.

Colostomy Surgical creation of opening into large bowel.

Compliance of lung Change in volume in response to change in pressure (ΔV/ΔP).
Normal: 0.09–0.40 l/cmH₂O.

Compliance of lung measured on IPPV
$$\frac{\text{tidal volume}}{\text{plateau airway pressure}} - \text{PEEP}.$$

Consolidation Replacement of alveolar air by substance of greater density than air.

COPD Chronic obstructive pulmonary disease.

CPAP Continuous positive airways pressure.

CPR Cardiopulmonary resuscitation.

Creatinine Electrolyte in plasma or urine, formed from muscle breakdown, excreted by kidneys.

Normal in plasma: 50–100 μmol/l, [0.6–1.2 mg/100 ml].

↑ in hypovolaemia or kidney failure, ↑↑ in septic shock.

CSF Cerebral spinal fluid.

CT Computed tomography.

CvO$_2$ Venous oxygen content.

Normal: 12–15 ml/100 ml.

CVP Central venous pressure.

Normal: 1–6 mmHg or 5–12 cmH$_2$O.

CXR Chest X-ray.

Dehydration low blood volume (*see also* hypovolaemia)

DIC Disseminated intravascular coagulation.

DNA Deoxyribonucleic acid.

DNR Do not rescusitate.

DO$_2$ *See* oxygen delivery.

Duty cycle *See* T_I/T_{TOT}.

DVT Deep vein thrombosis.

Dysphagia Pain and/or difficulty in swallowing.

ECCO$_2$R Extracorporeal carbon dioxide removal.

ECG Electrocardiogram.

ECMO Extracorporeal membrane oxygenation.

-ectomy Removal.

EIA Exercise-induced asthma.

ERO$_2$ *See* oxygen extraction ratio.

Left ventricular end-diastolic pressure Left ventricular preload.

Endotoxin Pyrogenic toxin in bacterial cell which increases capillary permeability.

Endotoxic shock Septic shock.

Eosinophil White blood cell associated with hypersensitivity reactions, ↑ in allergies such as extrinsic asthma.

Erythrocytosis Polycythaemia.

ETCO$_2$ End-tidal CO$_2$.

Normal: 4–6%.

ETT Endotracheal tube.

Eucapnia Normal $PaCO_2$.

FBC Full blood count.

FEF$_{25-75}$ Forced expiratory flow in middle half of expiration.

FET Forced expiration technique.

FEV$_1$ Forced expiratory volume in one second.

F$_I$O$_2$ Fraction of inspired oxygen ($F_I O_2$ of 0.6 = 60% inspired oxygen).

FRC Functional residual capacity.

FVC Forced vital capacity.

Glottis Vocal apparatus of the larynx.

Glucose level in blood

Normal: 3.0–5.5 mmol/l.

↑ in stress, ↑↑ in diabetis mellitus, ↓ in liver failure or starvation.

Goodpasture's syndrome Combination of lung haemorrhage and nephritis.

GOR Gastro-oesophageal reflux.

Haematocrit (packed cell volume) Concentration of red blood cells in blood, indicates oxygen-carrying capacity of blood.

Normal: 40–45%.

↓ in anaemia, i.e. < 38%, ↑ in polycythaemia, i.e. > 55%.

Haemoglobin (Hb) Respiratory pigment in red blood cells, combines reversibly with oxygen.

Normal for men: 14.0–18.0 g/100 ml.

Normal for women: 11.5–15.5 g/100 ml.

↓ in anaemia, ↑ in polycythaemia.

Hb Haemoglobin, *see* above.

HCO$^-_3$ Bicarbonate.

HDU High dependency unit.

HFV High frequency ventilation.

HFJV High frequency jet ventilation.

HFO High frequency oscillation.

HFPPV High frequency positive pressure ventilation.

HIV Human immunodeficiency virus.

HLT Heart lung transplant.

H:L ratio Ratio of power in high and low frequency bands of electromyogram of respiratory muscle, ↓ with respiratory muscle fatigue.

HME Heat moisture exchanger.

HR Heart rate.

Hypernatraemia ↑ serum sodium.

Hyperosmolar Containing high concentration of osmotically active ingredients.

Hyperreactivity of the airways Heightened sensitivity to a variety of stimuli, prominent in asthma, sometimes present in COPD, bronchiectasis, CF, sarcoidosis, LVF.

Hyperthermia Core temperature $> 40.5°C$.

Hyperventilation CO_2 removal in excess of CO_2 production, producing $PaCO_2 < 4.7$ kPa (35 mmHg).

Hypokalaemia ↓ potassium.

Hypopnoea Shallow slow breathing.

Hypoventilation CO_2 production in excess of CO_2 removal, producing $PaCO_2 > 6.0$ kPa (45 mmHg).

Hypovolaemia Low blood volume, with adverse haemodynamic outcome.

Hypoxia classifications

Hypoxaemic hypoxia: due to ↓ PaO_2,

Anaemic hypoxia: due to ↓ Hb in blood, or ↓ ability of Hb to carry oxygen e.g. anaemia, sickle cell anaemia,

Hypoperfusion or stagnant hypoxia: due to ↓ DO_2, e.g. heart failure, PVD, vasoconstriction.

Histotoxic hypoxia: due to inability of damaged tissues to accept oxygen delivered, e.g. cyanide poisoning, septic shock.

IABP Intra-aortic balloon pump.

Iatrogenic Causing or exacerbating a problem by medical intervention.

ICP Intracranial pressure.

ICU Intensive care unit.

I:E *See* inspiratory:expiratory ratio.

Ileostomy Surgical creation of an opening into the ileum.

Infection Presence of micro-organisms or their products invading normally sterile tissue (*see also* sepsis).

Inspiratory capacity Volume inspired during maximum inspiration from resting end-expiratory position.

Inspiratory:expiratory ratio Numerical expression of duration of inspiration relative to expiration.

Inspiratory force *See* MIP.

IMV Intermittent mandatory ventilation.

Intrapulmonary pressure Alveolar pressure (p. 4).

Intrathoracic pressure Pleural pressure (p. 4).

IPPB Intermittent positive pressure breathing.

IPPV Intermittent positive pressure ventilation.

IRT Immune reactive trypsin – antibody identified in CF screening.

IRV Inspiratory reserve volume.

IVOX Intravascular oxygenation

JVP Jugular venous pressure.

K *See* potassium.

Kartagena's syndrome Triad of bronchiectasis, sinusitis and dextrocardia, associated with primary ciliary dyskinesia.

kPa Kilopascal.

Kussmaul breathing Deep sighing breathing often seen in patients with metabolic acidosis.

l Litre

Lactate in blood (serum lactate)

Normal: < 1 mmol/l.

Severe oxygen debt, poor prognosis = 2.5–3.0.

Laparotomy Surgical incision through abdominal wall.

Larynx Cylindrical tube connecting pharynx and trachea, formed by cartilages and containing vocal cords.

Left ventricular end-diastolic volume (LVEDV) Determinant of preload, depends on venous return to left ventricle, circulating blood volume and efficiency of left atrial contraction.

LVEDV *See* above.

LVF Left ventricular failure.

μm Micron, i.e. 10^{-6} m.

MAP Mean arterial pressure.

Mast cells Connective tissue cells involved in hypersensitivity reactions, which release histamine in response to specific stimuli.

MDI Metered dose inhaler.

Mean arterial pressure Average arterial blood pressure.

   Normal: 65–100 mmHg.

Mean corpuscular haemoglobin (MCH) Amount of Hb in red blood cells.

Mean corpuscular volume (MCV) Reflects size of red blood cells.

   ↓ MCV (small RBCs): iron deficiency.

   ↑ MCV (large RBCs): vitamin B_{12} or folate deficiency.

MEF_{50} Maximum expiratory flow in mid-expiration.

MEP Maximal expiratory pressure.

   Normal: 100 cmH_2O.

   < 40 cmH_2O: inadequate cough.

MET (metabolic energy expenditure) Metabolic unit representing amount of oxygen consumed at rest.

   Normal 3.5 ml oxygen/kg body weight/min.

   Maximum MET levels (multiples of resting $\dot{V}O_2$) − estimated $\dot{V}O_2$ max ÷ resting $\dot{V}O_2$.

MI Myocardial infarction, i.e. death of portion of heart muscle due to myocardial ischaemia.

MIP Maximum inspiratory pressure (assessment of respiratory muscle strength).

   Normal: minus 100–130 cmH_2O (men), minus 70–100 cmH_2O (women).

   Typical value in hypercapnic COPD: minus 55 (men), minus 40 (women).

   Minus 20: poor weaning outcome, minus 0–20: inadequate cough.

MMEF Maximum mid-expiratory flow.

mmHg Millimetres of mercury.

MMV Mandatory minute ventilation.

Mucoviscidosis Cystic fibrosis.

Neutrophils Cells which release tissue-damaging enzymes as part of inflammatory process.

NFR Not for resuscitation.

NIPPV Nasal (or non-invasive) intermittent positive pressure ventilation.

NSAID Non-steroidal anti-inflammatory drug.

Occupational lung disease Disease due to inhalation of dust, particles, fumes or gases while working with industrial substances.

OHFO Oral high frequency oscillation.

Oliguria ↓ urine output, i.e. < 20 ml/h (normal 50–60 ml/h).

-oscopy Visual examination of interior of an organ.

Osmolality Number of osmotically active particles per kg of solvent.

Osmolarity Number of osmotically active particles per litre of solution.

-ostomy Formation of artificial opening on to skin surface.

-otomy Incision.

Oxygen consumption ($\dot{V}O_2$) Amount of oxygen consumed by tissues each minute.

   Normal at rest: 250 ml/min (if contributing values normal, i.e. CO 5 l/min, Hb 15 g/100 ml, SaO_2 97%, $S\bar{v}O_2$ 75%).

   600 ml/min: critical illness; 3600 ml/min: maximum exercise in unfit males; 5000 ml/min: maximum exercise in fit males.

Oxygen delivery (DO_2) Volume of oxygen delivered to tissues each minute.

   Normal: 550–1000 ml/min.

   Calculation: cardiac output × arterial oxygen content.

Oxygen demand Amount of oxygen needed by cells for aerobic metabolism, estimated by measurement of $\dot{V}O_2$.

Oxygen extraction ratio Ratio of oxygen consumption to oxygen delivery ($\dot{V}O_2/DO_2$), indicating efficiency of tissues in extracting oxygen.

   Normal: 25%.

   > 35% implies excessively high oxygen extraction to meet metabolic needs.

   Calculation: cardiac output ÷ CaO_2.

Oxygen flux % oxygen that reaches tissues.

Oxygen transport Oxygen delivery.

Oxygen uptake Oxygen consumption.

Ozone Gas that provides a protective layer to the earth's atmosphere, but at ground level it causes inflammation in people with hyperreactive airways.

P_{50} PO_2 at which 50% of haemoglobin in blood is saturated with oxygen, quantifies shift in dissociation curve (high value suggests slow affinity of Hb for oxygen). Normal: 27–28 mmHg.

PA Posteroanterior.

PA-aO$_2$ (alveolar to arterial oxygen gradient) Difference in partial pressures of alveolar oxygen (P_AO_2) and arterial oxygen (PaO_2).
    Normal on room air: < 10 mmHg (reflecting normal anatomical shunt).
        ↑ in respiratory disease (due to ↓ $\dot{V}_A/\dot{Q}$ mismatch),
        ↑ on exercise (up to 20–30 mmHg), ↑ in the elderly (up to 30 mmHg), ↑ on supplemental oxygen (up to 100 mmHg on 100% oxygen).

Pack years Number of years of smoking multiplied by number of packs smoked each day, e.g. smoking one pack a day for 30 years = 30 pack year history.

Packed cell volume *See* PCV.

Pancoast's tumour Tumour of upper lobe affecting brachial plexus, sometimes indicated by wasting of small muscles of the hand.

PaO$_2$ Partial pressure of oxygen in arterial blood.

PaCO$_2$ Partial pressure of CO$_2$ in arterial blood.

PAP Peak airways pressure (= peak inspiratory pressure).

PAP Pulmonary artery pressure. Normal: 10–20 mmHg.

Parenchyma Gas exchanging part of lung, largely alveolar tissue.

Parenchymal lung disease Disease affecting alveolar walls, e.g. interstitial lung disease, pneumonia, pulmonary TB, ARDS.

PAWP Pulmonary artery wedge pressure. Normal: 5–12 mmHg.

P̄aw Mean airway pressure.

PCA Patient controlled analgesia.

PCP *Pneumocystis carinii* pneumonia.

PCV Packed cell volume.
    Normal: 0.40–0.50 (men), 0.36–0.47 (women).
        ↑ in polycythaemia, ↓ in anaemia. Equivalent to haematocrit.

PCWP Pulmonary capillary wedge pressure (= PAWP).

PD Postural drainage.

PE Pulmonary embolus.

PEEP Positive end-expiratory pressure.

PEFR Peak expiratory flow rate (peak flow).

P$_{Emax}$ Maximum expiratory pressure at the mouth.

PEP Positive expiratory pressure.

pH Hydrogen ion.

Phlebotomy/venesection Therapeutic withdrawal of blood.

P$_{Imax}$ Maximum inspiratory pressure at the mouth (*see* MIP).

PIP Peak inspiratory pressure.

Plasma osmolarity Normal: 280–300 m osmol/l.

-plasty Reconstruction.

Platelet count *See* clotting studies.

Platypnoea Difficulty breathing while sitting up.

Plethoric Florid complexion due to excess red blood cells.

Pneumonitis Inflammation of lung tissue due to chemical or physical insult.

Polysomnography Recording of physiological parameters during sleep.

Polyuria ↑ urine output, i.e. > 100 ml/h.

POMR Problem oriented medical record.

Potassium (K) Electrolyte in plasma or urine. Normal in plasma: 3.5–5.0 mmol/l.
        ↓ K (hypokalaemia) predisposes to cardiac arrhythmias, ↑ K (hyperkalaemia) suggests kidney failure.

Poudrage Pleurodesis.

PP 'Pink puffer' patient.

Prader–Willi syndrome Combination of obesity, hypotonia and impaired cognitive ability, associated with respiratory problems due to reduced diaphragmatic excursion, upper airway soft-tissue collapse and sleep apnoea.

PT Prothrombin time (*see* clotting studies).

Psittacosis Infectious disease of birds transmitted to humans as atypical pneumonia.

PtcO$_2$ transcutaneous oxygen tension.

PtcCO$_2$ Transcutaneous carbon-dioxide tension.

PTT Partial prothrombin time (*see* clotting studies).

Pulmonary hypertension ↑ pulmonary artery pressure, i.e. > 25 mmHg (mean) atrest or 30 mmHg on exercise, in presence of cardiac output < 5 l/min.

Pulmonary vascular resistance Normal: 25–125 dyn.s.cm^{-5}.

Pulse pressure Difference between systolic and diastolic pressures (raised in hypertension), related to stroke volume, therefore gives indication of blood flow.
   Normal: 40–70 mmHg.
   20 mmHg: dangerously poor tissue perfusion.

Pulsus paradoxus Transient drop in systolic pressure on inspiration due to expansion of pulmonary vascular bed on inspiration.
   Normal: 10 mmHg.
   >10 mmHg = severe acute asthma (due to laboured breathing causing excess negative pressure in chest) or cardiac tamponade.

Pump (ventilatory/respiratory) Muscles and nerves of respiration, chest wall, respiratory centre.

PVD Peripheral vascular disease.

$P\bar{v}O_2$ mixed venous oxygen tension.
   Normal: 35–40 mmHg.
   Minimum acceptable: 28 mmHg.

$P\bar{v}CO_2$ mixed venous CO_2 tension,
   Normal: 46 mmHg.

$\dot{Q}$ blood flow.

$\dot{Q}O_2$ Oxygen delivery (alternative abbreviation to DO_2).

QRS complex The deflection of the ECG caused by depolarization of the ventricles, consisting of an upward, or positive deflection (R) preceded and followed by negative deflection (Q and S).

$\dot{Q}S$ shunted blood.

$\dot{Q}s/\dot{Q}t$ shunt, i.e. fraction of cardiac output not exposed to gas exchange in pulmonary capillary bed, measured by comparing arterial and mixed venous blood.
   Normal: 2–4%.
   20%: respiratory failure, 50%: ARDS

$\dot{Q}_T$ cardiac output.

Radiolabelling Monitoring of mucus clearance by inhalation of radiolabelled aerosoland following up its clearance by gamma camera.

RAP Right atrial pressure.

Raynaud's phenomenon of the lung Vasospasm in the lungs associated with Raynaud's syndrome.

REM (rapid eye movement) sleep Most restorative phase of sleep cycle.

Resection Surgical cutting out.

Respiratory inductive plethysmography Spirometry for ventilated patients, including measurement of lung volume to detect intrinsic PEEP.

Respiratory quotient (RQ) $\dfrac{CO_2 \text{ produced}}{\text{oxygen consumed}}$.
   Normal: 0.8, expired minute volume being slightly less than inspired minute volume because less CO_2 is excreted than O_2 absorbed.

RFTs Respiratory function tests.

RQ *See* respiratory quotient.

RR Respiratory rate.

RTA Road traffic accident.

SaO_2 Saturation of haemoglobin with oxygen.

Sepsis Clinical response characterized by ↑ temperature and WBC, caused usually but not always by infection.

Sepsis syndrome Preseptic shock state.

SGAW Specific airways conductance.

Shunt Perfusion without ventilation (*see* $\dot{Q}s/\dot{Q}t$).

SIMV Synchronized intermittent mandatory ventilation.

Small airways Terminal and respiratory bronchioles, i.e. less than 1 mm diameter, unsupported by cartilage and therefore influenced by transmitted pleural pressures.

SOB Shortness of breath.

Sodium (Na) Electrolyte in plasma or urine.
   Normal in plasma: 135–147 mmol/l, [135–147 mEq/l].
   ↓ Na (hyponatraemia): excess water administration or inappropriate ADH

secretion, ↑ Na (hypernatraemia): dehydration.

Standard bicarbonate Bicarbonate corrected for a normal $PaCO_2$, similar to bicarbonate in a person with normal acid-base status.

Sternotomy Surgical cutting through the sternum.

Surgical emphysema Subcutaneous emphysema.

Surfactant Phospholipid protein complex that lines alveoli, lowers surface tension and maintains patency.

SVR *See* systemic vascular resistance.

S$\bar{v}$O$_2$ Mixed venous oxygen saturation.
Normal: 75%.

Syncope Transient loss of consciousness, e.g. faint.

Systemic vascular resistance (SVR)
Normal: 800–1400 dyn.s.cm^{-5}.
Calculation: (MAP−CVP/cardiac output) × 79.9.
< 300 suggests septic shock.

TED Thromboembolic disease.

Tension-time index Measurement of inspiratory muscle fatigue (Ramonatxo 1995).

Thoracoplasty Surgery used historically for pulmonary TB, involving rib resection and localized lung collapse to allow healing.

Thrombocytopaenia ↓ platelet count.

T$_1$/T$_{TOT}$ Respiratory duty cycle, i.e. ratio of inspiratory to total respiratory cycle time, short T$_1$ in relation to T$_{TOT}$ indicating ↓ tidal volume and ↑ dead space, suggesting inspiratory muscle fatigue.

TLC Total lung capacity.

TLCO Total lung transfer capacity for carbon monoxide.

TPN Total parenteral nutrition.

Tracheal tube Endotracheal or tracheostomy tube.

Tracheostomy Artificial opening into the trachea.

Tracheotomy Operative formation of a tracheostomy.

Transairway pressure Pressure between mouth and alveoli.
Normal: 5 cmH$_2$O.

Transthoracic pressure Pressure across chest wall, i.e. pleural pressure minus atmospheric pressure.

Trendelenburg position Head down tilt.

Torr Measurement of pressure used in the USA, equivalent to mmHg.

U & E Urea and electrolytes.

Urea Electrolyte in plasma or urine, formed from protein breakdown and excreted by kidneys.
Normal in plasma: 3–7 mmol/l.
>8 dehydration; 18–20: hypovolaemia; 55: kidney failure.

V Volume of gas.

VAS Visual analogue scale.

v Venous.

v̇ Volume of gas per unit time, i.e. flow (dot indicates time derivative).

v̄ Mixed venous (line indicates mean or mixed value).

$\dot{V}_{50}$ Flow rate half-way through expiration.

$\dot{V}_A/\dot{Q}$ Ratio of alveolar ventilation to perfusion.
Normal: 0.8 (4 l/min for alveolar ventilation, 5 l/min for perfusion).

VC Vital capacity.

V$_D$ Volume of dead space gas.

V$_D$/V$_T$ Dead space in relation to tidal volume.
Normal: 0.3–0.4, i.e. 30–40% of each breath does not contribute to gas exchange.
0.6: critical increase in V_D.

VF Ventricular fibrillation.

$\dot{V}_E$ (Expired) minute volume.
Normal: 5–7 l/min.
200 l/min has been recorded on exercise.

$\dot{V}CO_2$ Carbon dioxide production.

$\dot{V}O_2$ *See* oxygen consumption.

$\dot{V}O_2/DO_2$ *See* oxygen extraction ratio.

$\dot{V}O_2$max Oxygen consumption at maximum exertion, reflecting aerobic capacity.
Increases with fitness, declines with advancing age but rate of decline is slower in physically active people.
Normal: > 25 ml/kg/min, or 25 times the resting level.
See also anaerobic threshold.

V_T Tidal volume.

Valsalva manoeuvre Expiration against closed glottis.

Vasopressor drug Drug that causes vasoconstriction of capillaries and arteries.

WBC *See* white blood cell count.

Wegener's granulomatosis Triad of upper respiratory tract lesions, pulmonary disease and glomerulonephritis.

Well-year of life Concept which includes morbidity and mortality, e.g. if disease reduces quality of life by a half over 2 years, patient has lost one full well-year.

White blood cell count (WBC)
  Normal: $4-10 \times 10^9$/l, [4000–10 000/mm^{-3}].

WOB Work of breathing.

Conversion of mmHg to kPa
mmHg = kPa × 7.5.

mmHg	*kPa*
150	20
120	16
105	14
90	12
75	10
60	8
40	5
30	4
15	2

Conversation of mmHg to cmH$_2$O

mmHg	*cmH$_2$O*
5	6.8
10	13.6
20	27.2
30	40.7
40	54.3

Appendix A: *Transatlantic dictionary*

British	North American
Adrenaline	Epinephrine
Accident and Emergency (A & E)	Emergency Room (ER)
ASAP (as soon as possible)	Stat
Cardiac arrest	Code
Chest drains	Chest tubes
Chronic obstructive airways diseases	Chronic obstructive pulmonary disease
Community care	Home care
Consultant	Staff person
Drip	IV
Drugs	Medication
Entonox	Nitronox (USA)
ECG	EKG
Frame	Walker
General practice	Primary care/family practice
Hospital	Health Sciences Center/Facility
Houseman/woman	Intern
Lignocaine	Lidocaine
mm of Hg (unit of pressure)	torr
Nil by mouth	NPO
Patient's notes	Patient's chart
Passive or active movements	Range of motion
Peak expiratory flow rate	Maximum expiratory flow rate
Queue	Line up
Referral	Consult
Registrar	Resident
Respiratory physiotherapist	Part physical therapist, part respiratory therapist (USA)
RTA (road traffic accident)	MVA (motor vehicle accident)
Salbutamol	Albuterol (USA)
Sluice	Utility room
Splint	Cast
Stick	Cane
Theatre	Operating room or OR
Walk or mobilize	Ambulate
Ward	Floor
1st floor	2nd floor

Appendix B: *Postural drainage positions*

1. UPPER LOBES

1(a) Apical segments of both upper lobes – sitting upright

1(b) Posterior segment of right upper lobe – left-side-lying, turned 45° towards prone

1(c) Posterior segment of left upper lobe – right-side-lying, turned 45° towards prone, shoulders raised 30 cm (12 ins)

1(d) Anterior segments of both upper lobes – supine

2. MIDDLE LOBE

Lateral and medial segments – supine, quarter turned to left, foot of bed raised 35 cm (14 ins)

3. LINGULA

Superior and inferior segments – supine, quarter turned to right, foot of bed raised 35 cm (14 ins)

4. LOWER LOBE

4(a) Apical segments of both lower lobes – prone, head turned to side

4(b) Anterior basal segments of both lower lobes – supine, foot of bed raised 46 cm (18 ins)

4(c) Posterior basal segments of both lower lobes – prone, head turned to side, foot of bed raised 46 cm (18 ins)

4(d) Medial basal segment – right-side-lying, foot of bed raised 46 cm (18 ins)

4(e) Lateral basal segment – left-side-lying, foot of bed raised 46 cm (18 ins)

From: Downie, P.A. (1987) (ed.) *Cash's Textbook of Chest Heart and Vascular Disorders for Physiotherapists*, Faber, London, with permission.

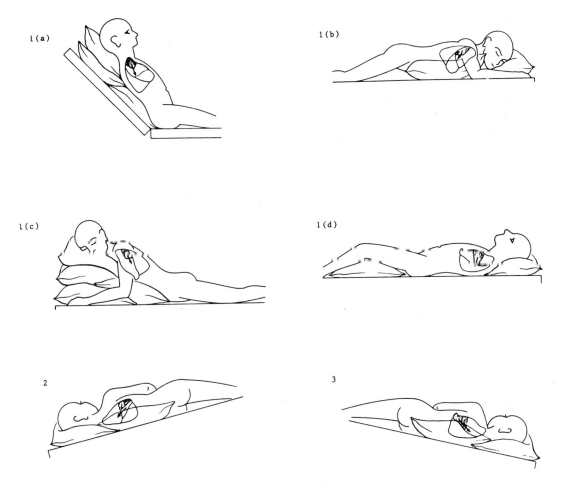

Appendix B Postural drainage positions.

4(a)

4(b)

4(c)

4(d)

4(e)

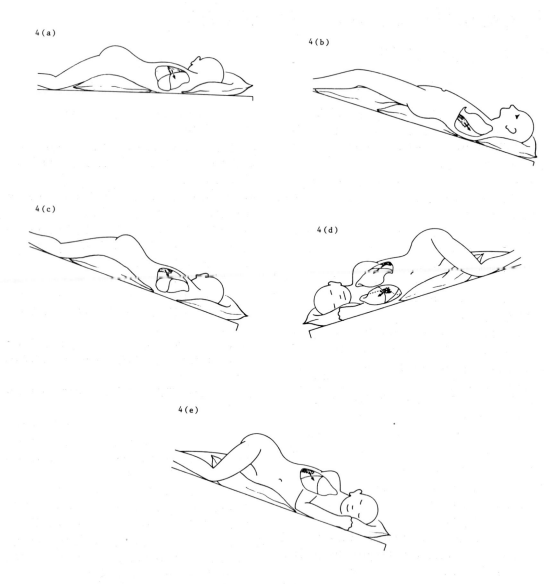

Appendix C: Resources and organizations

Action for Sick Children, Argyle House, 29–31 Euston Rd, London NW1 2SD, UK. (0171) 833 2041. Booklets and references on postoperative pain.

American Association for Respiratory Care, 11030 Ables Ln, Dallas, Texas, 75229. +1 (214) 243 2272.

American Lung Association and American Thoracic Society, 1740 Broadway, New York, NY 10019–4374. +1 (212) 315 8700. Includes 'Superstuff' children's asthma education programme.

ASH (Action on Smoking and Health), 109 Gloucester Place, London W1H 3DA, UK. (0171) 935 3519, fax (0171) 935 3463.

Association of Chartered Physiotherapists in Respiratory Care (ACPRC), c/o CSP, 14 Bedford Row, London WC1R 4ED, UK. (0171) 306 6666.

Asthma and Allergy Foundation of America, 1717 Massachusetts, Washington, DC, USA. +1 (202) 265 0265.

Asthma Society of Canada, PO Box 213, Station K, Toronto, Ontario M4P 2G5. +1 (416) 977 9684.

BACUP (British Association of Cancer United Patients), 3 Bath Place, London EC2A 3JR. (0171) 613 2121.

BiPAP equipment see CPAP.

British Lung Foundation, 72 Hatton Gardens, London EC1N 8JR, UK. (0171) 831 5831. Includes Breathe Easy Club (self-help club for patients) and Lung and Asthma Information Agency (epidemiological database for health staff).

British Snoring and Sleep Apnoea Association, The Steps, How Lane, Chipstead, Surrey, CR5 3LT. (01737) 557997, fax (01737) 556671.

Canadian Lung Association, Suite 908, 75 Albert St, Ottawa, Ontario, KIP 5E7. +1 (613) 237 1208.

Carbon monoxide biofeedback for smoking cessation, contact ASH, above.

Carers National Association, 20 Glasshouse Yard, London EC1A 4JS, UK. (0171) 490 8818, fax (0171) 490 8824.

CPAP and BiPAP equipment:
Medicaid, Hook Lane, Pagham, Sussex PO21 3PP, UK. (01243) 267321, fax (01243) 262556.
ResCare, 68 Milton Park, Abingdon, Oxon OX14 4RX, UK. (01235) 862997, fax (01235) 831336.
Respironics, 530 Seco Rd, Monroeville, PA 15146, USA.

Cystic Fibrosis Research Trust and Association of Cystic Fibrosis Adults, 5 Blyth Rd, Bromley, Kent BR1 3RS, UK. (0181) 464 7211, fax (0181) 313 0472.

Flutter: Clement Clarke, Airmed House, Edinburgh Way, Harlow, Essex CM20 2ED. (01279) 414969, fax (01279) 635232.

Guillain–Barré Syndrome Support Group, Foxley, Holdingham, Sleaford, Lincs, NG34 8NR, UK. (01529) 304615.

Headway (Head injuries association), 7 King Edward Court, King Edward Street, Nottingham NG1 1EW. (0115) 924 0800, support group (0115) 967 9669, fax (0115) 924 0432.

Inspiratory muscle trainers:
Medix, Medix House, Catthorpe, Lutterworth, Leics, L17 6DB, UK. (01788) 860366.
Healthscan, Cedar Grove, NJ 07009, USA.

Laryngectomy patients:
National Association of Laryngectomee Clubs, 6 Rickett Street, London SW6 1RU, UK. (0171) 381 9993.
International Association of Laryngectomees, 777 Third Ave, New York, NY 10017, USA. +1 (212) 371 2900.

Liver patients: The British Liver Trust, Central House, Central Avenue, Ransones Europark, Ipswich IP3 9QG, UK. (01473) 276326, fax (01473) 276327.

Manometer for testing bag-squeezing pressures: Vital Signs, 60 Gladstone Place, Brighton, Sussex BN2 3QD, UK. (01273) 625188, fax (01273) 624836.

MIP measurement – Precision Medical, Thornton Road Industrial Estate, Pickering, North Yorkshire, UK. (01751) 477577.

Motor Neurone Disease Association, PO Box 246, Northampton NN1 2PR, UK. (01604) 250505, helpline (0345) 626262, 24 hrs (01604) 22269, fax (01604) 24726. Supplies Breathing Space Kit to reduce fears in final stages of disease.

National Asthma Campaign, Providence House, Providence Place, London, N1 ONT, UK. (0171) 226 2260, helpline (0345) 010203, fax (0171) 704 0740.

National Heart, Lung and Blood Institute, Building 31, Room 4A18, National Institutes of Health, Bethesda, MD 20982, USA.

NIPPV equipment:
Medicaid, Respironics, Rescare, see CPAP.
Thomas Respiratory Systems, 33 Half Moon Lane, Herne Hill, London SE24 9JX, UK. (0171) 737 5881, fax (0171) 737 5234.
PneuPAC, Crescent Rd, Luton, Beds, LU2 OAH, UK. (01582) 453303, fax (01582) 453103.

Oscillator: Hayek oscillator, Medicom, 9 Burroughs Gardens, London NW4 4AU, UK. (0181) 203 9686, fax (0181) 203 4758.

Ozone alert (information on daily air pollution levels in UK), (0800) 556677.

Patient booklets:
Allen & Hanburys, Greenford, Middlesex UB6 OHB, UK. (0181) 990 9888, fax (0181) 990 4375.
Glaxo, Box 13398, Research Triangle Park, NC 27709, USA.

PEP masks:
Astra Tec, PO Box 13, Stroud, Glos G15 3DL, UK. (01453) 791763.
Astra Tec Inc, 1000 Winter St, Suite 2700, Waltham, MA 02154, USA.
Henleys, 39 Brownfields, Welwyn Garden City, Herts AL7 1AN, UK. (01707) 333164, fax (01707) 334795.

Primary Ciliary Dyskinesia Support Group, 67 Evendons Lane, Wokingham, Berks RG41 4AD, UK.

Pulmocare (low carbohydrate feed for respiratory patients): Abbott Laboratories, Abbott House, Moorbridge Rd, Maidenhead, Berks SL6 8JG, UK. (01628) 773355.

Ross Division, Abbott Park, N. Chicago, IL 60064–3500, USA.

Quitline (smoking cessation helpline in the UK); (0171) 487 3000.

Self Help Guide: directory of self-help groups in Britain, by Gann, R. and Knight, S. (1988), Chapman & Hall, London.

Shuttle audio tape and booklet: £25 to Respiratory Medicine Dept, Glenfields General Hospital, Groby Road, Leicester LE3 9QP, UK. (0116) 287 1471.

Spinal Injuries Association, Newpoint House, 76 St James Lane, London N10 3DF, UK. (0181) 444 2121.

Vibrator (electric chest pad): Niagara Manufacturing, Colomendy Industrial Estate, Rhyl Rd, Denbigh, Wales LL16 TS UK. (01745) 813666.

Appendix D: *Articles by patients*

Armstrong, A. (1977) Living on a mechanical respirator. *Guardian*, 6 Sept.

Bevan, P.G. (1964) Cholecystectomy in a surgeon. *Lancet*, **1**, 214–15.

Bevan, J.R. (1969) Polyneuropathy. *Lancet*, **1**, 1310.

Brooks, D.H.M. (1990) The route to home ventilation: a patient's perspective. *Care Crit. Ill*, **6**, 96–7.

Clark, K.J. (1985) Coping with Guillain–Barré syndrome. *Int. Care Nurs.*, **1**, 13–18.

Farrow, J. (1995) Cystic fibrosis – it's a funny name. *Respir. Dis. Pract.*, **12**(1), 5–6.

Gandy, A.P. (1968) An attack of tetanus. *Lancet*, **2**, 567–8.

Heath, J.V. (1989) What the patients say. *Int Care Nurs.*, **5**, 101–8.

Holden, T. (1980) Patiently speaking. *Nurs. Times*, **76**(24), 1035–6.

Houston, J.E. (1988) Physiotherapy from a patient's point of view. *S.A.J. Physiother.*, **44**, 38–41.

Kinnear, W.J.M. (1994) *Assisted Ventilation at Home – a Practical Guide*, Oxford Medical Publications, Oxford, Chapter 8: A patient's view of living with a ventilator, pp.85–93.

Lancet (1969) At the receiving end. *Lancet*, **2**, 1129–31.

Lancet (1969) Cardiac arrest. *Lancet*, **2**, 262–4.

Marsh, B. (1986) A second chance. *Br. Med. J.*, **292**, 675–6.

Nicholson, E.M. (1975) Personal notes of a laryngectomee. *Am. J. Nurs.*, **75** (12), 2157–8.

Neuberger, J. (1991) The patient's viewpoint. *Respir. Med.*, **85** (suppl.B), 53–6.

Nursing Times (1981) Who am I? Where am I? Why do I hurt so much? *Nurs. Times*, **77** (15), 633–5.

Redfern, S. (1985) Taking some of my own medicine. *Care Crit. Ill*, **1**, 6–7.

Ruiz, P A (1993) The needs of a patient in severe status asthmaticus. *Int. Crit. Care Nurs.*, **9**, 28–39.

Shovelton, D.S. (1979) Reflections on an intensive therapy unit. *Br. Med. J.*, **2**, 737–8.

Standing, C. (1987) The treatment of our son with cystic fibrosis. *J. Roy. Soc. Med.*, **80** (suppl. 15), 2–4.

Thomson, L.R. (1973) Sensory deprivation: a personal experience. *Am. J. Nurs.*, **73**, 266–8.

Villaire, M. (1995) ICU from the patient's point of view. *Crit. Care Nurse*, **15** (1), 80–7.

While, A. (1985) Personal View. *Br. Med. J.*, **291**, 343.

Wilkinson, J. (1987) The experience and expectations of parents of a child with cystic fibrosis. *J. Roy. Soc. Med.*, **80** (suppl. 15), 7–8.

Appendix E: Articles on outcome measures for pulmonary rehabilitation

Brannon, F.J., Foley, M.W., Starr, J.A. *et al* (1993) *Cardiopulmonary rehabilitation: Basic Theory and Application*, 2nd edn, F.A. Davis, Philadelphia.
(Outcomes: ↑ survival, ↑ exercise capacity, ↓ hospitalization, p.7.)

Bryant, A. (1993) Quality of life variables influenced by outpatient pulmonary rehabilitation. *Resp. Care*, **38**, 1230.

Cockcroft, A.E., Saunders, M.J. and Berry, G. (1981) Randomised controlled trial of rehabilitation in chronic respiratory disability. *Thorax*, **36**, 200–3.
(Outcomes: ↑ 12-minute distance, maintained on follow-up.)

Couser, J.I., Martinez, F.J., and Celli, B.R. (1993) Pulmonary rehabilitation that includes arm exercise reduces metabolic and ventilatory requirements for simple arm elevation. *Chest*, **103**, 37–41.

Donner, C.F. (1992) Pulmonary rehabilitation in COPD with recommendations for its use. *Eur. Respir. J.*, **5**, 266–75.
(Outcomes: 25% patients: > 10% ↓ SOB and/or > 10% ↑ 6-minute walk.)

Flanigan, K.S. (1991) Outcome of a 3-day pulmonary rehabilitation programme. *Respir. Care*, **36**, 1271.
(Short programme outcomes: ↑ ADL, ↑ confidence.)

Giddings, D.J. (1994) Outcome evaluation of a respiratory rehabilitation program. *Physiother. Can.*, **46**(2) (suppl.), 81.
(Outcomes: ↑ walking distance, ↑ ADL.)

Haas, F. and Axen, K. (1991) *Pulmonary Therapy and Rehabilitation*, Williams and Wilkins, London, p.336. (Cost savings > $2600/patient/year.)

Haggerty, M.C. (1991) Home care for the person with COPD, in *Pulmonary Therapy and Rehabilitation* (Eds F. Haas and K. Axen), Williams and Wilkins, London.
(Outcomes: ↓ hospitalization, ↓ A & E visits, ↑ quality of life.)

Hodgkin, J.E., Zorn, E.G. and Connors, G.L. (1993) *Pulmonary rehabilitation: guidelines to success*, 2nd edn, Lippincott, Philadelphia.
(Outcomes: ↓ costs by 1/5 (p.551), $217 610 saved in one hospital (p.533), 25% patients assumed full-time employment (p.555), ↓ hospitalization (p.550), chapter on cost effectiveness.)

Holden, D.A., Stelmach, K.D., and Curtis, P.S. (1990) The impact of a rehabilitation program on functional status of patients with chronic lung disease. *Respir. Care*, **35**, 332–41.
(Outcome: ↑ walking distance by average 27%.)

Hudson, L.D., Tyler, M.L. and Petty, T.L. (1976) Hospitalization needs during outpatient rehabilitation for severe chronic airway obstruction. *Chest*, **70**, 606–10.
(Outcome: ↓ hospitalization.)

Make, B. (1990) Pulmonary rehabilitation – what are the outcomes? *Respir. Care*, **35**, 329–31.
(Literature review of outcomes.)

Make, B. (1994) Collaborative self-management strategies for patients with respiratory disease. *Respir. Care*, **39**, 566–77.
(Outcomes: ↑ workload by 30%, ↑ $\dot{V}O_{2max}$ by 9.2%, 6-minute distance ↑ by 21%, ↑ ADL, ↑ social and emotional function.)

Murray, E. (1993) Anyone for pulmonary rehabilitation? *Physiotherapy*, **79**, 705–10.
(Outcomes: ↑ exercise capacity, ↓

hospitalization, ↓ symptoms, ↓ anxiety and depression, ↑ quality of life.)

Niederman, M.S., Clemente, P.H., Fein, A.M. *et al.* (1991) Benefits of a multidisciplinary pulmonary rehabilitation program. *Chest*, **99**, 798–804.
(Outcomes: ↑ endurance, ↓ SOB, ↓ oxygen consumption.)

Ojanen, M. (1993) Psychological changes in patients participating in a COPD rehabilitation program. *Respiration*, **60**, 96–102.
(Outcome: ↑ well-being, ↓ symptoms.)

Reardon, J. (1994) The effect of comprehensive outpatient pulmonary rehabilitation on dyspnea. *Chest*, **105**, 1046–52.
(Outcome: ↓ SOB.)

Petty, T.L. (1993) Pulmonary rehabilitation in perspective. *Thorax*, **18**, 855–62.
(Outcome: ↑ survival.)

Roselle, S. and Amico, F.J. (1982) The effect of home respiratory therapy on hospital readmission rates in patients with COPD. *Respir. Care*, **27**, 1194–9.

(Outcome: $2625 savings/patient/year.)

Schleifer, T.J. (1994) Patient responsibility in an innovative COPD therapy program. *Physiother. Can.*, **46**(2) (suppl), 81.
(Outcomes in severe disease: ↑ ADL, ↓ exacerbations, ↓ anxiety.)

Tougaard, L., Krone, T., Sorknaes, A. *et al.* (1992) Economic benefits of teaching patients with COPD about their illness. *Lancet*, **339**, 1517–20.
(Outcome: ↓ use of health services.)

Vale, F., Reardon, J.Z. and ZuWallack, R.L. (1993) The long term benefits of outpatient rehabilitation on exercise endurance and quality of life. *Chest*, **103**, 42–5.
(Outcomes: ↑ exercise capacity, ↑ quality of life.)

Zeballos, R.J. (1984) The effect of a 3-week physical rehabilitation program on exercise tolerance and performance in patients with COPD. *Am. Rev. Respir. Dis.*, **129**, 4(2), A275.
(Outcome: ↑ exercise capacity.)

Further reading

Armstrong, R.F., Bullen, C.L. Cohen, S.L. *et al.* (1991) *Critical Care Algorithms*. Oxford Medical Publications, Oxford.

Brannon, F.J., Foley, M.W., Starr, J.A. and Black, M.G. (1993) *Cardiopulmonary Rehabilitation: Basic Theory and Application*, 2nd edn, F.A. Davis, Philadelphia.

Cameron, I.R. and Bateman, N.T. (1990) *Respiratory Disorders*, Edward Arnold, London.

Carter, B. (1994) *Child and Infant Pain*, Chapman & Hall, London.

Cohen, M. and Hoskin, T.M. (1988) *Cardiopulmonary Symptoms in Physical Therapy*, Churchill Livingstone, New York.

Fried, R. (1993) *The Psychology and Physiology of Breathing*, Plenum Press, New York.

Frownfelter, D.L. (1987) *Chest Physical Therapy and Pulmonary Rehabilitation*, Year Book Medical Publishers, Chicago.

Irwin S. and Tecklin, J.S. (1995). *Cardiopulmonary Physical Therapy*, Mosby, Missouri.

Haas, F. and Axen, K. (1991) *Pulmonary Therapy and Rehabilitation*, Williams and Wilkins, London.

Hodgkin, J.E., Connors, G.L. and Bell, C.W. (1993) *Pulmonary Rehabilitation – Guidelines to Success*, Lippincott, Philadelphia.

Holmes, O. (1993) *Human Acid-base Physiology*, Chapman & Hall, London.

Kinnear, W.J.M. (1994) *Assisted Ventilation at Home – a Practical Guide*, Oxford Medical Publications, Oxford.

Landay, M.J. (1987) *Interpretation of the Chest Roentgenogram*, Little, Brown & Co, Boston.

Luce, J.M., Pierson, D.J. and Tyler, M.L. (1993) *Intensive Respiratory Care*, Saunders, London.

Mackenzie, C.F. (ed.) (1989) *Chest Physiotherapy in the Intensive Care Unit*, Williams and Wilkins, London.

Moser, K.M. Ries, A.L., and Sassi-Dambron, D.E. (1991) *Shortness of Breath: a Guide to Better Living and Breathing*, 4th edn, C.V. Mosby, Missouri.

Nunn, J.F. (1993) *Applied Respiratory Physiology*, Butterworth, London.

Petty, T.L. (1982) *Intensive and Rehabilitative Respiratory Care*, Lea and Febiger, Philadelphia

Petty, T.L. and Nett, L.M. (1984) *Enjoying Life with Emphysema*, Lea and Febiger, Philadelphia.

Pilbeam, S.P. (1992) *Mechanical Ventilation*, C.V. Mosby, Missouri.

Prasad, S.A. and Hussey, J. (1995) *Paediatric Respiratory Care*, Chapman & Hall, London.

Pryor, J.A. (ed.) (1991) *Respiratory Care*, Churchill Livingstone, Edinburgh.

Rees, J. and Price, J. (1995) *ABC of Asthma*, BMJ publications, London.

Schechter, L. Berde, C.B. and Yaster, M. (1993) *Pain in Infants, Children and Adolescents*, Williams and Wilkins, Baltimore.

Singleton, M.C. and Branch, E.F. (1990) *Advances in Cardiac and Pulmonary Rehabilitation*, Haworth Press, New York.

Spagnolo, S.V. (1994) *Handbook of Pulmonary Drug Therapy*, Little, Brown, New York.

Sykes, K. (1995) *Respiratory Support*, BMJ publications, London.

Timmons, B.H. and Ley, R. (1994) *Behavioral and Psychological Approaches to Breathing Disorders*, Plenum Press, New York.

Tobin, M.J. (1991) *Respiratory Monitoring*, Churchill, Livingstone, Edinburgh.

Webber, B.A. and Pryor, J.A. (1993) *Physiotherapy for Respiratory and Cardiac Problems*, Churchill Livingstone, Edinburgh.

Weinstock, D. (ed.) (1990) *Normal and Abnormal Breath Sounds*, Springhouse Audio, Pennsylvania (book and tape). ISBN 0–87434–201–5.

Wells, P.E., Frampton, V. and Bowsher, K. (1994) *Pain Management and Control in Physiotherapy*; 2nd edn, Heinemann, London.

West, J.B. (1995) *Respiratory Physiology*, 5th edn, Williams and Wilkins, Baltimore.

White, G.C. (1992) *Equipment Theory for Respiratory Care*, Delmar, New York.

Widdicombe, J. and Davies, A. (1991) *Respiratory Physiology*, Edward Arnold, London.

Wilkins, R.L., Sheldon, R.L. and Krider, S.J. (1995) *Clinical Assessment in Respiratory Care*, C.V. Mosby, Toronto.

Williams, S.J. (1993) *Chronic Respiratory Illness*, Routledge, London.

Zadai, C.C. (1992) *Pulmonary Management in Physical Therapy*, Churchill Livingstone, Edinburgh.

References

AARC (1992) Clinical Practice Guideline: exercise testing for evaluation of hypoxaemia. *Respir. Care*, **37**, 907–12.

AARC (1993a) Clinical Practice Guideline: intermittent positive pressure breathing. *Respir. Care*, **38**, 1189–94.

AARC (1993b) Clinical Practice Guideline: bland aerosol administration. *Respir. Care*, **38**, 1196–9.

AARC (1993c) Clinical Practice Guideline: directed cough. *Respir. Care*, **38**, 495–9.

Abbott, J., Dodd, M., Bilton, D. *et al.* (1994) Treatment compliance in adults with CF. *Thorax*, **49**, 115–20.

Abman, S.H. (1994) Acute effects of inhaled nitric oxide in children with severe hypoxemic respiratory failure. *J. Pediatr.*, **124**, 881–8.

Abu-Saad, H.H. (1994) Pain in children. *Disab. Rehabil.*, **16**, 45–50.

Acosta, F. (1988) Biofeedback and progressive relaxation in weaning the anxious patient. *Heart Lung*, **17**, 299–301.

Agnew, J.E., Vora, H. and Clarke, S.W. (1992) Effect of oral bronchodilator therapy on mucociliary clearance during sleep in asthma. *Am. Rev. Respir. Dis.*, **145**, 2(2), A769.

Ahmedzai, S. (1988) Respiratory distress in the terminally ill patient. *Respir. Dis. Pract.*, **5**(5), 20–6.

Aitkenhead, A.R. (1989) Analgesia and sedation in intensive care. *Br. J. Anaesth.*, **63**, 196–206.

Akyüz, G. (1993) Transcutaneous nerve stimulation in the treatment of pain and prevention of paralytic ileus. *Clin. Rehab.*, **7**, 218–21.

Albelda, M. (1983) Ventilator-induced subpleural air cysts. *Am. Rev. Resp. Dis.*, **127**, 360–5.

Aldrich, T.K. (1993) Intrinsic positive end-expiratory pressure in ambulatory patients with airways obstruction. *Am. Rev. Respir. Dis.*, **147**, 845–49.

Aldrich, T.K. (1989) Weaning from mechanical ventilation. *Crit. Care Med.*, **17**, 143–7.

Alison, J.A., Donnelly, P.M., Lennon, M. *et al.* (1994) The effect of a comprehensive intensive inpatient treatment program on lung function and exercise capacity in patients with CF. *Phys. Ther.*, **74**, 583–93.

Allen, P.W. and Hart, S.M. (1988) Minitracheotomy in children. *Anaesthesia*, **43**, 760–1.

Allen, J.K. (1990) Physical and psychosocial outcomes after coronary artery bypass graft surgery. *Heart Lung*, **19**, 49–54.

Allen, G.M., Hickie, I., Gandevia, S.C. *et al.* (1994) Impaired voluntary drive to breathe: a possible link between depression and unexplained ventilatory failure in asthmatic patients. *Thorax*, **49**, 881–4.

Allison, S.P. (1995) Malnutrition in hospital patients. *Hosp. Update*, **21**, 55–6.

Anand, K.J.S., Sippell, W.G. and Aynsley–Green, A. (1987). Randomised trial of fentanyl anaesthesia in preterm babies. *Lancet*, **1**, 243–7.

Andersen, J.B., Qvist, J. and Kann, T. (1979) Recruiting collapsed lung through collateral channels with PEEP. *Scand. J. Resp. Dis.*, **60**, 260–6.

Andersen, J.B., Oleson, K.P., Eikard, B. *et al.* (1980) Periodic CPAP by mask in the treatment of atelectasis. *Eur. J. Respir. Dis.*, **61**, 20–5.

Andersen, J.B. and Falk, M. (1991) Chest physiotherapy in the pediatric age group. *Respir. Care*, **36**, 546–54.

Anderson, H.L. (1994) Extracorporeal life support for respiratory failure after multiple trauma. *J. Trauma*, **37**, 266–74.

Andréasson, B., Jonson, B., Kornfält, R. *et al.* (1987) Long-term effects of physical exercise on working capacity and pulmonary function in CF. *Acta Paediatr. Scand.*, **76**, 70–5.

Anggärd, E. (1994) Nitric oxide: mediator, murderer, and medicine. *Am. J. Respir. Crit. Care Med.*, **343**, 1199–206.

Anon (1981) Who am I? Where am I? Why do I hurt so much? *Nurs. Times*, **77**(15), 633–5.

Anon (1985) Neonatal intensive care, *Care Crit. Ill*, **1**, 3.

Anon (1992) Maternal smoking increases squint risk in children. *Med. Monitor*, Nov. 27, 33.

Anzueto, A. (1992) Resistive breathing activates the glutathione redox cycle and impairs performance of rat diaphragm. *J. Appl. Phys.*, **72**, 529–34.

Anzueto, A., Tobin, M.J., Moore, G. *et al.* (1987) Effect of prolonged mechanical ventilation on diaphragmatic function. *Am. Rev. Respir. Dis.*, **135**, A201.

Arens, R., Gozal, D., Omlin, K.J. *et al.* (1994) Comparison of high frequency chest compression and conventional chest physiotherapy in hospitalized patients with CF. *Am. J. Respir. Crit. Care Med.*, **150**, 1154–7.

Argyropoulou, P. (1993) Buspirone effect on breathlessness and exercise in patients with COPD. *Respiration*, **60**, 216–20.

Armstrong, R.F., Bullen, C., Cohen, S.L. *et al.* (1991) *Critical Care Algorithms*. Oxford Medical, Oxford.

Armstrong, B.W. (1995) Pressure-controlled inverse ratio ventilation that avoids air trapping in ARDS. *Crit. Care Med.*, **23**, 279–85.

Arts, S.E. (1994) Age-related response to EMLA emulsion and effect of music distraction on pain. *Pediatrics*, **93**, 797–801.

Artucio, H. and Pereira, M. (1990) Cardiac arrhythmias in critically ill patients. *Crit. Care Med.*, **18**, 1383–8.

Ashby, E.C. (1995) Posture, blood velocity in femoral vein and prophylaxis of DVT. *Lancet*, **345**, 419–21.

Austin, J.H.M. and Ausubel, P. (1992) Enhanced respiratory muscular function in normal adults after lessons in proprioceptive musculoskeletal education. *Chest*, **102**, 486–90.

Austin, B. (1993) Study clears nitrous oxide. *Progress Notes*, **5**, 5–6.

Axen, K. (1991) Training for strength and endurance, in *Pulmonary Therapy and Rehabilitation*, (eds F. Haas and K. Axen), Williams and Wilkins, London, pp. 211 and 336.

Babineau, T.J. (1994) Time to consider early gut feeding. *Crit. Care Med.*, **22**, 191–2.

Bach, J.R. (1993) Airway secretion clearance by mechanical exsufflation. *Arch. Phys. Med. Rehab.*, **74**, 170–7.

Bach, J.R. (1994) Update and perspectives on noninvasive respiratory muscle aids. *Chest*, **105**, 1230–40.

Bachrach, L.K., Loutit, C.W. and Moss, R.B. (1994) Osteopenia in adults with cystic fibrosis. *Am. J. Med.*, **96**, 27–34.

Badr, M.S., Grossman, J.E. and Weber, S.A. (1994) Treatment of refractory sleep apnea with supplemental CO_2. *Am. J. Respir. Crit. Care Med.*, **150**, 561–4.

Baldwin, D.R. (1994) Effect of addition of exercise to chest physiotherapy on sputum expectoration and lung function in adults with CF. *Respir. Med.*, **88**, 49–53.

Balfour, C. (1993) Physiotherapists and smoking cessation. *Physiotherapy*, **79**, 247–50.

Ball, P. (1995) Acute infective exacerbations of chronic bronchitis. *Q.J.Med.*, **88**, 61–8.

Banner, A.S. (1994) Theophylline: should we discard an old friend? *Lancet*, **343**, 618.

Bardsley, P.A., Bentley, S., Hall, H.S. *et al.* (1993) Measurement of inspiratory muscle performance with incremental threshold loading. *Thorax*, **40**, 354–9.

Barker, S.J., Clarke, C., Trivedi, N. *et al.* (1993) Anesthesia for thoracoscopic laser ablation of bullous emphysema. *Anesthesiology*, **78**, 44–50.

Barker, D.P. (1995) Exposure to invasive procedures in neonatal ICU admissions. *Arch. Dis. Child.*, **72**, F47–8.

Barnas, G.M., Green, M.D., MacKenzie, C.F. *et al.* (1993) Effect of posture on lung and regional chest wall mechanics. *Anesthesiology*, **78**, 251–9.

Barratt, E. (1989) The management of pressure sores. *Int. Ther. Clin. Monit.*, **10**, 255–9.

Barrett, T.E. (1995) Inhaled β-adrenergic receptor agonists in asthma: more harm than good? *Am. J. Respir. Crit. Care Med.*, **151**, 574–7.

Barrow, P.M., Hughes, D.G., Redfern, N. *et al* (1994) Influence of droperidol on nausea and vomiting during patient-controlled analgesia. *Br. J. Anaesth.*, **72**, 460–1.

Barry, P.W. (1994) Inhaled steroid therapy. *Curr. Paediatr.* **4**, 114–17.

Bartlett, R.H., Gazzaniga, A.B. and Gerachty, T.R. (1973) Respiratory maneuvers to prevent postoperative pulmonary complications. *JAMA*, **224**, 1017–21.

Bartter, T. (1994) The evaluation of pleural effusion. *Chest*, **106**, 1209–14.

Bateman, J.R.M., Newman, S.P., Daunt, K.M. *et al.* (1979) Regional lung clearance of excessive bronchial secretions during chest physiotherapy. *Lancet*, **1**, 294–7.

Bateman, J.R.M., Newman, S.P., Daunt, K.M. *et al.* (1981) Is cough as effective as chest physiotherapy in the removal of excessive tracheobronchial secretions? *Thorax*, **36**, 683–7.

Bauer, M.L., McDougal, J. and Schoumacher, R.A. (1994) Comparison of manual and mechanical chest percussion in hospitalized patients with CF. *J. Pediatr.*, **124**, 250–4.

Baum, G.L. (1990) Mucociliary clearance from central airways in patients with and without primary ciliary dyskinesia. *Chest*, **98**, 608–12.

Baun, M.M. (1984) Cumulative effects of 3 sequential endotracheal suctioning episodes. *Heart Lung*, **13**, 148–54.

Baxter, J.N. (1995) Pathophysiology of laparoscopy. *Br. J. Surg*, **82**, 1–2.

Baxter, K., Nolan, K.M., Winyard, J.A. *et al.* (1993) Are they getting enough? Meeting the oxygen needs of postoperative patients. *Prof. Nurse*, **8**, 310–12.

Bayindir, O. (1991) Use of TENS in the control of postoperative chest pain after cardiac surgery. *J. Cardioth. Vasc. Anaesthesia*, **5**, 589–91.

Bazuaye, E.A., Stone, T.N., Corris, P.A. *et al.* (1992) Variability of inspired oxygen concentration with nasal cannulas. *Thorax*, **47**, 609–11.

Beale R., Grover, E.R., Smithies, M. *et al.* (1993) Acute respiratory distress syndrome *Br. Med. J.*, **307**, 1335–9.

Beck, K.C., Offord, K.P. and Scanlon, P.D. (1994) Bronchoconstriction occurring during exercise in asthmatic subject. *Am. J. Respir. Crit. Care Med.*, **149**, 352–7.

Bégin, P. (1991) Inspiratory muscle dysfunction and chronic hypercapnia in COPD. *Am. Rev. Respir. Dis.*, **143**, 905–12.

Bell, T. (1961) *In the Midst of Life*, Atheneum, New York.

Bellomo, R. (1994) Asthma requiring mechanical ventilation. *Chest*, **105**, 891–6.

Belman, M.J. (1993) Exercise in patients with COPD. *Thorax*, **48**, 936–46.

Belman, M.J., Brooks, L.R., Ross, D.J. *et al.* (1991) Variability of breathlessness measurement in patients with COPD. *Chest*, **99**, 566–71.

Bennett, N.T. (1991) Treatment of status asthmaticus with continuously aerosolized albuterol. *Respir. Care*, **36**, 1323.

Bertone, N. (1988) The role of physiotherapy in a neonatal intensive care unit. *Aust. J. Physiother.*, **34**, 27–34.

Berwick, D.M. (1991) The double edge of knowledge. *J. Am. Med. Ass.*, **266**, 841–2.

Bethune, D.D. (1991) Neurophysiological facilitation of respiration, in *Respiratory Care* (ed. J.A. Pryor), Churchill Livingstone, Edinburgh, pp.121–45.

Beyer, J.E. and Byers, M.L. (1985) Knowledge of paediatric pain. *Children's Health Care*, **13**, 150–9.

Biddle, C. (1992) Transdermal and transmucosal administration of pain-relieving and anxiolytic drugs. *Heart Lung*, **21**, 115–24.

Biley, F.C. (1989) Stress in high dependency units. *Int. Care Nursing*, **5**, 134–41.

Blanckenhagen, J. (1986) Unheard victims of breast cancer. *Independent*, 7 Oct.

BMJ Editorial (1978) Postoperative pain, *Br. Med. J.*, **6136**, 517–18.

Boeck, C.L. and Zinman, R. (1984) Cough versus chest physiotherapy. *Am. Rev. Respir. Dis.*, **129**, 182–4.

Bois, R.M. (1992) Management of fibrosing alveolitis. *Br. J. Hosp. Med.*, **47**, 680–3.

Bolgiano, C.S. (1990) Administering oxygen therapy. *Nursing* 90(20), 47–51.

Bolliger, C.T. and Van Eeden, S.F. (1990) Treatment of multiple rib fractures. *Chest*, **97**, 943–8.

Bond, D.M. (1994) Sustained inflations improve respiratory compliance during high-frequency oscillation. *Crit. Care Med.*, **22**, 1269–77.

Borak, J., Sliwinski, P. and Piasecki, Z. (1991) Psychological status of COPD patients on long term oxygen therapy. *Eur. Respir. J.*, **4**, 59–62.

Borel, C., Hanley, D., Diringer, M.N. *et al.* (1990) Intensive management of severe head injury. *Chest*, **98**, 180–9.

Bortoluzzi, G. (1994) Facing death: a personal perspective. *N.Z. J. Physiother.*, **22**(1), 6–9.

Borzotta, A.P. (1994) Enteral versus parenteral nutrition after severe head injury. *J. Trauma*, **37**, 459–68.

Bostick, J. and Wendelgass, S.T. (1987) Normal saline instillation as part of the suctioning procedure. *Heart Lung*, **16**, 532–6.

Bott, J., Keilty, S.E.J., Brown, A. *et al.* (1992) Nasal intermittent positive pressure ventilation. *Physiotherapy*, **78**, 93–6.

Bott, J., Carroll, M.P., Conway, J.H. *et al.* (1993) Randomised controlled trial of nasal ventilation in acute ventilatory failure due to COAD. *Lancet*, **341**, 1555–7.

Bouley, G.H. (1992) The experience of dyspnea during weaning. *Heart Lung*, **21**, 471–6.

Bower, L.K. (1995) Extracorporeal life support and high-frequency oscillatory ventilation. *Respir. Care*, **40**, 61–73.

Bradley, D. (1994) *Hyperventilation Syndrome*, Kyle Cathie, London.

Bradley, T.D. (1993) Unexpected presentations of sleep apnoea. *Br. Med. J.*, **306**, 1260–2.

Brannon, F.J., Foley, M.W., Starr, J.A. *et al.* (1993) *Cardiopulmonary Rehabilitation: Basic Theory and Application*, F.A. Davis, Philadelphia.

Branson R.D. (1993) The nuts and bolts of increasing oxygenation. *Respir. Care*, **38**, 672–89.

Branson R.D., Davis, K. and Campbell, R.S. (1993) Humidification in the ICU. *Chest*, **104**, 1800–5.

Branthwaite, M.A. (1985) The intensive care of asthma. *Br. J. Hosp. Med.*, **34**, 1–8.

Braun, N.M.T., Faulkner, J., Hughes, R.L. *et al.* (1983) When should respiratory muscles be exercised? *Chest*, **84**(1), 76–84.

Breathnach, A.S., Jenkins, D.R. and Pedler, S.J. (1992) Stethoscopes as possible vectors of infection by staphylococci. *Br. Med. J.*, **305**, 1573–4.

Breslin, E.H. (1992) The pattern of respiratory muscle recruitment during pursed lip breathing. *Chest*, **101**, 75–8.

Breslin, E.H., Garoutte, B.C., Kohlman–Carrieri, V. *et al.* (1990) Correlations between dyspnea, diaphragm and sternomastoid recruitment during inspiratory breathing. *Chest*, **98**, 298–302.

Brett, A. and Sinclair, D.G. (1993) Use of continuous positive airway pressure in the management of community acquired pneumonia. *Thorax*, **48**, 1280–1.

Briars, G. and Warner, J. (1993) Cystic fibrosis. *Practitioner*, **237**, 765–70.

Bright, L.D. (1994) How to protect your patient from DVT. *Am. J. Nurs.*, **94**(12), 28–32.

Britton, S., Bejstedt, M. and Vedin, L. (1985) Chest physiotherapy in primary pneumonia. *Br. Med. J.*, **290**, 1703–4.

Broad, S.H. (1991) An holistic approach to cardiac rehabilitation. *N.Z. J. Physioter*, **19**, 1, 6–10.

Brochard, L., Mion, G., Isabey, D. *et al.* (1991) Constant-flow insufflation prevents arterial oxygen desaturation during suctioning. *Am. Rev. Respir. Dis.*, **144**, 395–400.

Bromley, I. (1985) *Tetraplegia and Paraplegia*, Churchill Livingstone, Edinburgh.

Brooks, D.H.M. (1990) The route to home ventilation. *Care Crit. Ill*, **6**, 96–7.

Brooks-Brunn, J.A. (1995) Postoperative atelectasis and pneumonia. *Heart Lung*, **24**, 94–112.

Broome, M.E. (1990) Preparation of children for painful procedures. *Ped. Nurse*, **16**, 537–41.

Brown, S.E. (1983) Prevention of suction-related arterial oxygen desaturation. *Chest*, **83**, 621–8.

Brown K.K. (1994) Septic shock. *Am. J. Nurs.*, **94** (9) 20–7.

Browning, D. (1992) Treatment of acute severe asthma assisted by hyperthermia. *Anaesthesia*, **47**, 223–5.

Bruera, E., deStoutz, N., Velasco, A. *et al.* (1993) Effects of oxygen on dyspnoea in hypoxaemic terminal cancer patients. *Lancet*, **342**, 13–14.

Brunekreef, B. (1989) Home dampness and respiratory morbidity in children. *Am. Rev. Respir. Dis.*, **140**, 1363–7.

BTS: British Thoracic Society (1990) Guidelines for management of asthma in adults. *Br. Med. J.*, **301**, 797–800.

BTS: British Thoracic Society (1993) Guidelines for management of asthma: a summary. *Br. Med. J.*, **306**, 776–82.

BTS: British Thoracic Society (1994) Guidelines for the measurement of respiratory function. *Resp. Med.*, **88**, 165–94.

Burford, B.W. and Barton, S.J. (1993) Care of the dying patient, in *Physiotherapy for Respiratory and Cardiac Problems* (eds B.A. Webber and J.A. Pryor), Churchill Livingstone, Edinburgh.

Burge, P.S. (1992) Peak flow measurement. *Thorax*, **47**, 903.

Bush, G.H. (1963) Tracheobronchial suction in infants and children. *Br. J. Anaesth.*, **35**, 322–6.

Busse, W.W. (1995) Stress and asthma. *Am. J. Respir. Crit. Care Med*, **151**, 249–52.

Button, B.M., Heine, R.G., Catto, A.G. *et al.* (1994) Postural drainage exacerbates gastroesophageal reflux in patients with lung disease. *Ped. Research*, **36**(1), 2.

Bynum, L.J., Wilson, J.E. and Pierce, A.K. (1976) Comparison of spontaneous and positive-pressure breathing in supine normal subjects. *J. Appl. Physiol.*, **41**, 341–6.

Caldwell, M.T.P. (1993) Timing of extubation after oesophagectomy. *Br. J. Surg.*, **80**, 1537–9.

Callegari, G. (1994) Clinical effects of oscillating positive expiratory pressure. *Respir. Care*, **39**, 1104.

Cameron, I.R. and Bateman, N.T. (1990) *Respiratory Disorders*, Edward Arnold, London, p.75.

Campbell, E.J.M. and Howell, J.B.L. (1963) The sensation of dyspnea. *Br. Med. J.*, **2**, 868.

Campbell, E.J., Baker, M.D. and Crites, P. (1988) Subjective effects of humidification of oxygen for delivery by nasal cannula. *Chest*, **93**, 289–93.

Capen, C.L., Dedlow, E.R., Robillard, R.H. *et al.* (1994) The team approach to pediatric asthma education. *Ped. Nurs.*, **20**, 231–7.

Carmichael, R. (1981) Personal view. *Br. Med. J.*, **282**, 1388.

Carr, L. (1993) Manual therapy for patients with respiratory disease. *ACPRC J.*, **23**, 13–15.

Carr, L. (1994) A study into the effects of self chest clapping on oxygen saturation and patient perception of chest clapping. *ACPRC J.*, **25**, 4?

Carron, H. (1989) Extension of pain relief beyond the operating room. *Clin. J. Pain*, **5**(suppl. 1), S1–S4

Carruthers, D.M. and Harrison, B.D.W. (1995) Arterial blood gas analysis or oxygen saturation in the assessment of acute asthma? *Thorax*, **50**, 186–8.

Carson, M.M. (1994) Managing pain during mediastinal chest tube removal. *Heart Lung*, **23**, 500–5.

Carson, P. (1989) Rehabilitation after myocardial infarction. *Care Crit. Ill*, **5**, 192–4.

Casaburi, R. (1992) Principles of exercise training. *Chest*, **101**, 263S–75.

Cashman, J.N. (1993) Non-steroidal anti-inflammatory drugs versus postoperative pain. *J. Roy. Soc. Med.*, **88**, 464–7.

Castel, O. (1991) Evaluation of closed sterile prefilled humidification. *J. Hosp. Inf*, **17**, 53–9.

Celli, B.R., Rodriguez, K.S. and Snider, G.L. (1984) A controlled trial of IPPB, incentive spirometry and deep breathing exercises after abdominal surgery. *Am. Rev. Respir. Dis.*, **130**, 12–15.

Celli, B.R. (1993) Respiratory muscle strength after upper abdominal surgery. *Thorax*, **48**, 683–4.

Celli, B.R. (1994) Physical reconditioning of patients with respiratory diseases. *Respir. Care.* **39**, 481–99.

Chan, C.S. (1990) Eucapnia and hypercapnia in patients with chronic airflow limitation. *Am. Rev. Respir. Dis.*, **141**, 861–5.

Chang, M.C. (1994) Gastric tonometry supplements information provided by systemic indicators of oxygen transport. *J. Trauma*, **37**, 488–94.

Chang, S.-C., Shiao, G.-M. and Perng, R.-P. (1989) Postural effect on gas exchange in patients with unilateral pleural effusions. *Chest*, **96**, 60–3.

Chaouat, A. (1995) Association of COPD and sleep apnea. *Am. J. Respir. Crit. Care Med.*, **151**, 82–6.

Charbonneau, M. (1994) Changes in obstructive sleep apnea characteristics through the night. *Chest*, **106**, 1695–701.

Charpin, J. and Weibel, M.-A. (1990) Comparative evaluation of the antitussive activity of buta-mirate citrate linctus versus clobutinol syrup. *Respiration*, **57**, 275–9.

Chatburn, R.L. (1991) Principles and practice of neonatal and pediatric mechanical ventilation. *Respir. Care*, **36**, 569–95.

Chatham, K. (1995) Respiratory muscle training. *Br. J. Ther. Rehab.*, **2**(1), 31–6.

Chatham, K., Berrow, S., Beeson, C. *et al.* (1994) Inspiratory pressures in adult cystic fibrosis. *Physiotherapy*, **80**, 748–52.

Chauhan, A.J., Lindon, J.P., Dillon, P. *et al.* (1992) Regular balloon inflation for patients with chronic bronchitis. *Br. Med. J.*, **304**, 1668–9.

Chen, Y., Horne, S.L. and Dosman, J.A. (1993) Body weight and weight gain related to pulmonary function decline. *Thorax*, **48**, 375–80.

Chevrolet, J. (1991) Repeated vital capacity measurements as predictive parameters for mechanical ventilation and weaning in the Guillain–Barré syndrome. *Am. Rev. Respir. Dis.*, **144**, 814–18.

Choiniere, M. (1992) Patient-controlled analgesia in burn patients. *Anaesthesia*, **47**, 467–72.

Chouaid, C., Maillard, D., Housset, B. *et al.*, (1993) Cost effectiveness of noninvasive oxygen saturation measurement during exercise for the diagnosis of pneumocystis carinii pneumonia. *Am. Rev. Respir. Dis.*, **147**, 1360–3.

Christen, W.G. (1992) A prospective study of cigarette smoking and risk of cataract in men. *J. Am. Med. Ass.*, **268**, 989–93.

Christensen, E.F., Nedergaard, T. and Dahl, R. (1990) Long-term treatment of chronic bronchitis with PEP mask and chest physiotherapy. *Chest*, **97**, 645–50.

Christensen, H.R., Simonsen, K., Lange, P. *et al.* (1990) PEEP-masks in patients with severe obstructive pulmonary disease: a negative report. *Eur. Resp. J.*, **3**, 267–72.

Chudley, S. (1994) The effect of nursing activities on ICP. *Br. J. Nurs.*, **3**, 454–9.

Church, S.E. (1991) Bronchoconstricton caused by humidified oxygen in asthmatic patients. *Thorax*, **46**, 4 (abstract).

Ciesla, N.D. (1994) Chest physical therapy for the adult ICU trauma patient. *Phys. Ther. Pract.*, **3**, 92–108.

Clague, J.E. and Calverley, P.M.A. (1990) Management of COPD. *Hosp. Update*, **16**, 20–32.

Clark, K.J. (1985) Coping with Guillain–Barré syndrome. *Int. Care Nurs.*, **1**, 13–18.

Clarke, F. (1993) Terminal care. *Pulse*, Feb 6, 55–61.

Clarke, S.W. (1989) Rationale of airway clearance. *Eur. Respir. J.*, **2** (suppl. 7), 599s–604s.

Clarke, S.W. (1991) Chronic bronchitis in the 1990's. *Respiration*, **58** (suppl), 43–6.

Coates, A.L. (1992) Oxygen therapy, exercise and cystic fibrosis. *Chest*, **101**, 2–4.

Cochrane, G.M. (1995) Acute severe asthma. *Thorax*, **50**, 1–2.

Cochrane, G.M., Webber, B.A. and Clarke, S.W. (1977) Effects of sputum on pulmonary function. *Br. Med. J.*, **2**, 1181–3.

Cochrone, L.M., and Clark, C.J. (1990) Benefits and problems of a physical training programme for asthmatic patients. *Thorax*, **45**, 345–51.

Cockcroft, D.W., McParland, C.P., Britto, S.A. *et al.* (1993) Regular inhaled salbutamol and airway responsiveness to allergen. *Lancet*, **342**, 833–6.

Coffman, J.A. and McManus, K.P. (1984) Oxygen therapy via nasal catheter for infants with BPD. *Crit. Care Nurse*, **4**(3), 22–3.

Coghill, C.H., Haywood, J.L., Chatburn, R.L. *et al.* (1991) Neonatal and pediatric high-frequency ventilation. *Respir. Care*, **36**, 596–603.

Cogswell, J.J. (1994) Epidemiology of asthma. *Current Paed.*, **4**, 139–42.

Cole, J.G., Begish, A., Judas, M.L. *et al.* (1990) Changing the NICU environment. *Neonatal Network*, **9**, 15–23.

Coley, M.C. (1994) Criteria in the selection of organ transplant recipients. *Heart Lung*, **23**, 446–57.

Collins, J. (1976) Blood gases, rational oxygen therapy, air flow limitations. *Physiotherapy*, **62**, 48–52.

Collins, M.A. (1994) When your patient has an implantable cardioverter defibrillator. *Am. J. Nurs.*, **94**, 34–9.

Connors, A.F., Hammon, W.E., Martin, R.J. *et al.* (1980) Chest physical therapy: the immediate effect on oxygenation in acutely ill patients. *Chest*, **78**, 559–64.

Conway, J. (1992a) Chest physiotherapy – the way forward. *Physiotherapy*, **78**, 77–8.

Conway, J. (1992b) The effects of humidification for patients with chronic airways disease. *Physiotherapy*, **78**, 97–101.

Cormier, Y., Laviolette, M., Atton, L. *et al.* (1991) Influence of lung volume on collateral resistance. *Respir. Physiol.*, **83**, 179–88.

Corris, P.A. and Dark, J.H. (1993) Aetiology of asthma. *Lancet*, **341**, 1369–71.

Couriel, J.M. (1994a) Passive smoking and the health of children. *Thorax*, **49**, 731–4.

Couriel, J.M. (1994b) Patient education in childhood asthma. *Curr. Paediatr.*, **4**, 143–5.

Couser, J.I. (1995) Pulmonary rehabilitation improves exercise capacity in older elderly patients with COPD. *Chest*, **107**, 730–4.

Cousins, N. (1981) *Human Options*, W.W. Norton, New York, p. 210.

Cousins, M.J. (1989) Acute pain and the injury response. *Regional Anesth.*, **14**, 162–79.

Cowley, D.S. (1987) Hyperventilation and panic disorder. *Am. J. Med.*, **83**, 929–37.

Cowley, H.C. (1993) Management of liver disease on ICU. *Care Crit. Ill.*, **9**, 122–7.

Craig, D.B. (1981) Postoperative recovery of pulmonary function. *Anesth. Analg.*, **60**, 46–52.

Crane, L. (1994) The effect of exercise training on pulmonary function in persons with quadriplegia. *Paraplegia*, **32**, 435–41.

Crogan, K.J. (1991) Airway foreign body removal with CPT. *Respir. Care*, **36**, 1260

Cross, S. (1994) Asthma and the menstrual cycle. *Nurs. Standard*, **8**, 23–6.

Cupples, S.A. (1991) Effects of timing and reinforcement of pre-operative education for patients having coronary artery bypass graft surgery. *Heart Lung*, **20**, 654–60.

Currie, D.C., Gaskell, M.D., Cole, P.J. *et al.* (1986) Practice, problems and compliance with postural drainage. *Br. J. Dis. Chest*, **80**, 249–53.

Currie, A.E. and Gallagher, P.J. (1988) The pathology of clubbing. *Br. J. Dis. Chest.*, **82**, 382–5.

Curtis, J.R. (1994) Health-related quality of life among patients with COPD. *Thorax*, **49**, 162–70.

Czarnik, R.E., Stone, K.S., Everhart, C.C. *et al.* (1991) Differential effects of continuous versus intermittent suction on tracheal tissue. *Heart Lung*, **20**, 144–51.

Dall, J. (1992) Respiratory inductive plesmygraphy, in *Yearbook of Intensive Care and Emergency Medicine* (ed. J.L. Vincent), Springer-Verlag, Berlin.

Dar, K. (1995) Arterial versus capillary blood sampling. *Br. Med. J.*, **309**, 24–5.

Dargie, H.J. (1994) Diagnosis and management of heart failure. *Br. Med. J.*, **308**, 321–8.

Darin, J. (1982) An evaluation of water-vapor output from 4 brands of unheated prefilled bubble humidifiers. *Respir. Care*, **27**, 41–50.

David, A. (1991) Positive expiratory pressure, in *Respiratory Care* (ed. J.A. Pryor), Churchill Livingstone, Edinburgh, pp. 51–63.

Davies, R.J.O. and Hopkin, J.M. (1989) Nasal oxygen in exacerbations of ventilatory failure. *Br. Med. J.*, **299**, 13 1.

Davies, H., Helms, P. and Gordon, I. (1990) The effect of posture on regional ventilation in children and adults. *Thorax*, **45**, 313–14.

Davies, M.J., Wilson, R.G., Keston, M. *et al.* (1991) An implantable device for long term venous access in chronic lung conditions. *Br. Med. J.*, **302**, 570–1.

Davies, R.J.O. and Stradling, J.R. (1993) Acute effects of obstructive sleep apnoea. *Br. J. Anaesth.*, **71**, 725–9.

Davies, K. (1994) Prevention of pressure sores. *Br. J. Nurs.*, **3**, 1099–104.

Dean, M., Bell, E., Kershaw, C.R., *et al.* (1988) A short exercise and living course for asthmatics. *Br. J. Dis. Chest.*, **82**, 155–61.

Dean, E., and Ross, J. (1992) Mobilization and exercise conditioning, in *Pulmonary Management in Physical Therapy* (ed. C.C. Zadai), Churchill Livingstone, Edinburgh.

Dean, E. (1993) Physiotherapy skills: positioning and mobilization of the patient, in *Physiotherapy for Respiratory and Cardiac Problems* (eds B.A. Webber, and J.A. Pryor), Churchill Livingstone, Edinburgh.

Dean, D. (1994) Oxygen transport: a physiologically-based conceptual framework for the practice of cardiopulmonary physiotherapy. *Physiotherapy*, **80**, 347–54.

Deaves, D.M. (1993) An assessment of the value of asthma education in the prevention of childhood asthma. *J. Adv. Nurs.*, **18**, 354–63.

Dechman, C., Sato, J., Bates, J.H.T. (1993) Effect of pleural effusion on respiratory mechanics and the influence of deep inflation, in dogs. *Eur. Respir. J.*, **6**, 219–24.

Decramer, M. (1989) Effects of hyperinflation on the respiratory muscles. *Eur. Resp. J.*, **2**, 299–302.

DeGuire, S., Gevirtz, R., Kawahara, Y. *et al.* (1992) Hyperventilation syndrome and the assessment of treatment for functional cardiac symptoms. *Am. J. Cardiol.*, **70**, 673–7.

DeHoyos, A. (1995) Haemodynamic effects of CPAP in humans with normal and impaired left ventricular function. *Clin. Sci.*, **88**, 173–8.

Dekker, F.W., Schrier, A.C., Sterk, P.J. *et al.* (1992) Validity of peak expiratory flow measurement in assessing reversibility of airflow obstruction. *Thorax*, **47**, 162–6.

Delk, K.K., Gevirtz, R., Hicks, D.A. *et al.* (1993) The effects of biofeedback retraining on lung function in patients with CF. *Chest*, **105**, 23–8.

Demediuk, B.H., Manning, H., Lilly, J. *et al.* (1992) Dissociation between dyspnea and respiratory effort. *Am. Rev. Respir. Dis.*, **146**, 1222–5.

Dennis, A. (1994) Effects of passive and active smoking on induction of anaesthesia. *Br. J. Anaesth.*, **73**, 450–2.

Dettbarn, C.L. and Davidson, L.J. (1989) Pulmonary complications in the patient with acute head injury. *Heart Lung*, **18**, 583–91.

DeVito, A.J. (1990) Dyspnea during hospitalization for acute phase of illness as recalled by patients with COPD. *Heart Lung*, **19**, 186–91.

DiBenedetto, G., (1990) Effect of amiloride on human bronchial ciliary activity *in vitro*. *Respiration*, **57**, 37–9.

Dickey, J.L. (1989) Postoperative osteopathic manipulation of median sternotomy patients. *J. Am. Osteop. Ass.*, **89**, 1309–22.

Dilworth, J.P. and White, R.J. (1992) Postoperative chest infection after upper abdominal surgery. *Respir. Med.*, **86**, 205–10.

Dobb, G.J. and Coombs, L.J. (1987) Clinical examination of patients in the ICU. *Br. J. Hosp. Med.*, **38**, 102–8.

Dodd, M.E. (1991) Exercise in cystic fibrosis adults, in *Respiratory Care* (ed. J.A. Pryor) Churchill Livingstone, Edinburgh, pp.27–50.

DoII (1994) *The Evolution of Clinical Audit*, Department of Health.

Donahoe, M. and Rogers, R.M. (1990) Nutritional assessment and support in COPD. *Clin. Chest Med.*, **11**, 487–504.

Donahoe, M., Rogers, R.M. and Cottrell, J.J. (1992) Is loss of body weight in COPD patients with emphysema secondary to low tissue oxygenation? *Respiration*, **24** (suppl. 2), 33–9.

Donald, I. (1977) Pain – a patient's view, in *Pain – New Perspectives in Measurement and Management* (ed. A.W. Harcus), Churchill Livingstone, Edinburgh, p.1.

Donchin, Y. (1995) A look into the nature and causes of human errors in the ICU. *Crit. Care Med.*, **23**, 294–300.

Donner, C.F. and Howard, P. (1992) Pulmonary rehabilitation in COPD with recommendations for its use. *Eur. Resp. J.*, **5**, 266–75.

Douglas, N.J. (1993) Nocturnal asthma. *Thorax*, **48**, 100–2.

Downs, J.A. (1989) Endotracheal suction: a method of tracheal washout. *Physiotherapy*, **75**, 454.

Downs, J.A., Edwards, A.D., McCormick, D.C. *et al.* (1991) Effect of intervention on development of hip posture in very preterm babies. *Arch. Dis. Child.*, **66**, 797–801.

Dreher, M.C., Nugent, K. and Hudgins, R. (1994) Prenatal marijuana exposure and neonatal outcomes in Jamaica. *Pediatrics*, **93**, 254–260.

Driscoll, J. (1994) Reflective practice for practise. *Sen. Nurse*, **13**(7), 47–50.

Dulfano, M.J. (1973) Physical properties of sputum. *Am. Rev. Respir. Dis.*, **107**, 130–3.

Dunlevy, C.D. and Tyl, S.E. (1992) The effect of oral versus nasal breathing on oxygen concentrations from nasal cannulas. *Respir. Care*, **37**, 357–60.

Durand, M., Sangha, B. and Cabal, L.A. (1989) Cardiopulmonary and intracranial pressure changes related to endotracheal suctioning in preterm infants. *Crit. Care Med.*, **17**, 506–10.

Duranti, R. (1995) Mechanical loading and control of breathing in patients with severe COPD. *Thorax*, **50**, 127–33.

Durbin, C.G. (1993) Oxygen toxicity in the critically ill patient. *Respir. Care*, **38**, 739–53.

Durbin, C.G. (1994) Monitoring gas exchange. *Respir. Care*, **39**, 123–37.

Eales, C.J., Shapiro, A., Edelman, D. *et al.* (1991) A study to compare the ventilation patterns with intermittent positive pressure breathing to those by deep breathing. *S. Afr. J. Physiother.*, **41**, 63–7.

Eales, C.J., Barker M and Cubberley, N.J. (1995) Evaluation of a single chest physiotherapy treatment to postoperative, mechanically ventilated cardiac surgery patients. *Physiother. Theory Pract.*, **11**, 23–8.

East, T.D. (1993) The magic bullets in the war on ARDS. *Respir. Care*, **38**, 690–704.

Eaton, T.D., Bannister, P., Mulley, G.P. *et al.* (1994) Axillary sweating in clinical assessment of dehydration in ill elderly patients. *Br. Med. J.*, **308**, 1271.

Egbert, L.D., Battit, G.E., Welch, C.E. *et al.* (1964) Reduction of postoperative pain by encouragement and instruction of patients. *N. Engl. J. Med.*, **270**, 825–7.

Eggleston, P.A. (1991) A controlled trial of long term bronchodilator therapy in CF. *Chest*, **99**, 1088–92.

Eid, N. (1991) Chest physiotherapy in review. *Respir. Care*, **36**, 270–82.

Eigen, H., Clark, N.M. and Wolle, J.M. (1987) Clinical-behavioral aspects of CF. *Am. Rev. Respir. Dis.*, **136**, 1509–13.

Eland, J.M. (1985) The role of the nurse in children's pain, in *Perspectives in Pain* (ed. L.A. Copp), Churchill Livingstone, New York.

Elborn, J.S., Johnston, B., Allen, F. *et al.* (1992) Inhaled steroids in patients with bronchiectasis. *Respir. Med.*, **86**, 121–4.

Elliott, M.W., Simonds, A.K., Carroll, M.P. *et al.* (1992) Domiciliary nocturnal NIPPV in hypercapnic respiratory failure due to COLD. *Thorax*, **47**, 542–8.

Elliott, M.W., Aquilina, R., Green, M. *et al.* (1994) A comparison of different modes of noninvasive ventilatory support. *Anaesthesia*, **49**, 279–83.

Ellis, B. (1995) Cardiac transplantation. *Physiotherapy*, **81**, 157–62.

Emergency Care Research Institute (1977) Suction catheters. *Health Devices*, **6**, 132–41.

Empey, D. (1992) International consensus on diagnosis and treatment of asthma. *Resp. Dis. Pract.*, **9**(3), 13–20.

Empey, D. (1993a) Tuberculosis – a killer returns. *Resp. Dis. Pract.*, **10**(1), 4–5.

Empey, D. (1993b) The appliance of science. *Resp. Dis. Pract.*, **10**(3), 4.

Enderby, P. (1995) The effect of dairy products on the viscosity of saliva. *Clin. Rehab*, **9**, 61–4.

Engdahl, O. (1993) Chest radiograph – a poor method for determining the size of a pneumothorax. *Chest*, **103**, 26–9.

Enright, S. (1992) Cardiorespiratory effects of chest physiotherapy. *Intensive Care Britain*, Greycoat, 1 Harley St, London, 118–23.

Epstein, C.D. (1993) Oxygen transport variables in the identification and treatment of tissue hypoxia. *Heart Lung*, **22**, 328–48.

Ernst, E. (1993) Smoking and physical medicine. *Eur. J. Phys. Med. Rehab.*, **3**, 181.

Everard, M.L., Clark, A.R., Milner, A.D. *et al.* (1992) Drug delivery from holding chambers with attached facemask. *Arch. Dis. Child.*, **67**, 580–5.

Everard, M.L., Evans, M. and Milner, A.D. (1994) Is tapping jet nebulisers worthwhile? *Arch. Dis. Child.*, **70**, 538–9.

Everhart, M.A. and Pearlman, R.A. (1990) Stability of patient preferences regarding life-sustaining treatments. *Chest*, **97**, 159–64.

Everly, G.S. (1989). *A Clinical Guide to the Treatment of the Human Stress Response*, Plenum Press, New York.

Fahrenfort, M. (1987) Patient emancipation by health education. *Patient Education Council, USA*, **10**, 25.

Faling, L.J. (1986) Pulmonary rehabilitation – physical modalities. *Clin. Chest Med.*, **7**, 599–618.

Fallowfield, L. (1993) Giving sad and bad news. *Lancet*, **341**, 476–8.

Fanta, C.H. (1992) Emergency management of acute severe asthma. *Respir. Care*, **37**, 551–63.

Fawcett, D.D. (1995) Inhaled anti-inflammatory agents in childhood asthma. *Respir. Care*, **40**, 108–13.

Feldman, Z. (1992) Effect of head elevation on head-injured patients. *J. Neurosurg.*, **76**, 207–11.

Ferguson, J.A. (1992) Pain following coronary artery bypass grafting. *Int. Crit. Care Nurs.*, **8**, 153–62.

Fernandez, E. (1991) Sustained improvement in gas exchange after negative pressure ventilation. *Am. Rev. Respir. Dis.*, **144**, 390–4.

Ferrer, A., Roca, J., Wagner, P.D. *et al.* (1993) Airway obstruction and ventilation perfusion relationships in acute severe asthma. *Am. Rev. Respir. Dis.*, **147**, 579–84.

Fiatarone, M.A. (1994) Exercise training and nutritional supplementation for physical frailty in very elderly people. *N. Engl. J. Med.*, **330**, 1769–75.

Finfer, S.R. and Garrard, C.S. (1993) Ventilatory support in asthma. *Br. J. Hosp. Med.*, **49**, 357–60.

Fiel, S.B. (1993) Clinical management of pulmonary disease in CF. *Lancet*, **341**, 1070–4.

Fink, M.P., Helsmoortel, C.M., Stein, K.L. *et al.* (1990) The efficacy of an oscillating bed in the prevention of lower respiratory tract infection in critically ill victims of blunt trauma. *Chest*, **97**, 132–7.

Fiore, M.C., Kenford, S.L. and Jorenby, D.E. (1994) Two studies of the clinical effectiveness of the nicotine patch with different counselling treatments. *Chest*, **105**, 524–33.

Fiorentini, A. (1992) Potential hazards of tracheobronchial suctioning. *Int. Crit. Care Nurs.*, **8**, 217–26.

Fisher, E.B., Haire-Joshu, K., Morgan, G.D. *et al.* (1990) Smoking and smoking cessation. *Am. Rev. Respir. Dis.*, **142**, 702–20.

Fishman, A.P. (1981) Down with the good lung. *N. Engl. J. Med.*, **304**, 537–8.

Fitting, J.-W. (1992) Nutritional support in chronic obstructive lung disease. *Thorax*, **47**, 141–3.

Fixley, M.S. (1978) Flow dependence of gas distribution and the pattern of inspiratory muscle contraction. *J. Appl. Phys.*, **45**, 733–41.

Flanigan, K.S. (1991) Outcome of a 3-day pulmonary rehabilitation programme. *Respir. Care*, **36**, 1271.

Fletcher, E.C. (1992) A double-blind trial of nocturnal supplemental oxygen for sleep desaturation in patients with COPD. *Am. Rev. Resp. Dis.*, **145**, 1070–6.

Fletcher, E.C. (1994) Controversial indications for long-term oxygen therapy. *Respir. Care*, **39**, 333–41.

Fong, S.L.C. (1994) Compliance among adults with CF. *Ann. Pharmacother.*, **24**, 689–91.

Forbes, C. (1994) Management of deep vein thrombosis. *Practitioner*, **238**, 168–75.

Fourrier, F. (1992) Septic shock, multiple organ failure and DIC. *Chest*, **101**, 816–23.

Fraser, J. and Kerr, J.R. (1993) Psychophysiological effects of back massage on elderly institutionalized patients. *J. Adv. Nurs.*, **18**, 238–45.

Freedberg, P.D., Hoffman, L.A., Light, W.C. *et al.* (1987) Effect of progressive muscle relaxation on asthma. *Heart Lung*, **16**, 24–30.

Freeman, J.A. and Armstrong, I.R. (1994) Pulmonary function tests before and after laparoscopic cholecystectomy. *Anaesthesia*, **49**, 579–82.

Freitag, L., Bremme, J. and Schroer, M. (1989) High frequency oscillation for respiratory physiotherapy. *Br. J. Anaesth.*, **63**, 44S–6S.

Freshman, S. (1993) Hypertonic saline versus mannitol. *J. Trauma*, **35**, 344–8.

Fried, R. (1987) *The Hyperventilation Syndrome*, Johns Hopkins University Press, Baltimore.

Fried, R. (1993) *The Psychology and Physiology of Breathing*, Plenum Press, New York.

Frischer, T. (1995) Variability of peak expiratory flow rate in children. *Thorax*, **50**, 35–9.

Frischknecht, E. (1991) Treatment of bronchial asthma with terbutaline inhaled by conespacer combined with PEP mask. *Chest*, **100**, 317–21.

Froese, A.B. and Bryan, C. (1974) Effects of anesthesia and paralysis on diaphragmatic mechanics in man. *Anesthesiology*, **41**, 242–55.

Frownfelter, D.L. (1987) *Chest Physical Therapy and Pulmonary Rehabilitation*, Year Book Medical Pubishers, Chicago, p.738.

Fulmer, J.D. (1984) ACCP-NHLBI National conference on oxygen therapy. *Chest*, **86**, 234–47.

Gallagher, R. and Trenchard, J. (1986) *Movements of Life*, Redemptionist Publications, Alton.

Gallagher, C.G. (1994) Respiratory steroid myopathy. *Am. J. Respir. Crit. Care Med.*, **150**, 4–6.

Gallego, J. and Perruchet, P. (1991) Effect of practice on the voluntary control of a learned breathing pattern. *Physiol. Behaviour*, **49**, 315–19.

Gandy, A.P. (1968) An attack of tetanus. *Lancet*, **2**, 567–8.

Garden, G.M.F. and Ayres, J.G. (1993) Psychiatric and social aspects of brittle asthma. *Thorax*, **48**, 501–5.

Garradd, J. and Bullock, M. (1986) The effect of respiratory therapy on ICP in ventilated neurosurgical patients. *Aust. J. Physiother.*, **32**, 107–11.

Gelb, A.F., Schein, M. and Kuei, J. (1993) Limited contribution of emphysema in advanced COPD. *Am. Rev. Respir. Dis.*, **147**, 1157–61.

Gersin, K. (1994) The efficacy of sequential compression devices in multiple trauma patients with severe head injury. *J. Trauma*, **37**, 205–8.

Gidding, S. (1994) Active and passive tobacco exposure. *Pediatrics*, **94**, 750–1.

Gilbert, V.E. (1989) Detection of pneumonia by auscultation of the lungs in the lateral decubitus positions. *Am. Rev. Respir. Dis.*, **140**, 1012–16.

Gill, J. and Slater, J. (1991) Building barriers against infection. *Nurs. Times*, **87** (50), 53–4.

Gillespie, D. (1989) Let's listen to the children. *Respir. Dis. Pract.*, **6** (5), 23.

Girard, J.P. and Terki, N. (1994) The Flutter as an adjunct to drug therapy in the management of bronchial asthma. *J. Invest. Allerg. Clin. Immun.*, **4**, 23–7.

Girodo, M., Ekstrand, K.A. and Metivier, G.J. (1992) Deep diaphragmatic breathing for the asthmatic patient. *Arch. Phys. Med. Rehab.*, **73**, 717–20.

Goldhaber, S.Z. and Morpurgo, M. (1992) Diagnosis, treatment and prevention of pulmonary embolism. *JAMA*, **268**, 1727–33.

Golding, J. (1994) The consequences of smoking in pregnancy. *Smoking in Pregnancy Conference*, University of Bristol, Bristol.

Goldman, J.M. (1986) Effect of abdominal binders on breathing in tetraplegic patients. *Thorax*, **41**, 940–5.

Goldman, J.M., Teale, C. and Muers, M.F. (1992) Simplifying the assessment of patients with chronic airflow limitation for home nebulizer therapy. *Respir. Med.*, **86**, 33–8.

Goldstein, R.S. (1993) Ventilatory muscle training. *Thorax*, **48**, 1025–33.

Golster, M. (1995) Blood volume and colloid osmotic pressure. *Crit. Care Med.*, **23**, A88.

Goldstone, J. and Moxham, J. (1991) Weaning from mechanical ventilation. *Thorax*, **48**, 56–62.

Gong, H. (1992) Breathing easy: exercise despite asthma. *Phys. Sports Med.*, **120**, 159–67.

Goodnough, S.K. (1985) The effects of oxygen and hyperinflation on arterial oxygen tension after suction. *Heart Lung*, **14**, 11–17.

Gordon, S. (1994) What's in a name? *J. Emerg. Nurs.*, **20**, 170–1.

Goresky, G.V. (1994) Psychological preparation of children for surgery. *Can. J. Anaesth.*, **41**, 1033–5.

Gosselink, R.A.A.M. (1995) Diaphragmatic breathing reduces efficiency of breathing in patients with COPD. *Am. J. Respir. Crit. Care Med.*, **151**, 1136–42.

Gould, T.H., Crosby, D.L., Harmer, M. *et al.* (1992) Policy for controlling pain after surgery. *Br. Med. J.*, **305**, 1187–93.

Gounden, P. (1993) The effect of posture on pectoralis major and latissimus dorsi in expiration in tetraplegia. *S.A. J. Physiother.*, **49**, 25–7.

Gourlay, G.K. and Boas, R.A. (1992) Fatal outcome with use of rectal morphine for postoperative pain control in an infant. *Br. Med. J.*, **304**, 766–7.

Govan, J.R.W., Brown, P.H., Maddison, J. *et al.* (1993) Evidence for transmission of *Pseudomonas cepacia* by social contact in CF. *Lancet*, **342**, 15–19.

Grace, D. and Orr, D.A. (1993) Continuous spinal anaesthesia in acute respiratory failure. *Anaesthesia*, **48**, 226–8.

Gradwell, G. (1994) Emergency room asthma treatment with PEP. *Resp. Care*, **39**, 1072.

Graff, T.D. and Benson, D.W. (1969) Systemic and pulmonary changes with inhaled humid atmospheres. *Anaesthesiology*, **30**, 199–207.

GRASSIC: Grampian Asthma Study of Integrated Care (1994) Integrated care for asthma. *Br. Med. J.*, **308**, 559–64.

Gray, B.A. and Blalock, J.M. (1991) Interpretation of the alveolar–arterial oxygen difference in patients with hypercapnia. *Am. Rev. Resp. Dis.*, **143**, 4–8.

Gray, J.F., MacIntyre, N.R., Kronenberger, W.G. *et al.* (1990) The effects of bolus normal saline instillation with endotracheal suctioning. *Respir. Care*, **35**, 785–90.

Gray, H.H. (1992) Management of pulmonary embolism. *Thorax*, **47**, 825–32.

Green, M. and Moxham, J. (1993) Respiratory muscles in health and disease, in *Respiratory Medicine: Recent Advances* (ed. P.J. Barnes), Butterworth Heineman, London.

Greenough, A. (1990) Bronchopulmonary dysplasia. *Arch. Dis. Child.*, **65**, 1082–8.

Greenough, A. (1994) Pulse oximetry. *Curr. Paed.*, **4**, 196–9.

Greenwald, B.M. (1993) CPAP to treat profound hypoxaemia associated with acute severe asthma. *Crit. Care Med.*, **21** (suppl.), S154.

Gribbins, H.R. (1993) Management of respiratory failure. *Br. J. Hosp. Med.*, **49**, 461–77.

Groen, J.J. (1979) The psychosomatic theory of bronchial asthma. *Psychother. Psychosom.*, **31**, 38–48.

Gronkiewicz, C.A. (1983) Effect of end-inspiratory pause on pulmonary compliance following endotracheal suctioning. *Am. Rev. Respir. Dis.*, **127**, 147.

Groom, L., Frisch, S.R. and Elliott, M. (1990) Reproducibility and accuracy of pulmonary artery pressure measurement in supine and lateral. *Heart Lung*, **19**, 147–51.

Gross, D. and King, M. (1984) High frequency chest wall compression. *Physiother. Can.*, **36**, 137–9.

Grunberg, G. (1991) Facilitation of mechanical ventilation in status asthmaticus with continuous intravenous thiopental. *Chest*, **99**, 1216–19.

Haake, R., Schlichtig, R., Ulstad, D.R. *et al.* (1987) Barotrauma. *Chest*, **91**, 608–13.

Haas, F. and Axen, K. (1991) *Pulmonary Therapy and Rehabilitation*, Williams and Wilkins, London.

Haas, F. and Haas, S.S. (1990) *The Chronic Bronchitis and Emphysema Handbook*, Wiley, Chichester.

Hall, O. (1984) Physical and social problems of CF in the young adult. *ACPRC Newsletter*, **7**, 29–33.

Hall, P.A. (1995) Parents in the recovery room. *Br. Med. J.*, **310**, 163–4.

Hallsworth, M. (1995) Positioning the pre-term infant. *Paed. Nurs.*, **7**(1), 18–20.

Hammon, W.E., Connors, A.F., McCaffree, D.R. *et al.* (1992) Cardiac arrhythmias during postural drainage and chest percussion of critically patients. *Chest*, **102**, 1836–41.

Hanley, M.V. and Tyler, M.L. (1987) Ineffective airway clearance related to airway infection. *Nurs. Clin. N. Am.*, **22**, 135–49.

Hanning, C.D. (1992) Prolonged oxygen therapy. *Br. J. Anaesth.*, **69**, 115–16.

Hansen, N.C.G. (1994) Orally administered N-acetylcysteine may improve general well-being in patients with mild chronic bronchitis. *Respir. Med.*, **88**, 531–5.

Haponik, E.F. (1992) Smoke inhalation injury. *Respir. Care*, **37**, 609–29.

Harcus, A.W. (1977) *Pain – New Perspectives in Measurement and Management*, Churchill Livingstone, Edinburgh, p. 39.

Hardinge, F.M. (1995) Effects of short term high frequency negative pressure ventilation. *Thorax*, **50**, 44–9.

Hardy, K.A. (1993) Advances in our understanding and care of patients with CF. *Respir. Care*, **38**, 282–9.

Hargreaves, M.R. (1995) Inhaled sodium cromoglycate in ACE-inhitor cough. *Lancet*, **345**, 13–15.

Harrington, G.R. (1993) Noninvasive monitoring. *Am. J. Med.*, **95**, 221–7.

Harris, P. (1989) Are pulmonary haemodynamics of importance to survival in chronic obstructive lung disease? *Eur. Respir. J.*, **2** (suppl.7), 674–7s.

Harris, A. (1991) *Cystic Fibrosis: the Facts*, Oxford University Press, Oxford, p.29.

Harris, D.N.F., Bailey, S.M., Smith, P.L.C. *et al.* (1993) Brain swelling in the first hour after coronary artery bypass surgery. *Lancet*, **342**, 586–7.

Harrison, D.A., Breen, D.P., Harris, N.D. *et al.* (1993) The performance of two intensive care humidifiers at high gas flows. *Anaesthesia*, **48**, 902–5.

Harrison, K.S. and Laube, B.L. (1994) Bronchodilator pretreatment improves aerosol deposition uniformity in HIV-positive patients who cough while inhaling aerosolized pentamidine. *Chest*, **106**, 421–6.

Harvey, C.J. (1995) Effect of a spacer on pulmonary aerosol deposition from a jet nebuliser during mechanical ventilation. *Thorax*, **50**, 50–3.

Hasani, A., Pavia, D., Agnew, J.E. *et al.* (1994) Regional lung clearance during cough and FET. *Thorax*, **49**, 557–61.

Hazinski, M.F. (1984) *Nursing Care of the Critically Ill Child*, C.V. Mosby, Missouri, p.263.

Hayden, R.A. (1993) Trend-spotting with the SvO_2 monitor. *Am. J. Nurs.*, **93**(1), 26–33.

HEA (1995) *Passive Smoking*, Health Education Authority, London.

Hecht, S. (1993) A tobacco-specific carcinogen in the urine of men exposed to cigarette smoke. *N. Engl. J. Med.*, **329**, 1543–6.

Hedbäck, B.E.L., Perk, J., Engwall, J. *et al* (1990) Cardiac rehabilitation after coronary artery bypass grafting. *Arch. Phys. Med. Rehabil.*, **71**, 1069–73.

Heidjra, Y.F. (1994) Effects of body position, hyperinflation and blood gas tensions on maximal respiratory pressures in patients with COPD. *Thorax*, **49**, 453–8.

Heijerman, H.G.M. (1993) Chronic obstructive lung disease and respiratory muscle function. *Respir. Med.*, **87** (suppl.B), 49–51.

Hellman, E.A. (1994) Outpatient cardiac rehabilitation in elderly patients. *Heart Lung*, **23**, 506–12.

Henderson, A. (1994) Chronic respiratory failure. *Practitioner*, **238**, 345–50.

Henke, K.G. (1992) Load compensation and respiratory muscle function during sleep. *J. Appl. Phys.*, **72**, 1221–34.

Herring, D. King, A.I and Connelly, M. (1987) New rehabilitation concepts in management of radical neck dissection syndrome. *Phys. Ther.*, **67**, 1095–9.

Hertanu, J.S. (1986) Cardiac rehabilitation exercise program. *Arch. Phys. Med. Rehab.*, **67**, 431–5.

Hess, D. (1991) Neonatal and pediatric respiratory care. *Respir. Care*, **36**, 489–505.

Hess, D. (1994) Inhaled bronchodilators during mechanical ventilation *Respir. Care*, **39**, 105–21.

Heulitt, M.J. (1995) Acute respiratory distress syndrome in pediatric patients. *Respir. Care*, **40**, 74–85.

Heyland, D.K. (1994) Selective decontamination of the digestive tract. *Chest*, **105**, 1221–9.

Hickey, P.R., Hansen, D.D., Wessel, D.L. *et al.* (1985) Blunting of stress responses in the pulmonary circulation of infants by fentanyl. *Anesth. Analg*, **64**, 1137–42.

Hickling, K.G. (1994) Low mortality in ARDS using permissive hypercapnia. *Crit. Care Med.*, **22**, 1568–78.

Hill, S. (1989) *Family*, Michael Joseph, London.

Hill, N.S. (1994) Use of negative pressure ventilation, rocking beds and pneumobelts. *Respir. Care*, **39**, 532–49.

Hirsch, E. (1991) Work of breathing during CPAP and PSV. *Respir. Care*, **36**, 815–28.

Hirschberg, A.J. (1994) Use of doxapram hydrochloride as an alternative to intubation for COPD patients with hypercapnia. *Ann. Emerg. Med*, **4**, 701–3.

Hodge, D. (1991) Endotracheal suctioning in the infant. *Neonatal Network*, **9**, 7–14.

Hodgkin, J.E. and Petty, T.L. (1987) *Chronic Obstructive Pulmonary Disease*, Saunders, London.

Hodgkin, J.E., (1993) *Pulmonary Rehabilitation: Guidelines to Success*, Butterworth, London.

Hodgkinson, D.W., O'Driscoll, B.R., Driscoll, P.A. *et al.* (1993) Chest radiographs. *Br. Med. J.*, **307**, 1202–6.

Hoffman, L.A. (1994) Novel strategies for delivering oxygen. *Respir. Care*, **39**, 363–77.

Hoffman, G.M. (1995) Airway complications of instrumentation. *Respir. Care*, **40**, 97–107.

Holden, T. (1980) Patiently speaking. *Nurs. Times*, **76**(24), 1035–6.

Holland, L. (1991) Breathlessness, in *Respiratory Care* (ed. J.A. Pryor), Churchill Livingstone, Edinburgh, pp. 5–26.

Holmes, P.W., Barter, C.E. and Piera, R.J. (1992) Chronic persistent cough: use ipratropium bromide in undiagnosed cases following upper respiratory tract infection. *Respir. Med.*, **86**, 425–9.

Holt, W.J. (1995) Pulmonary response to an inhaled bronchodilator in chronically ventilated preterm infants. *Respir. Care*, **40**, 145–51.

Honkavaara, P. (1995) Effect of transdermal hyoscine on nausea and vomiting after surgical correction of prominent ears under general anaesthesia. *Br. J. Anaesth.*, **74**, 647–50.

Horiuchi, K. (1995) Propofol attenuates the metabolic and cardiopulmonary responses to stressful ICU procedures. *Crit. Care Med.*, **23**, A36 (suppl).

Hormann, C. (1994) Effect of kinetic therapy in patients with severe ARDS. *Crit. Care Med.*, **22**, A87.

Horseman, T.O. (1989) Expert systems. *Respir. Care*, **34**, 993–1001.

Hosker, H.S.R. (1995) Assessment and provision of home nebulizers for COPD. *Respir. Med.*, **89**, 47–52.

Howard, F. (1994) Endotracheal suctioning and the neonate. *Paediatr. Nurs.*, **6**(7), 14–17.

Howard–Glenn, L. and Koniak–Griffin, D. (1990) Evaluation of manometer use in mechanical ventilation of infants. *Heart Lung*, **19**, 620–7.

Howes, T.Q., Deane, C.R., Levin, G.E. *et al.* (1995) The effects of oxygen and dopamine on renal and aortic blood flow in COPD. *Am. J. Respir. Crit. Care Med.*, **151**, 378–83.

Hsia, C.C.W. (1993) Respiratory muscle limitation in patients after pneumonectomy. *Am. Rev. Respir. Dis.*, **147**, 744–52.

Hsiang, J. (1993) Paralysis for ICP control in severe head injury. *Crit. Care Med.*, **21**, S236.

Hsieh, A.H., Bishop, M.J., Kubilis, P.S. *et al.* (1992) Pneumonia following closed head injury. *Am. Rev. Respir. Dis,* **146**, 290–4.

Huang, D., Ades, P.A. and Weaver, S. (1990) Cardiac rehospitalizations and costs are reduced following cardiac rehabilitation. *J. Cardiopulmon. Rehab.,* **10**, 108.

Hudes, E.T. (1989) Recovery room oxygenation. *Can. J. Anaesth,* **36**, 20–4.

Hughes, R.L. (1980) Do no harm – cheaply. *Chest,* **77** (5), 582–3.

Hull, C.J. (1988) Control of pain in the perioperative period. *Br. Med. Bull.,* **4**, 341–56.

Hund, E.F. (1993) Intensive management and treatment of severe Guillain–Barré syndrome. *Crit. Care Med.,* **21**, 433–46.

Hung, P. (1992) Pre-operative fasting. *Nurs. Times,* **88** (48), 57–60.

Hurewitz, A.N. (1985) Obesity alters regional ventilation in lateral decubitus position. *J. Appl. Phys.,* **59**, 774–83.

Hussey, J. (1992) Effects of chest physiotherapy for children in intensive care after surgery. *Physiotherapy,* **78**, 109–13.

Hyland, M.E. (1991) The living with asthma questionnaire. *Respir. Med.,* **85** (suppl. B), 13–16.

Ibañez, J., Raurich, J.M., Abinanda, R. *et al.* (1981) The effect of lateral positions on gas exchange in patients with unilateral lung disease during mechanical ventilation. *Int. Care Med.,* **7**, 231–4.

Imai, Y. (1994) Inflammatory chemical mediators during conventional and high frequency oscillatory ventilation. *Am. J. Respir. Crit. Care Med.,* **150**, 1550–4.

Ing, A.J., Meng C., Ngu, M.B. *et al.* (1992) Chronic persistent cough and clearance of esophageal acid. *Chest,* **102**, 1668–71.

Ingram, R.H. (1967) Effect of pursed lips expiration on the pulmonary pressure-flow relationship in obstructive lung disease. *Am. Rev. Resp. Dis.,* **96**, 381–8.

Innocenti, D.M. (1966) Breathing exercises in the treatment of emphysema. *Physiotherapy,* **52**, 437–41.

Innocenti, D.M. (1974) Physiotherapy in the management of acute asthma. *Nurs. Mirror,* **139**, 77–9

Irsfeld, S., Klement, W. and Lipfert, P. (1993) Dermal anaesthesia. *Br. J. Anaesth.* **71**, 375–8.

Isaacs, D. (1995) Bronchiolitis. *Br. Med. J.,* **310**, 4–5.

Isea, J.O. (1993) Controlled trial of a continuous irrigation suction catheter. *Chest,* **103**, 1227–30.

Jack, C.I.A. (1995) Simultaneous tracheal and oesophageal pH measurements in asthmatic patients. *Thorax,* **50**, 201–4.

Jackson, M., Flower, C.D.R. and Shneerson, J.M. (1993) Treatment of symptomatic pulmonary aspergillomas. *Thorax,* **48**, 928–30.

Jacox, A., Carr. D. and Chapman, C.R. (1992) Clinician's quick reference guide to postoperative pain management in adults. *J. Pain Symptom. Manag.,* **7**, 214–28.

Jacques, A. (1994) Epidural analgesia. *Br. J. Nurs.,* **3**, 734–8.

Jalleh, R., Fitzpatrick, M.F., Jan, M.A. *et al.,* (1993) Alcohol and cor pulmonale in chronic bronchitis and emphysema. *Br. Med. J.,* **306**, 374.

James, I. (1991) Respiratory management in paediatrics. *Care Crit. Ill,* **7**, 47–50.

James, P.B., Scott, B. and Allen, M.W. (1993) Hyperbaric oxygen therapy in sports injuries. *Physiotherapy,* **79**, 571–2.

Jarvis, M.J. (1986) Low cost carbon monoxide monitor in smoking assessment. *Thorax,* **41**, 886–7.

Jederlinic, P., Muspratt, J.A. and Miller, M.J. (1984) Inspiratory muscle training in clinical practice. *Chest,* **86**, 870–3.

Jenkins, S.C., Soutar, S.A. and Moxham, J. (1988) The effects of posture on lung volumes in normal subjects and in patients pre- and post-coronary artery surgery. *Physiotherapy,* **74**, 492–6.

Jenkins, S.C. and Moxham, J. (1991) The effects of mild obesity on lung function. *Respir. Med.,* **85**, 309–11.

Jette, A.M. (1993) Tobacco use; a modifiable risk factor for dental disease among the elderly. *Am. J. Public Health,* **83**, 1271–4.

Jindani, A. (1993) Postoperative cardiac surgical care. *Br. Heart. J.,* **69**, 59–64.

Jobst, K., McPherson, K., Brown, V. *et al.* (1986) Controlled trial of acupuncture for disabling breathlessness. *Lancet,* **2**, 1416–18.

Johnson, K.L. (1994) Closed versus open endotracheal suctioning. *Crit. Care Med.,* **22**, 658–66.

Johnston, T.D. (1993) Lung injury from gut ischemia. *J. Trauma,* **5**, 508–11.

Johnstone, M. (1994) Children visiting members of their family receiving treatment in ICUs. *Int. Crit. Care Nurs.,* **10**, 289–92.

Jones, P.D.E. (1992) Depression of salivary epidermal growth factor by smoking. *Br. Med. J.,* **304**, 480–1.

Jones, A. and Bowen, M. (1994) Screening for childhood asthma using an exercise test. *Br. J. Gen. Pract.,* **44**, 127–31.

Jones, A. (1994) An introduction to meta-analysis. *Respir. Care,* **39**, 34–48.

Jones, A. (1995) A brief overview of the analysis of lung sounds. *Physiotherapy,* **81**, 37–42.

Jubran, A. (1994) Use of flow-volume curves in detecting secretions in ventilator-dependent patients. *Am. J. Respir. Crit. Care Med.*, **150**, 766–9.

Judson, M.A. (1994) Mobilization of secretions in ICU patients. *Respir. Care*, **39**, 213–25.

Jung, R.C. and Gottleib, L.S. (1976) Comparison of tracheobronchial suction catheters in humans. *Chest*, **69**, 179–81.

Juniper, E.F. (1993) Measuring quality of life in asthma. *Am. Rev. Respir. Dis.*, **147**, 832–8.

Justins, D.M. and Richardson, P.H. (1991) Clinical management of acute pain. *Br. Med. Bull.*, **47**, 561–83.

Kacmarek, R.M. and Hess, D. (1991) The interface between patient and aerosol generator. *Respir. Care*, **36**, 952–73.

Kallenbach, J.M., Frankel, A.H., Lapinsky, S.E. *et al.* (1993) Determinants of near fatality in acute severe asthma. *Am. J. Med.*, **95**, 265–72.

Kam, A.C., O'Brien, M., and Kam, P.C.A. (1993) Pleural drainage systems. *Anaesthesia*, **48**, 154–61.

Kam, P.C.A. (1994) Noise pollution in the anaesthetic and intensive care environment. *Anaesthesia*, **49**, 982–6.

Kang, B. (1974) Evaluation of postural drainage with percussion in COLD. *J. All. Clin. Immunol.*, **53**, 109 (abstract).

Kaplan, D.K. (1994) Treatment of empyema thoracis. *Thorax*, **49**, 845–6.

Karper, W.B. and Boschen, M.B. (1993) Effects of exercise on acute respiratory tract infections and related symptoms. *Geriat. Nurs.* **14**, 15–18.

Kass, J.E. (1995) Heliox therapy in acute severe asthma. *Chest*, **107**, 757–60.

Katz, J., Clairoux, M. and Kavanagh, B.P. (1994) Preemptive lumber epidural anaesthesia reduces postoperative pain. *Pain*, **59**, 395–403.

Kauffmann, (1993) The ageing lung. *Respir. Med.*, **87**, 5–7.

Kavanagh, B.P. (1994) Pain control after thoracic surgery. *Anesthesiology*, **81**, 737–59.

Kawagoe, Y. (1994) Hyperinflation with intrinsic PEEP. *J. Appl. Phys.*, **77**, 2440–8.

Keeley, D. (1994) Managing elderly patients with asthma in general practice. *Care of Elderly*, **6**, 289.

Keilty, S.E.J. and Bott, J. (1992) Continuous positive airways pressure. *Physiotherapy*, **78**, 90–2.

Keilty, S.E.J. (1993) Inhalation burn injured patients and physiotherapy management. *Physiotherapy*, **79**, 87–90.

Keilty, S.E.J. (1994) Effect of inspiratory pressure support on exercise tolerance and breathlessness in patients with severe stable COPD. *Thorax*, **49**, 990–4.

Kellner, R., Samet, J. and Pathak, D. (1992) Dyspnea, anxiety and depression in chronic respiratory impairment. *Gen. Hosp. Psychiatry*, **14**, 20–8.

Kemper, M.S. (1992) The effect of increasing mechanical ventilation during chest physical therapy. *Respir. Care*, **37**, 1313.

Kemper, M. (1993) The effects of adding pressure support during chest physical therapy. *Respir. Care*, **38**, 1245.

Kennedy, L. (1994) Talc pleurodesis for the treatment of pneumothorax and pleural effusion. *Chest*, **106**, 1215–20.

Khajotia, R.R. (1991) Induced sputum and cytological diagnosis of lung cancer. *Lancet*, **338**, 976–7.

Kikuchi, R., Watabe N., Konno, T. *et al.* (1994) High incidence of silent aspiration in elderly patients with community-acquired pneumonia. *Am. J. Respir. Crit. Care Med*, **150**, 251–3.

Killian, K.J. (1992) Exercise capacity and ventilatory, circulatory and symptom limitation in patients with chronic airflow limitation. *Am. Rev. Resp. Dis.*, **146**, 935–40.

Kimmel, P.L., Miller, G., Washington, W.B. *et al.* (1989) Sleep apnoea syndrome in chronic renal disease. *Am. J. Med.*, **86**, 308–14.

King, J.C. and Nixon, P.G.F. (1988) A system of cardiac rehabilitation: psychophysiological basis and practice. *Br. J. Occup. Ther.*, **51**, 378–83.

King, D. and Morrell, A. (1992) A survey on manual hyperinflation as a physiotherapy technique in intensive care units. *Physiotherapy*, **78**, 747–50.

King, T.K. and Simon, R.H. (1987) Pulse oximetry for tapering supplemental oxygen in hospitalized patients. *Chest*, **92**, 713–16.

Kinsella, J., Carter, R., Reid, W.H. *et al.* (1991) Increased airways reactivity after smoke inhalation. *Lancet*, **337**, 595–6.

Kinsman, R.A., Yaroush, R.A., Fernandez, E. *et al.* (1983) Symptoms and experiences in chronic bronchitis and emphysema. *Chest*, **83**, 755–61.

Kleiber, C., Krutzfield, N. and Rose, E.F. (1988) Acute histologic changes in the tracheobronchial tree associated with different suction catheter insertion techniques. *Heart Lung*, **17**, 10–14.

Klein, P., Kemper, M., Weissman, C. *et al.* (1988) Attenuation of the hemodynamic responses to chest physical therapy. *Chest*, **93**, 38–42.

Klingstedt, C., Hedenstierna, G., Lundquist, H., *et al.* (1991) The influence of body position and differential ventilation on lung dimensions and atelectasis. *Respir. Care*, **36**, 12.

Kollef, M.H. (1994) Antibiotic use and resistance in the ICU. *Heart Lung*, **23**, 363–7.

Koltyn, K.F. and Morgan, W.P. (1992) Efficacy of perceptual versus heart rate monitoring in the development of endurance. *Br. J. Sp. Med.*, **26**, 132–4.

Konstan, M.W., Vargo, K.M. and Davis, P.B. (1990) Ibuprofen attenuates the inflammatory response in a rat model of chronic pulmonary infection. *Am. Rev. Respir. Dis.*, **141**, 186–92.

Konstan, M.W. (1994) Efficacy of the flutter device for airway mucus clearance in patients with CF. *J. Pediatr.*, **124**, 689–93.

Koretz, R.L. (1995) Nutritional supplementation in the ICU. *Am. J. Respir. Crit. Care Med.*, **151**, 570–3.

Kraft, A.R. (1984) The hyperventilation syndrome. *Br. J. Psych.*, **145**, 538–42.

Kramer, M.R. (1994) Bronchiolitis obliterans following heart–lung and lung transplantation. *Respir. Med.*, **88**, 9–15.

Kripke, B.J., Justice, R.E. and Hechtman, H.B. (1983) Postoperative nitrous oxide analgesia and the FRC. *Crit. Care Med.*, **11**, 105–9.

Kübler-Ross, E. (1973) *On Death and Dying*, Tavistock, London.

Kuo, C.-D., Shiao, G.-M. and Lee, J.-D. (1993) The effects of high-fat and high-carbohydrate diet loads on gas exchange and ventilation in COPD patients and normal subjects. *Chest*, **104**, 189–96.

Kuwahira, I. (1993) Changes in regional blood flow distribution and oxygen supply during hypoxia in conscious rats. *J. Appl. Phys.*, **74**, 211–14.

Lamm, W. (1994) Mechanism by which the prone position improves oxygenation in acute lung injury. *Am. J. Respir. Crit Care Med.*, **150**, 184–93.

Lancet editorial (1992) Pacifiers, passive behaviour and pain. *Lancet*, **339**, 275–6.

Landa, J.F., Kwoka, M.A., Chapman, G.A. *et al.* (1980) Effects of suctioning on mucociliary transport. *Chest*, **77**, 202.

Landau, L.I. and Geelhoed, G.C. (1994) Aerosolized steroids for croup. *New. Eng. J. Med.*, **331**, 322–3.

Lander, J. (1993) TENS for children's procedural pain. *Pain*, **52**, 209–16.

Lane, D.J. (1991) Chronic persistent asthma. *Respir. Med.*, **85**, 359–63.

Lane, D.J. and Lane, T.V. (1991) Alternative and complementary medicine for asthma. *Thorax*, **46**, 787–97.

Lang, C. (1991) Using relaxation and exercise for people living with HIV/AIDS. *Physiotherapy*, **79**, 379–84.

Lannefors, L. (1992) Mucus clearance with three chest physiotherapy regimes in CF. *Eur. Respir. J.*, **5**, 748–53.

Lapidus, R., Kintzel, J.S. and Courtright, T.M. (1993) Non-invasive mask ventilation as an alternative to intubation. *Respir. Care*, **38**, 1221.

Lavie, C.J., Milani, R.V., Squires, R.W. *et al.* (1992) Exercise and the heart. *Postgrad. Med.*, **91**, 130–50.

Lavies, N. (1992) Identification of patient, medical and nursing staff attitudes to postoperative opioid analgesia. *Pain*, **48**, 313–19.

Lawler, K. (1995) Entonox: too useful to be limited to childbirth? *Prof. Care Mother Child*, **5**(1), 19–21.

Lawrence, G. (1995) Asthma self-management programs can reduce the need for hospital-based care. *Respir. Care*, **40**, 39–43.

Laws, A.K. and McIntyre, R.W. (1969) Chest physiotherapy: a physiological assessment during IPPV in respiratory failure. *Can. Anaes. Soc. J.*, **16**, 487–92.

Leach, C.L. (1993) Perfluorocarbon-associated gas exchange. *Crit. Care Med.*, **21**, 1270–8.

Leach, R.M. and Bateman, N.T. (1993) Acute oxygen therapy. *Br. J. Hosp. Med.* **49**, 637–44.

Leach, R.M. and Bateman, N.T. (1994) Domiciliary oxygen therapy. *Br. J. Hosp. Med.*, **51**, 47–54.

Lee, S.-T. (1989) Intracranial pressure changes during positioning of patients with severe head injury. *Heart Lung*, **18**, 411–14.

Lehrer, P.M., Hochron, S.M., McCann, B. *et al.* (1986) Relaxation decreases large-airway but not small-airway asthma. *J. Psychosom. Res.*, **30**, 13–25.

Levine, S. (1988) *Who Dies?*, Gateway, Bath, p.134.

Levy, M. and Bell, L. (1984) General practice audit of asthma in childhood. *Br. Med. J.*, **289**, 1115–18.

Lewandowski, K. (1992) Approaches to improve survival in severe ARDS, in *Yearbook of Intensive Care and Emergency Medicine* (ed. J.L. Vincent), Springer-Verlag, Berlin.

Lewis, R.A. (1985) Fractional deposition from a jet nebuliser. *Br. J. Dis. Chest*, **79**, 361–6.

Lewith, G.T. (1995) Asthma: complementary approaches. *Update*, **50**, 371–5.

Light, R.W. (1989) Effects of oral morphine on breathlessness and exercise tolerance in patients with COPD. *Am. Rev. Respir. Dis.*, **139**, 126–33.

Light, R.W. (1993) Management of spontaneous pneumothorax. *Am. Rev. Respir. Dis.*, **148**, 245–8.

Lim, T.K., Ang, S.M., Rossing, T.H. *et al.* (1989) The effects of deep inhalation on maximal expiratory flow during spontaneous asthmatic episodes. *Am. Rev. Respir. Dis.*, **140**, 340–3.

Lindeman, C.A. (1971) Nursing intervention with the presurgical patient. *Nurs. Res.*, **20**, 319–32.

Lingnau, W. (1995) Continuous hemofiltration improves multiple organ failure outcome. *Crit. Care Med.*, **23**, A106.

Link, W.J., Spaeth, E.E., Wahle, W.M. *et al.* (1976) The influence of suction catheter tip design on tracheobronchial trauma and fluid aspiration. *Anesth. Analg.*, **55**, 290–7.

Linsenbardt, S.T., Thomas, T.R. and Madsen, R.W. (1992) Effect of breathing techniques on blood pressure response to resistance exercies. *Br. J. Sp. Med.*, **26**, 97–100.

Liposky, J. M. (1994) Ventilatory response to high calorie loads. *Crit. Care Med.*, **22**, 796–802.

Lipworth, B.J. (1995) New perspectives on inhaled drug delivery. *Thorax*, **50**, 105–10.

Liu, R. (1994) Effects of background stress and anxiety on postoperative recovery. *Anaesthesia*, **49**, 382–6.

Loffert, D.T. (1994) A comparison of commercial jet nebulizers. *Chest*, **106**, 1788–93.

Lomholt, N. (1982a) The new NL tracheal suction catheter. *Acta Anaesth. Scand.*, **26**, 4–8.

Lomholt, N. (1982b) Design and function of tracheal suction catheters. *Acta Anaesth. Scand.*, **26**, 1–3.

Lowell, J.A. (1990) Postoperative fluid overload. *Crit. Care Med.*, **18**, 728–33.

Luce, J.M., Tyler, M.T. and Pierson D.J. (1984) *Inten. Respir. Care*, W.B. Saunders, London.

Ludington, S.M. (1990) Energy conservation during skin-to-skin contact between infants and mothers. *Heart Lung*, **19**, 445–51.

Ludwig, C. (1984) When you learn that you are a myasthenic. *Remedial Therapist*, Feb. 24, 8.

Lynch, J.J. (1978) The simple art of touching. *Nursing*, **8**, 32–6.

MacDougald, I. (1994) Laser therapy for OSA. *Nurs. Times*, **90**(19), 32–4.

MacKay, L.E. (1992) Early intervention in severe head injury. *Arch. Phys. Med. Rehab.*, **73**, 635–41.

MacKay–Lyons, M. (1994) Shoulder pain in patients with acute quadriplegia. *Physiother. Can.*, **46**, 255–8.

MacKellaig, J.M. (1990) A review of the psychological effects of intensive care on the isolated patient and family. *Care Crit. Ill.*, **6**, 100–2.

MacKenzie, C.F. and Shin, B. (1985) Cardiorespiratory function before and after chest physiotherapy in mechanically ventilated patients. *Crit. Care Med.*, **13**, 483–6.

Macklem, P.T. and Eidelman, D. (1990) Reexamination of the elastic properties of emphysematous lungs. *Respiration*, **57**, 187–92.

Mador, M.J. (1991) Respiratory muscle fatigue and breathing pattern. *Chest*, **100**, 1430–5.

Mador, M.J. (1992) Weaning parameters. *Chest*, **102**, 1642–3.

Magarian, G.J. (1982) Hyperventilation syndromes. *Medicine*, **61**, 219–35.

Mahler, D.A. (1995) Changes in dyspnea, health status and lung function in chronic airway disease. *Am. J. Respir. Crit. Care Med.*, **151**, 61–5.

Main, P. (1993) Prescribing in terminal illness. *Practitioner*, **237**, 361–4.

Mainous, M.R. and Deitch, E.A. (1994) Nutrition and infection. *Surg. Clin. N. Am.*, **74**, 659–76.

Majid, A.A. (1992) Pain control after thoracotomy. *Chest*, **101**, 981–4.

Mak, V.H.F., Bugler, J.R., Roberts, C.M. *et al.* (1993) Effect of arterial desaturation on 6-minute walk, effort and breathlessness in patients with airflow limitation. *Thorax*, **48**, 33–8.

Make, B.M. (1994) Collaborative self-management strategies for patients with respiratory disease. *Respir. Care*, **39**, 566–77.

Mann, N.P. (1986) Effect of night and day on preterm infants. *Br. Med. J.*, **293**, 1265–7.

Manne, S.L., Jacobsen, P.B. and Redd, W.H. (1992) Assessment of acute pediatric pain. *Pain*, **48**, 45–52.

Manthous, C.A. (1994) Administration of therapeutic aerosols to mechanically ventilated patients. *Chest*, **106**, 560–71.

Manthous, C.A. (1995) The effect of mechanical ventilation on oxygen consumption in critically ill patients. *Am. Rev. Respir. Dis.*, **151**, 210–14.

Manzano, J.L. (1993) Verbal communication of ventilator-dependent patients. *Crit. Care Med.*, **21**, 512–17.

Marcus, C.L. (1992) Supplemental oxygen and exercise performance in patients with CF. *Chest*, **101**, 52–7.

Marini, F.J., Tyler, M.L., Hudson, L.D. *et al.* (1984) Influence of head-dependent positions on lung volume and oxygen saturation in chronic air-flow limitation. *Am. Rev. Respir. Dis.*, **129**, 101–5.

Marino, J. (1995) Neuromuscular blockade in the ICU. *Crit. Care Med*, **23**, A240.

Marsh, B. (1986) A second chance. *Br. Med. J.*, **292**, 675–6.

Marshall, P. (1991) TENS in chronic angina. *Prof. Nurse*, **7**, 20–2.

Martin, C.J., Ripley H., Reynolds, J. *et al.* (1976) Chest physiotherapy and the distribution of ventilation. *Chest*, **69**, 174–8.

Martin, L. (1990) How much reduced haemoglobin is necessary to generate central cyanosis? *Chest*, **97**, 182–4.

Martin, T.J. (1995) Noninvasive BiPAP to prevent endotracheal intubation in acute respiratory failure. *Crit. Care. Med.*, **23**, A129.

Martinez, F. (1994) Increased resistance of hygroscopic condenser humidifiers when using closed circuit suction. *Crit. Care Med.*, **22**, 1668–73.

Martinez, F., Epstein, S., Roe, J. *et al.* (1991) Determinants of respiratory muscle strength in CAO. *Am. Rev. Respir. Dis.*, **143**(4), A161.

Mathewson, H.S. (1993) Combined drug therapy in asthma. *Respir. Care*, **38**, 1340.

McCaffery, M. and Ferrell, B.R. (1992) Does the gender gap affect your pain control decisions? *Nursing*, **92**(22), 49–51.

McCarren, B. (1992) Dynamic pulmonary hyperinflation. *Austr. Physiother. J.*, **38**, 175–9.

McConnochie, K. and Chatham, K. (1991) Double blind controlled study of inspiratory muscle training. *Thorax*, **46**, 755P.

McEvoy, R.D., Davies, J.H., Hedenstierna, G. *et al.* (1982) Lung mucociliary transport during high-frequency ventilation. *Am. Rev. Respir. Dis.*, **126**, 452–6.

McGowan, H. (1994) Siblings and death. *Paed. Nurs.*, **6**(5), 10–13.

McIlwaine, M., Davidson, A.G.F., Wong, L.T.K. *et al.* (1991) The effect of chest physiotherapy by postural drainage and autogenic drainage on oxygen saturation in CF. *Pediatr. Pulmonol.*, **6**, 291.

McIntosh, A. (1989) Sleep deprivation in critically ill patients. *Nursing*, **3**, 44–5.

McIntosh, N., Van Veen, L. and Brameyer, H. (1993) The pain of heelprick and its measurement in preterm infants. *Pain*, **52**, 71–4.

McKenzie, D.K. (1994) Dynamic changes in the zone of apposition and diaphragm length during maximal respiratory efforts. *Thorax*, **49**, 634–8.

McLaren, P. (1991) The right to know. *Br. Med. J.*, **303**, 937–8.

McMichan, J.C., Michel, L. and Westbrook, P.R. (1980) Pulmonary dysfunction following traumatic quadriplegia. *JAMA*, **243**, 528–9.

McMillan, C. (1994) Transcutaneous electrical stimulation of anti-emetic acupuncture point in controlling sickness. *Physiotherapy*, **80**, 5–9.

McNamara, R.M. (1992) Utility of the peak expiratory flow rate in the differentiation of acute dyspnea. *Chest*, **101**, 129–32.

Melendez, J.A. (1992) Postthoracotomy respiratory muscle mechanics during incentive spirometry. *Chest*, **101**, 432–6.

Mellins, R.B., Zimmerman, B and Clark, N.M. (1992) Patient compliance. *Am. Rev. Respir. Dis.*, **146**, 1376–7.

Menier, R.J. (1994) Benefits of a multidisciplinary pulmonary rehabilitation program [letter]. *Chest*, **105**, 640–1.

Menkes, H. and Britt, J. (1980) Rationale for physical therapy. *Am. Rev. Respir. Dis.*, **122**, 127–32.

Mezzanotte, W.S. (1994) Nocturnal nasal CPAP in patients with COPD. *Chest*, **106**, 1100–8.

Michie, J. (1994) An introduction to lung cancer. *Physiotherapy*, **80**, 844–7.

Middleton, P.G., Geddes, D.M. and Alton, E.W.F.W. (1993) Effect of amiloride and saline on nasal mucociliary clearance in CF. *Thorax*, **48**, 812–16.

Mier, A., Laroche, C. and Agnew, J.E. (1990) Tracheobronchial clearance in patients with bilateral diaphragmatic weakness. *Am. Rev. Respir. Dis.* **142**, 545–8.

Mihm, F.G. (1989) Recovery of cardiopulmonary reflexes in monkeys undergoing heart lung transplantion. *J.Thorac. Card. Surg.*, **98**, 510–16.

Miles, J. and Ayres, J. (1993) Gastro-oesophageal reflux and asthma. *Respir. Dis. Pract.*, **10**(3), 18–21.

Miljeteig, H. and Hoffstein, V. (1993) Determinants of continuous positive airway pressure levels for treatment of OSA. *Am. Rev. Respir. Dis.*, **147**, 1526–30.

Miller, K.M. and Perry, P.A. (1990) Relaxation techniques and postoperative pain in patients undergoing cardiac surgery. *Heart Lung*, **19**, 136–46.

Miller, R.F. and Semple, S.J.G. (1991) Continuous positive airways pressure for pneumocystis carinii pneumonia. *Respir. Med.*, **85**, 133–8.

Miller, R.F., Kocjan, G., Buckland, J. *et al.* (1991) Sputum induction for diagnosis of pulmonary disease in HIV-positive patients. *J. Inf.*, **23**, 5–15.

Miller, R.F., Tomlinson, M.C., Cottrill, C.P. *et al.* (1992) Bronchopulmonary Kaposi's sarcoma in patients with AIDS. *Thorax*, **47**, 721–5.

Miller, S., Hall, D.O., Clayton, C.B. *et al.* (1995) Chest physiotherapy in cystic fibrosis. *Thorax*, **50**, 165–9.

Milner, A.D. and Murray, M. (1989) Acute bronchiolitis in infancy. *Thorax*, **44**, 1–5.

Milner, E.A. (1994) A longitudinal study of resting energy expenditure in thermally injured patients. *J. Trauma*, **37**, 167–70.

Mitchell, L. (1987) *Simple Relaxation*, John Murray, London.

Mitchell, P.H. and Mauss, N.K. (1978) Relationship of patient–nurse activity to ICP variations. *Nurs. Res.*, **27**, 4–10.

Mitchell, P.H., Ozuna, J. and Lipe, H.P. (1981) Moving the patient in bed: effects on ICP. *Nurs. Res.*, **30**, 212–18.

Mogan, J., Wells, N. and Robertson, E. (1985) Effects of preoperative teaching on postoperative pain. *Int. J. Nurs. Studies*, **22**, 267–85.

Mohsenifar, Z., Horak, D., Brown, H.V. *et al.* (1983) Sensitive indices of improvement in a pulmonary rehabilitation program. *Chest*, **83**, 189–92.

Mohsenin, V. (1994) Daytime oxygen saturation does not predict nocturnal desaturation in patients with COPD. *Arch. Phys. Med. Rehab.*, **75**, 285–9.

Moinard, J. (1994) Effect of inhaled nitric oxide on hemodynamics and $\dot{V}_A/\dot{Q}$ inequalities in patients with COPD. *Am. J. Respir. Crit. Care Med.*, **149**, 1482–7.

Moore, F.D. (1994) The effect of length of stay on complications. *Ann. Surg*, **220**, 738–9.

Morgan, A.D., Peck, D.F., Buchanan, D.R. *et al.*

(1983) Effect of attitudes and beliefs on exercise tolerance in chronic bronchitis. *Br. Med. J.*, **286**, 171–3.

Morgan, M.D.L. (1992) Detection and quantification of pulmonary emphysema by computed tomography. *Thorax*, **47**, 1001–4.

Morrell, N.W. (1994) Collateral ventilation and gas exchange in emphysema. *Am. J. Respir. Crit. Care Med.*, **150**, 635–41.

Morrison, J.B. (1988a) Chronic asthma and improvement with relaxation induced by hypnotherapy. *J. Roy. Soc. Med.*, **81**, 701–4.

Morrison, S.A. (1988b) Biofeedback to facilitate unassisted ventilation in individuals with high-level quadriplegia. *Phys. Ther.*, **68**, 1378–80.

Mortensen, J., Falk, M., Groth, S. *et al.* (1991) The effects of postural drainage and PEP in cystic fibrosis. *Chest*, **100**, 1350–7.

Moseley, A.M. (1993) The effect of a regimen of casting and prolonged stretching in traumatic head-injured adults. *Physiother. Theory Pract.*, **9**, 215–21.

Moser, K.M., Ries, A.L. and Sassi–Dambron, D.E. (1991) *Shortness of Breath: A Guide to Better Living and Breathing*, 4th edn, C.V. Mosby, Missouri, p. 82.

Moss, E. and McDowall, D.G. (1979) ICP increases with 50% nitrous oxide in severe head injuries. *Br. J. Anaesth.*, **51**, 757–60.

Moxham, J. (1993) Diaphragmatic pacing. *Am. Rev. Respir. Dis.*, **148**, 533–6.

Muers, M. (1993) Understanding breathlessness. *Lancet*, **342**, 1190–1.

Muir, J.-F. (1993) Home mechanical ventilation. *Thorax*, **48**, 1264–73.

Muir, J.-F., Girault, C., Cardinaud, J.-P. *et al.* (1994) Survival and long-term follow-up of tracheostomized patients with COPD treated by home mechanical ventilation. *Chest*, **106**, 201–9.

Mukhopadhyay, S., Staddon, G.E., Eastman, C. *et al.* (1994) The quantitative distribution of nebulised antibiotic in CF. *Respir. Med.*, **88**, 203–11.

Mulholland, C., Lennon, S. and Graham, R. (1994) Does prone positioning improve oxygen saturation in a patient with CF? *Physiother. Theory Pract.*, **10**, 223–33.

Mulley, G. (1993) Nursing elderly patients out of bed. *Br. Med. J.*, **307**, 80.

Mulloy, E. (1993) Theophylline improves gas exchange during rest, exercise and sleep in severe COPD. *Am. Rev. Respir. Dis.*, **148**, 1030–6.

Munday, I.T., Desai, P.M., Marshall, C.A. *et al.* (1993) The effectiveness of preoperative advice to stop smoking. *Anaesthesia*, **48**, 816–18.

Munro, N.C. (1992) Radiological evidence of progression of bronchiectasis. *Respir. Med.*, **86**, 397–401.

Murphy, F.M. (1991) The high-risk infant. *Physiotherapy*, **77**, 367–70.

Murray, E. (1993) Anyone for pulmonary rehabilitation? *Physiotherapy*, **79**, 705–10.

Natale, J.E., Pfeifle, J. and Homnick, D.N. (1994) Comparison of intrapulmonary percussive ventilation and chest physiotherapy. *Chest*, **105**, 1789–93.

Neilly, J.B. (1992) Effects of selective sleep deprivation on ventilation during recovery sleep in normal humans. *J. Appl. Physiol.*, **72**, 100–9.

Neville, E., Gribbins, H. and Harrison, B.D.W. (1991) Acute severe asthma. *Respir. Med.*, **85**, 463–74.

Neville, S. and French, S. (1991) Clinical education. *Physiotherapy*, **77**, 351–4.

Newman, K.B., Lynch, D.A., Newman, L.S. *et al.* (1994) Quantitative computed tomography detects air trapping due to asthma. *Chest*, **106**, 105–9.

Newton, D.A.G. and Stephenson, A. (1978) Effect of physiotherapy on pulmonary function. *Lancet*, **2**, 228–30.

Ng, G.Y. and Stokes, M.J. (1992) EMG recordings of respiratory muscles during unilateral and bilateral chest expansion. *Austr. Phys. J.*, **38**, 203–8.

Nichols, D.G. (1993) Disposition and respiratory effects of intrathecal morphine in children. *Anesthesiology*, **79**, 733–6.

Nicholson, C. (1993) Are you ready for video thoracoscopy? *Am. J. Nurs.*, **93**, 54–7.

Nickoladze, G.D. (1992) Functional results of surgery for bullous emphysema. *Chest*, **101**, 119–22.

Niederman, M.S., Clemente, P.H., Fein, A.M. *et al.* (1991) Benefits of a multidisciplinary pulmonary rehabilitation program. *Chest*, **99**, 798–804.

Ninan, T.K., Reid, I.W., Carter, P.E. *et al.* (1993) Effects of high doses of inhaled corticosteroids on adrenal function in children with severe persistent asthma. *Thorax*, **48**, 599–602.

Ninane, V., Yernault, J.-C. and deTroyer, A. (1993) Intrinsic PEEP in patients with COPD. *Am. Rev. Respir. Dis.*, **148**, 1037–42.

Ninane, V., Rypens, F., Yernault, J.-C. *et al.* (1992) Abdominal muscle use during breathing in patients with CAO. *Am. Rev. Resp. Dis.*, **146**, 16–21.

Noppen, M., Dhondt, E., Mahler, T. *et al.* (1994) Successful management of recurrent pneumothorax in CF by localized apical thoracoscopic talc poudrage. *Chest*, **106**, 262–4.

Nosworthy, J., Barter, C., Thomas, S. *et al.* (1992) An evaluation of three elements of pulmonary rehabilitation. *Austr. Physiother.*, **38**, 189–93.

Novak, R.A., Shumaker, L., Snyder, J.V. *et al.* (1987) Do periodic hyperinflations improve gas exchange in patients with hypoxemic respiratory failure? *Crit. Care Med.*, **15**, 1081–5.

Nunn, J.-F., Coleman, A.J., Sachithanandan, T. *et al.* (1965) Hypoxaemia and atelectasis produced by forced expiration. *Br. J. Anaesth.*, **37**, 3–11.

Nunn, J.F. (1987) *Applied Respiratory Physiology*, 3rd edn, Butterworth-Heinemann, Oxford.

O'Callaghan, C. (1993) Improvement in sodium cromoglycate delivery from a spacer device. *Thorax*, **48**, 603–6.

Odell, J.A. (1994) Management of empyema. *J. Roy. Soc. Med.*, **87**, 466–70.

O'Donnell, D.E. and Webb, K.A. (1992) Breathlessness in patients with severe chronic airflow limitation. *Chest*, **102**, 824–31.

O'Donnell, D.E. (1994) Breathlessness in patients with chronic airflow a limitation. *Chest*, **106**, 904–12.

Ogura, H. (1994) The effect of inhaled nitric oxide on smoke inhalation. *J. Trauma*, **37**, 294–302.

Okabe, S. (1995) Role of hypoxia on increased BP in patients with obstructive sleep apnoea. *Thorax*, **50**, 28–34.

Olds, D.L. (1994) Intellectual impairment in children of women who smoke cigarettes during pregnancy. *Pediatrics*, **93**, 221–7.

Olséni, L. (1994) Chest physiotherapy in COPD: FET combined with either postural drainage or PEP. *Respir. Med.*, **88**, 435–40.

O'Nunain, S. (1993) Cardiac arrest. *Lancet*, **341**, 1641–7.

Onuoha, A.R.A. (1994) Effective clinical teaching from the perspectives of students, supervisors and teachers. *Physiotherapy*, **80**, 208–14.

Orenstein, D.M., and Kaplan, R.M. (1991) Measuring the quality of well-being in and lung transplantation. *Chest*, **100**, 1016–18.

Osman, L.M., Abdalla, M.I., Beattie, J.A.G. *et al.* (1994) Reducing hospital admission through computer supported education for asthma patients. *Br. Med. J.*, **308**, 568–71.

O'Sullivan, G., Harvey, I., Bass, C. *et al.* (1992) Psychophysiological investigations of patients with unilateral symptoms in the hyperventilation syndrome. *Br. J. Psych.*, **160**, 664–7.

Owen, S., Morganstern, M., Hepworth, J. *et al.* (1990) Control of house dust mite antigen in bedding. *Lancet*, **335**, 396–7.

Owen, H., Kluger, M.T., Ilsley, A.H. *et al.* (1993) The effect of fentanyl administered epidurally. *Anaesthesia*, **48**, 20–5.

Palange, P. (1994) Cardiopulmonary exercise testing in the evaluation of patients with ventilatory vs circulatory causes of reduced exercise tolerance. *Chest* **105**, 1122–6.

Papastamelos, C. (1995) Developmental changes in chest wall compliance in infancy and early childhood. *J. Appl. Phys.*, **78**, 179–84.

Papazian, L. (1993) Effect of bolus doses of midazolam on ICP and CPP in patients with severe head injury. *Br. J. Anaesth.*, **71**, 267–71.

Paratz, J. (1993) The effect of respiratory physiotherapy on ventilated neurosurgical patients. *Physiother. Theory Pract.*, **9**, 3–11.

Park, G.R. (1994) What changes drug metabolism in critically ill patients? *Anaesthesia*, **49**, 188–91.

Parker, A. (1993) Paediatrics, in *Physiotherapy for Respiratory and Cardiac Problems* (eds B.A., Webber and J.A. Pryor), Churchill Livingstone, Edinburgh.

Parker, J.C. and Hernandez, L.A. (1993) Mechanisms of ventilator-induced lung injury. *Crit. Care Med.*, **21**, 131–42.

Parker, S., and Middleton, P.G. (1993) Assessment, in *Physiotherapy for Respiratory and Cardiac Problems* (eds, B.A. Webber and J.A. Pryor), Churchill Livingstone, Edinburgh.

Parker, M.M., Schubert, W., Shelhamer, J.H. *et al.* (1984) Perceptions of a critically ill patient experiencing therapeutic paralysis in an ICU. *Int. Care Med.* **12**, 69–71.

Parry, G.W. (1992) Surgical intervention in spontaneous pneumothorax. *Respir. Med.*, **86**, 1–2.

Partridge, M.R. (1992) Smoking and the young. *Br. Med. J.*, **305**, 2.

Pasero, C.L. (1994) Avoiding opioid-induced respiratory depression. *Am. J. Nurs.*, **94**, 25–31.

Patel, M. (1993) Optimal time for measuring the cardiorespiratory effects of PEEP. *Chest*, **104**, 139–42.

Paterson, D.H. (1992) Effects of ageing on the cardiorespiratory system. *Can. J. Sport Sci.*, **17**, 171–7.

Pavia, D., Thomson, M.L. and Clarke, S.W. (1978) Enhanced clearance of secretions from the human lung after administration of hypertonic saline aerosol. *Am. Rev. Resp. Dis.*, **117**, 199–203.

Pavia, D. (1991) Bronchoalveolar clearance. *Respiration*, **58** (suppl.), 13–17.

Payne, R. (1995) *Relaxation Techniques: a Handbook for the Health Care Professional*, Churchill Livingstone, Edinburgh.

Peach, H. and Pathy, M.S. (1981) Follow-up study of disability among elderly patients discharged from hospital with exacerbations of chronic bronchitis. *Thorax*, **36**, 585–9.

Pearce, A.C., and Jones R.M. (1984) Smoking and anaesthesia. *Anesthesiology*, **61**, 576–84.

Pearl, R.G. (1993) Inhaled nitric oxide. *Anesthesiology*, **78**, 413–16.

Pehrsson, K. (1994) Quality of life of patients treated by home mechanical ventilation due to restrictive ventilatory disorders. *Respir. Care*, **88**, 21–6.

Pennock, B.E. (1994) Distressful events in the ICU. *Heart Lung*, **23**, 323–7.

Pentland, B. (1994) Pain in Guillain–Barré syndrome. *Pain*, **59**, 159–64.

Peper, E. (1992) Fifteen-month follow up with asthmatics utilizing EMG/incentive inspirometer feedback. *Biofeedback Self-regulation*, **17**, 143–51.

Pesenti, A. and Pelosi, P. (1992) Respiratory resistance in mechanically ventilated patients, *Yearbook of Intensive Care and Emergency Medicine* (ed. J.L. Vincent), Springer–Verlag, Berlin.

Petersen, G.M., Pierson, D.J. and Hunter, P.M. (1979) Arterial oxygen saturation during nasotracheal suctioning. *Chest*, **76**, 283–7.

Peto, R., Speizer, E., Cochrane, A.L. *et al.* (1983) The relevance in adults of airflow obstruction but not of mucus hypersecretion to mortality from chronic lung disease. *Am. Rev. Resp. Dis.*, **128**, 491–500.

Petty, T.L. (1990) The national mucolytic study. *Chest*, **97**, 75–83.

Petty, T.L. and O'Donohue, W.J. (1994) Further recommendations for prescribing and research in long-term oxygen therapy. *Am. J. Respir. Crit. Care Med.*, **150**, 875–7.

Phelan, P.D. (1994) Asthma in children: epidemiology. *Br. Med. J.*, **308**, 1584–5.

Philip, C. (1987) Mastectomy – an approach to total rehabilitation. *S.A.J. Physiother*, **43**, 77–80.

Philips, B.J. (1992) Surgical face masks are effective in reducing bacterial contamination. *Br. J. Anaesth.*, **69**, 407–8.

Phillips, S. (1993) Zingiber officinale (ginger): an antiemetic for day surgery. *Anaesthesia*, **48**, 715–17.

Phillips, S., Hutchinson, S. and Davidson, T. (1993) Preoperative drinking does not affect gastric contents. *Br. J. Anaesth.*, **70**, 6–9.

Phillips, S., Daborn, A.K. and Hatch, D.J. (1994) Preoperative fasting for paediatric anaesthesia. *Br. J. Anaesth.*, **73**, 529–36.

Phillips, G.D. and Millard, F.J.C. (1994) The therapeutic use of ultrasonic nebulizers in acute asthma. *Respir. Med.*, **88**, 387–9.

Phillipson, E.A. (1993) Effect of aging on metabolic respiratory control in sleeping dogs. *Am. Rev. Resp. Dis.*, **147**, 1521–5.

Pierson, D.J. (1988) Alveolar rupture during mechanical ventilation. *Respir. Care*, **33**, 472–86.

Pierson, D.J. and Lakshminarayan, S. (1984) Postoperative ventilatory management. *Respir. Care*, **29**, 603–11.

Pietropauli J.A., Rogers, F.B., Shackford, S.R. *et al.* (1992) The deleterious effects of intraoperative hypotension in patients with severe head injuries. *J. Trauma*, **33**, 403–7.

Piirilä, P., Sovijärvi, A.R.A., Kaisla, T. *et al.* (1991) Crackles in patients with fibrosing alveolitis, bronchiectasis, COPD and heart failure. *Chest*, **99**, 1076–83.

Pilbeam, S.P. (1992) *Mechanical Ventilation*, C.V. Mosby, Missouri.

Pinn, S. (1992) Paediatric asthma. *Resp. Dis. in Pract.*, **9**(2), 10–11.

Pinney, S., Freeman, L.J. and Nixon, P.G.F. (1987) Role of the nurse counsellor in managing patients with the hyperventilation syndrome. *J. Roy. Soc. Med.*, **80**, 216–18.

Piper, A.J., Parker, S., Torzillo, P.J. *et al.* (1992) Nocturnal nasal IPPV stabilizes patients with CF and hypercapnic respiratory failure. *Chest* **102**, 846–50.

Pitcher, W.D. (1993) Oxygen cost of increasing tidal volume and diaphragm flattening in obstructive pulmonary disease. *J. Appl. Physiol.*, **74**, 2750–6.

Pitts, M. and Healey, S. (1989) Factors influencing the inferences of pain made by three health professions. *Physiother. Pract.*, **5**, 65–8.

Poelaert, J., Lannoy, B., Vogelaers, D. *et al.* (1991) Influence of chest physiotherapy on arterial oxygen saturation. *Acta Anaesth. Belg*, **42**, 165–70.

Polacek, T.L., Barth, L., Mestad, P. *et al.* (1992) The effect of positioning on arterial oxygenation in children with atelectasis after cardiac surgery. *Heart Lung*, **21**, 457–62.

Pollock, M., Roa, J., Benditt, J. *et al.* (1993) Estimation of ventilatory reserve by stair climbing. *Chest*, **104**, 1378–83.

Ponte, J. (1990) Indications for mechanical ventilation. *Thorax*, **45**, 885–90.

Postma, D.S. (1991) Inhaled therapy in COPD. *Respir. Med.*, **85**, 447–49.

Potempa, K.M., Folta, A., Braun, L.T. *et al.* (1991) The relationship of resting and exercise blood pressure in subjects with essential hypertension before and after propranolol. *Heart Lung*, **21**, 509–14.

Potts, M. (1994) Grief has to be. *Lancet*, **343**, 279–80.

Prabhu, M.B., Mink, J.T., Graham, B.L. *et al.* (1990). Effect of a deep breath on gas mixing and diffusion in the lung. *Resp. Physiol.*, **79**, 195–204.

Prasad, S.A. (1993) Current concepts in physiotherapy. *J. Roy. Soc. Med.*, **86** (suppl. 20), 23–9.

Prasad, S.A. and Hussey, J. (1995) *Paediatric Respiratory Care*, Chapman & Hall, London.

Preston, I.M., Matthews, H.R. and Ready, A.R. (1986) Minitracheotomy. *Physiotherapy*, **72**, 494–6.

Pullan, R.D., Rhodes, J., Ganesh, S. *et al.* (1994) Transdermal nicotine for active ulcerative colitis. *N. Engl. J. Med.*, **330**, 811–15.

Purssel, E. (1994) Telling children about their impending death. *Br. J. Nurs.*, **3**, 119–20.

Purtilo, R.B. (1976) Similarities in patient response to chronic and terminal illness. *Phys. Ther.*, **56**, 279–84.

Qureshi, J. (1994) A pain assessment tool for all children. *Paed. Nurs.*, **6**(7), 11–13.

Radford, R. (1982) A rational basis for percussion-augmented mucociliary clearance. *Respir. Care*, **27**, 556–63.

Ramonatxo, M. (1995) Validation of a non-invasive tension-time index of inspiratory muscles. *J. Appl. Physiol.*, **78**, 646–53.

Ramsay, J. (1994) The psychology of childhood asthma. *Paed. Nurs.*, **6**(8), 17–18.

Raphael, J.H. (1993) Combined high frequency ventilation. *Anaesthesia*, **48**, 596–8.

Raphael, J.H. (1994) Effects of the cervical collar on CSF pressure. *Anaesthesia*, **49**, 437–9.

Ras, G.J., Staden, M.V., Schultz, C. *et al.* (1994) Respiratory manifestations of rigid spine syndrome. *Am. J. Respir. Crit. Care Med.*, **150**, 540–6.

Ray, J.F. (1974) Immobility, hypoxemia, and pulmonary arteriovenous shunting. *Arch. Surg.*, **109**, 537–41.

Reardon, J. (1994) The effect of comprehensive outpatient pulmonary rehabilitation on dyspnea. *Chest*, **105**, 1046–52.

Redfern, S. (1985) Taking some of my own medicine. *Care Crit. Ill*, **1**, 6–7.

Rees, J. (1987) Cough. *Update*, **34**, 1110–19.

Regnis, J.A. (1994) Benefits of nocturnal nasal CPAP in patients with CF. *Chest*, **106**, 1717–24.

Reid, W.D. and Loveridge, B.M. (1983) Physiotherapy management of patients with COPD. *Physiother. Can.*, **35**, 183–95.

Reid, P.T. and Rudd, R.M. (1993) Management of malignant pleural effusion. *Thorax*, **48**, 779–80.

Reid, P. (1994) Management of massive haemoptysis. *Respir. Dis. Pract*, **11**(4), 10–11.

Reisman, J.J. (1988) Role of conventional physiotherapy in CF. *J. Pediatr.*, **113**, 632–6.

Renston, J.P. (1994) Respiratory muscle rest using nasal BiPAP ventilation in patients with stable severe COPD. *Chest*, **105**, 1053–60.

Resende, T.L. and O'Neill, P.A. (1992) Effects of exercise and abdominal massage on constipation and faecal incontinence. *Physiotherapy*, **78**, 589.

Restrick, L.J. (1993) Nasal intermittent positive pressure ventilation in weaning intubated patients. *Respir. Med.*, **87**, 199–204.

Rice, L.J. (1989) Management of acute pain in pediatric patients. *Clin. J. Pain*, **5** (suppl. 1), S42–50.

Ricour, C. (1989) Stress-induced disturbances of the gastro-intestinal tract in children. *Int. Care Med.*, **15**, S32–S36.

Riegel, B. (1985) A review and critique of the literature on preoxygenation for endotracheal suctioning. *Heart Lung*, **14**, 507–18.

Rimington, L.D., Spence, D.P.S., Ryland, I. *et al.* (1994) Is the order and timing of drugs used in assessing bronchodilators in COPD important? *ACPRC Annual Conference Proceedings*, **1**, 3.

Rivara, D. (1984) Positional hypoxemia during artifical ventilation. *Crit. Care Med.*, **12**, 436–8.

Rivington-Law, B. (1981) Review of literature in chest physical therapy. *Physiother. Can.*, **33**, 269–75.

Roa, J. (1991) Work of breathing and ventilatory muscle recruitment during pursed lip breathing. *Am. Rev. Resp. Dis.*, **143**, 4.

Roberts, C.J., Parke, T.J. and Sykes, M.K. (1993) Effects of intraoperative inspired gas mixtures on postoperative nocturnal oxygen saturation. *Br. J. Anaesth.*, **71**, 476–80.

Robertson, C.S. (1995) Reduced blood glucose concentration with a carbohydrate-free diet in head injured patients. *Crit. Care Med.*, **23**, A71.

Robinson, D.M., Egglestone, D.M., Hill, P.M. *et al.* (1992) Effects of a physical conditioning programme on asthmatic patients. *N.Z. Med.J.*, **105**, 253–6.

Rochester, D.F. and Arora, N.S. (1983) Respiratory muscle failure. *Med. Clin. N. Am.*, **67**, 573–97.

Rochester, D.F. (1991) The diaphragm in COPD. *N. Engl. J. Med.*, **325**, 961–2.

Rolla, G. (1994) Effect of pleurotomy on pulmonary function after CABG with IMA. *Respir. Med.*, **88**, 417–20.

Rosenberg, M. (1992) Patient-controlled analgesia. *J. Oral. Maxillofac. Surg.*, **50**, 386–9.

Rosner, M.J. and Coley, I.B. (1986) Cerebral perfusion pressure, ICP, and head elevation. *J. Neurosurg.*, **65**, 636–41.

Ross, J., Dean, E. and Abboud, R.T. (1992) The effect of postural drainage on ventilation homogeneity in healthy subjects. *Phys. Ther.*, **72**, 794–9.

Rossi, O.V.J., Kinnula, V.L., Tienari, J. *et al.* (1993) Association of severe asthma attacks with weather, pollen and air pollutants. *Thorax*, **48**, 244–8.

Rossi, A. (1994) Effects of PEEP on $\dot{V}_A/\dot{Q}$ mismatching in ventilated patients with chronic airflow limitation. *Am. J. Respir. Crit. Care Med.*, **149**, 1077–84.

Roth, G. (1990) *Maps to Ecstasy*, Crucible, London.

Rothen, H.U. (1993) Re-expansion of atelectasis during general anaesthesia. *Br. J. Anaesth.*, **71**, 788–95.

Rothen, J.U. (1995) Prevention of atelectasis during general anaesthesia. *Lancet*, **345**, 1387–91.

Rouby, J.J. (1990) High frequency ventilation, in *Update in Intensive Care and Emergency Medicine* (ed. J.L. Vincent), Springer-Verlag, Berlin.

Rowbotham, E. (1990) *ACPRC Study Day*, London.

Rowe, B.H. (1993) Performance of an asthma quality of life questionnaire. *Am. Rev. Respir. Dis.*, **148**, 675–81.

Rowland, E. (1994) Arrhythmias. *J. Roy. Soc. Med.*, **87**, 87–90.

Rudd, R. (1994) Endobronchial therapy for lung cancer. *Respir. Dis. Pract.*, **11**(2), 10–13.

Rudy, E.B., Turner, B.S., Baun, M. *et al.* (1991) Endotracheal suctioning in adults with head injury. *Heart Lung*, **20**, 667–74.

Ruggier, R., Bailey, C.R. and Grounds, R.M. (1994) A simple method for maintenance of oxygen saturation following intravenous induction of anaesthesia. *Anaesthesia*, **49**, 759–61.

Ruiz, P.A. (1993) The needs of a patient in severe status asthmaticus. *Int. Crit. Care Nurs.*, **9**, 28–39.

Russell, P.Q., Epstein, L.H., Johnston, J.J. *et al.* (1988) The effects of physical activity as maintenance for smoking cessation. *Add. Behaviors*, **13**, 215–18.

Russell, G. (1994) Fluticasone propionate in children. *Respir. Med.*, **88**(A), 25–9.

Rustom, R. (1993) Quality of life after intensive care. *Br. J. Nurs.*, **2**, 316–20.

Rusznak, C. (1991) Influence of salbutamol and salmeterol on ciliary beat frequency. *Thorax*, **46**, 782P.

Ruta, T.S. (1993) The effect of acute hypocapnia on local cerebral blood flow. *Anesthesiogy*, **78**, 134–40.

Ryan, C.F., Road, R.D., Buckley, P.A. *et al.* (1993) Energy balance in stable malnourished patients with COPD. *Chest*, **103**, 1038–44.

Ryan-Wenger, N.M. (1994) Children's perspectives on coping with asthma. *Pediatr. Nurs.*, **20**, 224–8.

Sacchetti, A. (1994) Pediatric analgesia and sedation. *Ann. Emerg. Med.*, **23**, 237–49.

Sahebjami, H. (1993) Anthropometric and pulmonary function test profiles of outpatients with stable COPD. *Am. J. Med.*, **94**, 469–74.

Salazar, J. (1991) Exercise physiology, in *Pulmonary Therapy and Rehabilitation* (eds F. Haas and K. Axen), Williams and Wilkins, Baltimore, pp.58 and 63.

Salmon, B., Wilson, N.M. and Silverman, M. (1990) How much aerosol reaches the lungs of wheezy infants and toddlers? *Arch. Dis. Child*, **65**, 401–3.

Salmon, P. (1992) Surgery as a psychological stressor. *Stress Med.*, **8**, 193–8.

Saltin, B., Blomqvist, G., Mitchel, J.H. *et al.* (1968) Response to bed rest after exercise and after training. *Circulation*, **38** (suppl 7), 1–76.

Salyer, J.W. (1991) Pulse oximetry in the neonatal unit. *Respir. Care*, **36**, 17–20.

Sammon, M.P. (1994) Entrainment of respiration to rocking in premature infants. *J. Appl. Phys.*, **77**, 1548–54.

Samuels, M.P. and Southall, D.P. (1989) Negative extrathoracic pressure in infants and young children. *Br. Med. J.*, **299**, 1253–7.

Samuels, S., Samuels M., Dinwiddie, R. *et al.* (1995) A survey of physiotherapy techniques used in specialist clinics for cystic fibrosis. *Physiotherapy*, **81**, 279–83.

Sandler, H. (1988) The hemodynamic effects of repeated bed rest exposure. *Aviation, Space Environ. Med.*, **54**, 1047–54.

Sara, C. (1965) The management of patients with a tracheostomy. *Med. J. Aust.*, **1**, 99–103.

Sato, P., Sargur, M.K. and Schoene, R.B. (1986) Hypnosis effect on carbon dioxide chemosensitivity. *Chest*, **89**, 828–31.

Savage, J. (1992) Advice to take home. *Nurs. Times*, **88**(38), 24–7.

Sawyer, E.H. and Clanton, T.L. (1993) Improved pulmonary function and exercise tolerance with inspiratory muscle conditioning in children with cystic fibrosis. *Chest*, **104**, 1490–7.

Scalea, T.M. (1994) Resuscitation of multiple trauma and head injury. *Crit. Care Med.*, **22**, 1610–15.

Schleifer, T.J., Gleason, J. and Grady, L. (1994) Patient responsibility in an innovative COPD program. *Physiother. Can.*, **46** (2) (suppl), 81.

Schlichtig, R. and Sargent, S.C. (1990) Nutritional support of the mechanically ventilated patient. *Crit. Care Clin.*, **6**, 767–77.

Schnapp, L.M. (1994) Frequency and importance of barotrauma in 100 patients with acute lung injury. *Crit. Care Med.*, **23**, 272–8.

Schols, A.M., Mostert, R., Soeters, P.B. *et al.* (1991) Body composition and exercise performance in patients with COPD. *Thorax*, **46**, 695–9.

Schöni, M.H. (1989) Autogenic drainage. *J. Roy. Soc. Med.*, (suppl. 16), 32–7.

Schreur, H.J.W., Sterk, P.J., Vanderschoot, J. *et al.* (1992) Lung sound intensity in patients with emphysema and in normal subjects. *Thorax*, **47**, 674–9.

Schumann, L. and Parsons, G.H. (1985) Tracheal suctioning and ventilator tube changes in ARDS. *Heart Lung*, **14**, 362–7.

Schwartz, S.Z. (1987) Effects of blood volume and discontinuance of ventilation on pulmonary vascular pressures. *Crit. Care Med.*, **15**, 671–5.

Schwartzstein, R.M. (1992) Asthma: to run or not to run? *Am. Rev. Resp. Dis.*, **145**, 739–40.

Schweitzer, J.A. (1994) Specific breathing exercises for the patient with quadriplegia. *Phys. Ther. Pract.*, **3**, 109–22.

Sciaky, A.J. (1994) Mobilizing the intensive care unit patient. *Phys. Ther. Pract.*, **3**, 69–80.

Sears, M.R. (1994) Growing up with asthma. *Br. Med. J.*, **309**, 72–3.

Seaton, A. (1994) Management of allergic bronchopulmonary aspergillosis without maintenance oral corticosteroids. *Q. J. Med.*, **87**, 529–37.

Seche, L.A. (1992) The thermo cardiosystems implantable left ventricular assist device. *Heart Lung*, **21**, 112–14.

Sell, L., Devlin, B., Bourke, S.J. *et al.* (1993) Communicating the diagnosis of lung cancer. *Respir. Med.*, **87**, 61–3.

Senekal, M. (1994) The optimal physiotherapeutic approach to penetrating stab wounds of the chest. *S.A. J. Physiother.*, **50**, 29–36.

Shah, P.L., Scott, S.F. and Hodson, M.E. (1994) Lobar atelectasis in CF and treatment with recombinant human DNase. *Respir. Med.*, **88**, 313–15.

Shaheen, S.O., Barker, D.J.P., Shiell, A.W. *et al.* (1994) The relationship between pneumonia in early childhood and impaired lung function in late adult life. *Am. J. Respir. Crit. Care Med.*, **149**, 616–19.

Shapiro, S.H., Ernst, P., Gray-Donald, K. *et al.* (1992) Effect of negative pressure ventilation in severe COPD. *Lancet*, **340**, 1425–9.

Shelledy, D.C. (1995) A comparison of the effects of assist-control, SIMV and SIMV with pressure support. *Heart Lung*, **24**, 67–75.

Shelly, M.P., Lloyd, G.M. and Park, G.R. (1988) A review of the mechanisms and methods of humidification of inspired gases. *Int. Care Med.*, **14**, 1–9.

Shelly, M.P. (1992) Intensive care sedation, in *Yearbook of Intensive Care and Emergency Medicine* (ed. J.L. Vincent), Springer-Verlag, Berlin.

Sherman, C.B., Hubert, M. and Fogel, B.S. (1992) Unrecognized respiratory disease in the elderly. *Am. Rev. Respir. Dis.*, **145**, 2(2), A763.

Shivaram, U., Donath, J. and Khan, F.A. (1987) Effects of continuous positive airway pressure in acute asthma. *Respiration*, **52**, 157–62.

Shum, M.I.D., Lauder, I., Lam, W.K. *et al.* (1993) Effect of antibiotics on sputum inflammatory contents in acute exacerbations of bronchiectasis. *Respir. Med.*, **87**, 449–54.

Sibuya, M., Yamada, M., Kanamaru, A. *et al.* (1994) Effect of chest wall vibration on dyspnea. *Am. J. Resp. Crit. Care Med.*, **149**, 1235–40.

Signorile, J.F. (1995) Increased muscle strength in paralyzed patients after spinal cord injury. *Arch. Phys. Med. Rehab.*, **76**, 55–8.

Silver, J.A. and Foster, W.M. (1990) Effect of short term vitamin C therapy on mucociliary function. *Am. Rev. Resp. Dis.*, **141**, 2/2, A523.

Sim, J. (1986) Truthfulness in the therapeutic relationship. *Physiother. Pract.*, **2**, 121–7.

Sim, K.M. (1994) Ventilation in severe acute asthma. *Thorax*, **49**, 297–9.

Sim, J. (1995) The external validity of group comparative and single system studies. *Physiotherapy*, **81**, 263–70.

Similowski, T. (1991) Contractile properties of the human diaphragm during chronic hyperinflation. *N. Engl. J. Med.*, **325**, 917–23.

Simpson, F.G. (1993) Home nebulisers – do we know what we are doing? *ACPRC J.*, **22**, 36–7.

Simpson, K., Killian, K., McCartney, N. *et al.* (1992) Randomised controlled trial of weightlifting exercise in patients with chronic airflow limitation. *Thorax*, **47**, 70–5.

Singer, M., Vermaat, J. and Hall, G. (1994) Hemodynamic effects of manual hyperinflation in critically ill mechanically ventilated patients. *Chest*, **106**, 1182–7.

Singh, V., Wisniewski, A., Britton, J. *et al.* (1990) Effect of yoga breathing exercises on airway reactivity in subjects with asthma. *Lancet*, **335**, 1381–3.

Singh, S. (1992) The use of field walking tests for assessment of functional capacity in patients with CAO. *Physiotherapy*, **78**, 102–4.

Sisson, R. (1990) Effects of auditory stimuli on comatose patients with head injury. *Heart Lung*, **19**, 373–8.

Sloan, J.P., Muwanga, C.L., Waters, E.A. *et al.* (1986) Multiple rib fractures: TNS versus conventional analgesia. *J. Trauma*, **26**(12), 1120–2.

Slutsky, A.S. (1993) Mechanical ventilation. *Respir. Care*, **38**, 1389–19.

Small, S.P. and Graydon, J.E. (1992) Perceived uncertainty, physical symptoms and negative mood in hospitalized patients with COPD. *Heart Lung*, **21**, 568–74.

Smalldone, G.C. (1993) Regional impairment of mucociliary clearance in COPD. *Chest*, **103**, 1390–6.

Smedstad, K.G. (1992) Postoperative pain relief and hospital stay after total esophagectomy. *Clin. J. Pain*, **8**, 149–53.

Smith, K., Cook, D., Guyatt, G.H. *et al.* (1992) Respiratory muscle training in CAL. *Am. Rev. Resp. Dis.*, **145**, 533–9.

Smith, G. (1991) Pain after surgery. *Br. J. Anaesth.*, **67**, 233–4.

Snider, G.L. (1995) Withholding and withdrawing life-sustaining therapy. *Am. J. Respir. Crit. Care Med.*, **151**, 279–81.

Sommers, M.S. (1991) Potential for injury: trauma after cardio-pulmonary resuscitation. *Heart Lung*, **20**, 287–95.

Sottile, F.D. (1986) Nosocomial pulmonary infection. *Crit. Care Med.*, **14**, 265–70.

Sparsholt, M. (1989) Pain and the special care baby unit. *Nurs. Times*, **85** (41), 61–4.

Speidel, B.D. (1978) Adverse effects of routine procedures on preterm infants. *Lancet*, **1**, 864–6.

Spence, D.P.S. (1991) Effect of nebulised salbutamol on walking distance. *Thorax*, **46**, 305P.

Spence, D.P.S. and Hay, J.G. (1993) Oxygen saturation and breathlessness in corridor walking in COPD. *Thorax*, **48**, 1145–50.

Spence, D.P.S., Graham, D.R., Ahmed, J. *et al.* (1993) Does cold air affect exercise capacity and dyspnea in stable COPD? *Chest*, **103**, 693–6.

Sperry, S.J. (1992) Fentanyl and sufentanil increase ICP in head trauma patients. *Anesthesiology*, **77**, 416–20.

Spiro, S. (1993) Management of lung cancer. *Practitioner*, **237**, 778–81.

Sporik, R. (1994) Why block a small hole? *Arch. Dis. Child.*, **71**, 393–4.

Spragg, R.G. (1994) Acute effects of a single dose of porcine surfactant on patients with ARDS. *Chest*, **105**, 195–202.

Sridhar, M.K. (1995) Nutrition and lung health. *Br. Med. J.*, **310**, 75–6.

Starke, I.D., Webber, B.A. and Branthwaite, M.A. (1979) IPPB and hypercapnia in respiratory failure. *Anaesthesia*, **34**, 283–7.

Sterk, P.J. (1993) Airway responsiveness. *Eur. Respir. J.*, **6**(suppl.) 53–83.

Steven, M.H., Pryor, J.A., Webber, B.A. *et al.* (1992) Physiotherapy versus cough alone in the treatment of cystic fibrosis. *N.Z. J. Physioth.*, **20**, 31–7.

Stevensen, C.J. (1994) The psychophysiological effects of aromatherapy massage following cardiac surgery. *Complementary Ther. Med.*, **2**, 27–35.

Stewart, T. (1993) Barotrauma in severe ARDS is greatest in non dependent lung zones. *Crit. Care Med.*, **21**, S284.

Stewart, A.G. and Howard, P. (1992) Indications for long term oxygen therapy. *Respiration*, **59** (suppl. 2), 8–13.

Stewart, T. and Shields, C.R. (1985) Grief in chronic illness. *Arch. Phys. Med. Rehabil.*, **66**, 447–50.

Stewart, T.D. and Rossier, A.B. (1978) Psychological considerations in the adjustment of spinal cord injury. *Rehab. Lit.*, **39**, 75–80.

Stiller, K.R. and Munday, R.M. (1992) Chest physiotherapy for the surgical patient. *Br. J. Surg.*, **79**, 745–9.

Stiller, K., Montarello, J., Wallace, M. *et al.* (1994) Are breathing and coughing exercises necessary after coronary artery surgery? *Physiother. Theory Pract.*, **10**, 143–52.

Stone, R.A. and DeLeo, J. (1976) Psychotherapeutic control of hypertension. *N. Engl. J. Med.*, **294**, 80–4.

Strachan, D.P. (1991) Ventilatory function and winter fresh fruit consumption. *Thorax*, **46**, 624–9.

Strickland, J.H. (1993) A computer-controlled ventilator weaning system. *Chest*, **103**, 1120–6.

Striebel. H.W. (1993) Intranasal fentanyl titration for postoperative pain management. *Anaesthesia*, **48**, 753–7.

Strunk, R.C. (1993) Death due to asthma. *Am. Rev. Respir. Dis.*, **148**, 550–2.

Sun, W.-Z. (1992) Successful cardiopulmonary resuscitation in the prone position. *Am. Rev. Respir. Dis.*, **77**, 202 4.

Susini, G., Sisillo, E., Bortone, F. *et al.* (1992) Postoperative atelectasis reexpansion by selective insufflation through a ballon-tipped catheter. *Chest*, **102**, 1693–6.

Sutton, P.P., Lopez, M.T., Pavia, D. *et al.* (1985) Assessment of percussion, vibratory shaking and breathing exercises in chest physiotherapy. *Eur. J. Resp. Dis.*, **66**, 147–52.

Swann, P. (1989) Stress management for pain control. *Physiotherapy*, **75**, 295–8.

Swanston, M. (1993) Pain assessment with interactive computer animation. *Pain*, **53**, 347–51.

Swerts, P.M.J. (1990) Exercise reconditioning in the rehabilitation of patients with COPD. *Arch. Phys. Med. Rehab.*, **71**, 570–3.

Swinamer, D.L. (1987) Twenty-four hour energy expenditure in critically ill patients. *Crit. Care Med.*, **15**, 637–43.

Swingle, H.M., Eggert, L.D. and Bucciarelli, R.L. (1984) New approach to management of unilateral tension pulmonary interstitial emphysema in premature infants. *Pediatrics*, **74**, 354–7.

Szaflarski, N.L. (1989) Use of pulse oximetry in critically ill adults. *Heart Lung*, **18**, 444–55.

Szaflarski, N.L. and Cohen, N.H. (1991) Use of capnography in critically ill adults. *Heart Lung*, **20**, 363–74.

Szasz, T.S. (1968) The psychology of persistent pain, in *Pain* (ed. A. Soulairac), Academic Press, London.

Tamaoki, J. (1992) Effect of indomethacin on bronchorrhea. *Am. Rev. Resp. Dis.*, **145**, 548–52.

Tamaoki, J. (1994) Effect of long term treatment with oxitropium bromide on airway secretion in chronic bronchitis. *Thorax*, **49**, 545–8.

Tashkin, D.P., Coulson, A.H., Clark, V.A. *et al.* (1987) Respiratory symptoms and lung function in habitual heavy smokers of marijuana. *Am. Rev. Resp. Dis.*, **135**, 209–16.

Tashkin, D.P., Simmons, M.S., Chang, P. *et al.* (1993) Effects of smoked substance abuse on nonspecific airway hyperresponsiveness. *Am. Rev. Respir. Dis.*, **147**, 97–103.

Teague, W.G. (1995) Noninvasive ventilatory support in pediatric respiratory failure. *Respir. Care*, **40**, 86–96.

Thomas, E.A. (1987) Pre-operative fasting – a question of routine? *Nurs. Times*, **83**(49), 46–7.

Thomas, S., O'Doherty, M. and Bateman, N. (1990) *Pneumocystis carinii* pneumonia. *Br. Med. J.*, **300**, 211–12.

Thomas, A.N., Ryan, J.P., Doran, B.R.H. *et al.* (1992) Nasal CPAP after coronary artery surgery. *Anaesthesia*, **47**, 316–19.

Thomas, V. (1995) Psychological characteristics and the effectiveness of patient-controlled analgesia. *Br. J. Anaesth.*, **74**, 271–6.

Thorax editorial (1989) Acute bronchiolitis in infancy. *Thorax*, **44**, 1–5.

Tidwell, S.L. (1990) Effects of position changes on mixed venous oxygen saturation in patients after coronary revascularization. *Heart Lung*, **19**, 574–8.

Tillett, J.M. (1993) Effect of continuous rotational therapy on ICP in the severely brain-injured patient. *Crit. Care Med.*, **21**, 1005–11.

Timmons, B.H. and Ley, R. (1994) *Behavioral and Psychological Approaches to Breathing Disorders*, Plenum Press, London.

Tobin, M.J. (1988) Respiratory muscles in disease. *Clin. Chest Med.*, **9**, 263–86.

Tobin, M.J. and Yang, J. (1990) Weaning from mechanical ventilation. *Crit. Care Clin.*, **6**, 725–46.

Tobin, M.J. (1991) What should the clinician do when a patient fights the ventilator? *Resp. Care*, **36**, 395–406.

Tokioga, H. (1992) The effect of pressure support ventilation on auto-PEEP in a patient with asthma. *Chest*, **101**, 285–6.

Torres, A. (1992) Pulmonary aspiration of gastric contents in patients receiving mechanical ventilation. *Ann. Int. Med.*, **116**, 540–3.

Torrington, K., Sorenson, D. and Sherwood, L. (1984) Postoperative chest percussion with postural drainage in obese patients following gastric stapling. *Chest*, **86**, 891–5.

Tougaard, L., Krone, T., Sorknaes, A. *et al.* (1992) Economic benefits of teaching patients with COPD about their illness. *Lancet*, **339**, 1517–20.

Trochtenberg, S. (1994) Nebulized lidocaine in refractory cough. *Chest*, **105**, 1592–3.

Truwit, J.D. (1992) Validation of a technique to assess maximal inspiratory pressure in poorly co-operative patients. *Chest*, **102**, 1216–19.

Tucker, E.Z. (1991) Tracheostomy speaking valve in pediatric ventilator-assisted patients. *Respir. Care*, **36**, 1271.

Tweeddale, P.M., Rowbottom, I., and McHardy, G.J.R. (1994) Breathing retraining. *J. Psychosom. Res*, **38**, 11–21.

Twycross, R. and Lack, S. (1984) *Therapeutics in Terminal Cancer*, Pitman, Bath.

Twycross, R., and Lack, S. (1990) *Oral Morphine in Advanced Cancer*, Beaconsfield Ltd, Beaconsfield.

Tyler, D., Fitzgerald, M., McGrath, P. *et al.* (1991) Second international symposium on pediatric pain. *Pain*, **47**, 3–4.

Ueda, T. (1994) Distribution of surfactant and ventilation in surfactant-treated preterm lambs. *J. Appl. Phys*, **76**, 45–55.

Ulrich, R.S. (1984) View through a window may influence recovery from surgery. *Science*, **224**, 420–1.

Underwood, M.J. (1993) Current concepts in the use of intra-aortic balloon counterpulsation. *Br. J. Hosp. Med*, **50**, 391–7.

Ungeman–deMent, P., Bemis, A. and Siebens, A. (1986) Exercise program for patients after cardiac surgery. *Arch. Phys. Med. Rehabil.*, **67**, 463–6.

Valacio, R. and Lie, M. (1994) Diuretics and ACE inhibitors. *Care of the Elderly*, **6**, 294–6.

Vallés, J. (1995) Continuous aspiration of subglottic secretions in preventing ventilator-associated pneumonia. *Ann. Int. Med*, **122**, 179–86.

Van Dixhoorn, J., Duivenvoordent, H.J., Staal, J.A. *et al.* (1987) Cardiac events after myocardial infarction: possible effect of relaxation therapy. *Eur. Heart J.*, **8**, 1210–14.

Van Mieghem, W. (1989) Cardiopulmonary function after lobectomy or pneumonectomy. *Respir. Med.*, **83**, 199–206.

Vansteenkiste, J., Rochette, F., Demedts, M. *et al.* (1991) Diagnostic tests of hyperventilation syndrome. *Eur. Resp. J.*, **4**, 393–9.

Veddeng, O.J. (1992) Selective PEEP and intracardiac dimensions in dogs. *J. Appl. Phys.*, **73**, 2016–20.

Venables, T. (1994) Helping patients who want to quit smoking. *Respir. Dis. Pract.*, **11**(2), 6–8.

Vender, R.L. (1994) Chronic hypoxic pulmonary hypertension. *Chest*, **106**, 236–43.

Verbeken, E.K., Cauberghs, M., Mertens, I. *et al.* (1992) The senile lung. *Chest*, **101**, 793–9.

Verboon, J.M.L., Bakker, W., Sterk, P.J. *et al.* (1986) The value of the forced expiration technique with and without postural drainage. *Eur. J. Respir. Dis.*, **69**, 169–74.

Vickers, M.D. (1992) Tramadol: pain relief by an opioid without depression of respiration. *Anaesthesia*, **47**, 291–6.

Villaire, M. (1995) ICU from the patient's point of view. *Crit. Care Nurse*, **15**(1), 80–7.

Vos, H.R. (1993) Making headway with intracranial hypertension. *Am. J. Nurs.*, **93**(2), 28–36.

Wagg, A. (1995) Cardiopulmonary resuscitation: doctors and nurses expect too much. *J. Roy. Coll. Phys. London*, **29**, 20–4.

Wagner, P.D. (1992) Ventilation-perfusion matching during exercise. *Chest*, **101**, 192S–85.

Wald, S.L. (1993) The effect of secondary insults on mortality and disability after severe head injury. *J.Trauma*, **34**, 377–81.

Walker, A. (1995) Patient compliance and the placebo effect. *Physiotherapy*, **81**, 120–6.

Walsh, J.M., Vanderwarf, C., Hoscheit, D. *et al.* (1989) Unsuspected hemodynamic alterations during endotracheal suctioning. *Chest*, **95**, 162–5.

Wanner, A. (1990) The role of mucus in COPD. *Chest*, **97**, 11S–15S.

Watcha, M.F. and White, P.F. (1992) Postoperative nausea and vomiting. *Anaesthesiology*, **77**, 162–84.

Watts, N.T. (1985) Decision analysis, in *Clinical decision making in Physical Therapy* (ed. S. Wolf), F.A. Davis, Philadelphia, pp. 7–23.

Webber, B.A. and Pryor, J.A. (1993) *Physiotherapy for Respiratory and Cardiac Problems*, Churchill Livingstone, Edinburgh.

Weil, J.V., Castro, O., Malik, A.B. *et al.* (1993) Pathogenesis of lung disease in sickle hemoglobinopathies. *Am. Rev. Respir. Dis.*, **148**, 249–56.

Weiner, P. (1991) Stressful experience and cardiorespiratory disorders. *Circulation*, **83** (suppl. II), II–2–II–8.

Weiner, P. (1992) Inspiratory muscle training combined with general exercise reconditioning in patients with COPD. *Chest*, **102**, 1351–6.

Weiner, P., Azgad, Y., Ganam, R. *et al.* (1992) Inspiratory muscle training in patients with bronchial asthma. *Chest*, **102**, 1357–61.

Weissleder, A. (1976) Physical therapeutic approach to the control of an acute asthmatic attack. *Phys.Ther.*, **56**, 681–3.

Weissman, C., Kemper, M., Damask, M.C. *et al.* (1984) Effect of routine intensive care interactions on metabolic rate. *Chest*, **86**, 815–8.

Weissman, C. and Kemper, M. (1991) The oxygen uptake oxygen delivery relationship during ICU interventions. *Chest*, **99**, 430–5.

Weissman, C. (1993) Stressing the critically ill patient. *J. Crit. Care*, **8**, 100–8.

Wenger, N.K. (1982) Early ambulation. *Adv. Cardiol.*, **31**, 138–41.

Wessel, D.L. (1993) Hemodynamic responses to perioperative pain and stress in infants. *Crit. Care Med.*, **21**, S361–S362.

West, J.B. (1995) *Respiratory Physiology*, 5th edn, Williams and Wilkins, Baltimore.

Westbrook, J.L. and Sykes, M.K. (1992) Peroperative arterial hypoxaemia. The interaction between intrapulmonary shunt and cardiac output. *Anaesthesia*, **47**, 307–10.

Wetter, D.W. (1994) Smoking as a risk factor for sleep-disordered breathing. *Arch. Intern. Med.*, **154**, 2219–24.

Wheatley, J.R. (1990) The effect of hyperinflation on respiratory muscle work in acute induced asthma. *Eur. Respir. J.*, **3**, 625–32.

White, K.L. (1988) Foreword, in *Medicine and Culture* (ed. L. Payer), Henry Holt, New York.

White, K.M., Winslow, E.H., Clark, A.P. *et al.* (1990) The physiologic basis for continuous mixed venous oxygen saturation monitoring. *Heart Lung*, **19**, 548–51.

Whitehead, B.F. and Leval, M.R. (1994) Paediatric lung transplantation: the agony and the ecstasy. *Thorax*, **49**, 437–9.

Whitney, J.D. (1989) Physiologic effects of tissue oxygenation on wound healing. *Heart Lung*, **18**, 466–76.

Widdicombe, J. and Davies, A. (1991) *Respiratory Physiology*, Edward Arnold, London.

Widdicombe, J. (1992) Tracheobronchial vasculature. *Br. Med. Bull.*, **48**, 108–19.

Wiener, C.M., McKenna, W.J., Myers, M.J. *et al.* (1990) Left lower lobe ventilation is reduced in patients with cardiomegaly in the supine but not the prone position. *Am. Rev. Resp. Dis.*, **141**, 150–5.

Wiener, J.P. (1992) Postoperative pleural and pulmonary abnormalities in patients undergoing CABG. *Chest*, **102**, 1313–4.

Wiggins, J. (1991) Steroid trials in the assessment of air flow limitation. *Resp. Med.*, **85**, 295–9.

Wijkstra, P.J. (1994) Relation of lung function, maximal inspiratory pressure, dyspnoea and quality of life with exercise capacity in patients with COPD. *Thorax*, **49**, 468–72.

Wiles, F.W. and Hnizdo, E. (1991) Relevance of airflow obstruction and mucus hypersecretion to mortality. *Respir. Med.*, **85**, 27–35.

Wilkes, L. (1983) *Nightmare*, quoted in *The Oxford Book of Death*, Oxford University Press, Oxford.

Wilkins, R.L., Sheldon, R.L. and Krider, S.J. (1990) *Clinical Assessment in Respiratory Care*, C.V. Mosby, Toronto.

Williams, S.J. (1993) *Chronic Respiratory Illness*, Routledge.

Williams, A.R., Hind, M. and Sweeney, B.P. (1994) The incidence and severity of postoperative nausea and vomiting in patients exposed to positive intra-operative suggestions. *Anaesthesia*, **49**, 340–2.

Williamson, I.J. (1993) Role of oxygen during recovery from exercise in patients with COPD. *Thorax*, **48**, 1056.

Wilson, R. (1988) Secondary ciliary dysfunction. *Clin. Sci.*, **75**, 113–20.

Wilson, R.C. and Jones, P.W. (1991) Differentiation between the intensity of breathlessness and the distress it evokes in normal subjects during exercise. *Clin. Sci.*, **80**, 65–70.

Windsor, J.A. and Hill, G.L. (1988) Risk factors for postoperative pneumonia. *Ann. Surg.*, **208**, 209–14.

Winkelmann, B.R. (1994) Low-dose almitrine bismesylate for hypoxemia due to COPD. *Chest*, **105**, 1383–91.

Winslow, E.H., Clark, A.P., White, K.M. *et al.* (1990) Effects of a lateral turn on mixed venous oxygen saturation and heart rate. *Heart Lung*, **19**, 557–61.

Wollam, P.J. (1994) Prediction and assessment of bronchodilator response in mechanically ventilated patients. *Respir. Care*, **39**, 730–5.

Wollmer, P., Ursing, K., Midgren, B. *et al.* (1985) Inefficiency of chest percussion in the physical therapy of chronic bronchitis. *Eur. J. Resp. Dis.*, **66**, 233–9.

Wood, D.E. (1993a) Thoracoscopic surgery. *Respir. Care*, **38**, 388–97.

Wood, A.M. (1993b) A review of literature relating to sleep in hospital. *Int. Crit. Care Nurs.*, **9**, 129–36.

Woodhead, M. and Tattersfield, A. (1987) The unacceptable face of tipping. *Br. Med. J.*, **294**, 921–2.

Worcester, M.C., Hare, D.L., Oliver. R.G. *et al.* (1993) Early programmes of high and low intensity exercise and quality of life after acute myocardial infarction. *Br. Med. J.*, **307**, 1244–7.

Wren, W.S. (1989) Anaesthetic technique in the newborn. *Int. Care Med.*, **15**, S46–S49.

Wright, A.L. (1989) Breast feeding and lower respiratory tract illness. *Br. Med. J.*, **299**, 946–9.

Wright, J. (1990) Auto-PEEP: incidence, magnitude and contributing factors. *Heart Lung*, **19**, 352–7.

Wuyam, B., Payen, J.F., Levy, P. *et al.* (1992) Metabolism and aerobic capacity of skeletal muscle in chronic respiratory failure related to COPD. *Eur. Respir. J.*, **5**, 157–62.

Yan, S. (1992) Effect of fatigue on diaphragmatic function at different lung volumes. *J. Appl. Phys.*, **72**, 1064–7.

Yang, Q.-H. (1991) Effect of lung inflation on regional lung expansion in supine and prone rabbits. *J. Appl. Phys.*, **71**, 76–82.

Yaster, M., Tobin, J.R., Billett, C. *et al.* (1994) Epidural analgesia for severe vaso-occlusive sickle cell crisis. *Paediatrics*, **93**, 310–15.

Yaster, M. (1995) Pain relief. *Paediatrics*, **95**, 427–8.

Yoon, R., McKenzie, D.K., Bauman, A. *et al.* (1993) Controlled trial evaluation of an asthma education programme for adults. *Thorax*, **48**, 1110–16.

York, E.L., Lewall, D.B., Hirji, M. *et al.* (1990) Endoscopic diagnosis and treatment of postoperative bronchopleural fistula. *Chest*, **97**, 1390–2.

Young, S., Bitsakou, H., Caric, D. *et al.* (1991) Coughing can relieve or exacerbate symptoms in asthmatic patients. *Resp. Med.*, **85** (suppl. A), 7–12.

Yuksel, B. (1994) Comparison of the effects on lung function of two methods of bronchodilator administration. *Respir. Med.*, **88**, 229–33.

Zadai, C. (1991) Cardiopulmonary ageing and exercise, in *Respiratory Care* (ed. J.A. Pryor), Churchill Livingstone, Edinburgh, p.199–226.

Zapleta, A., Stefanova, J., Horak, J. *et al.* (1983) Chest physiotherapy and airway obstruction in patients with cystic fibrosis – a negative report. *Eur. J. Resp. Dis.*, **64**, 426–33.

Zhuang, J., Schmoker, J.D., Shackford, S.R. *et al.* (1992) Focal brain injury results in severe cerebral ischemia despite maintenance of cerebral perfusion pressure. *J. Trauma*, **33**, 83–8.

Zibrack, J.D., Rossetti, P. and Wood, E. (1986) Effect of reduction in respiratory therapy. *N. Engl. J. Med.*, **315**, 292–5.

Zideman, D.A. (1994) Guidelines for paediatric life support. *Br. Med. J.*, **308**, 1349–55.

Zidulka, A., Braidy, T.F., Rizzi, M.C. *et al.* (1982) Position may stop pneumothorax progression in dogs. *Am. Rev. Resp. Dis.*, **126**, 51–3.

Zidulka, A., Chrome, J.F., Wight, D.W. *et al.* (1989) Clapping or percussion causes atelectasis. *J. Appl. Physiol.*, **66**, 2833–8.

Ziegler, D.W. (1994) The morbidity and mortality of rib fractures. *J. Trauma*, **37**, 975–9.

Index

Page numbers appearing in **bold** represent figures, page numbers appearing in *italic* represent tables.